QUICK LOOK
METABOLISM

D1295263

QUICK LOOK

METABOLISM

Carole J. Coffee, Ph.D.

Professor of Biochemistry
Department of Molecular Genetics and Biochemistry
University of Pittsburgh School of Medicine
Pittsburgh, Pennsylvania

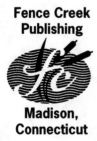

**Fence Creek
Publishing**

**Madison,
Connecticut**

© 1999 by Fence Creek Publishing, LLC, Madison, Connecticut

Production by Karen Feeney, Derra
Typeset by Pagesetters, Brattleboro, VT
Printed by Port City Press, Baltimore, MD
Illustrations by Oxford Illustrators, Oxford, UK

Distributors:

USA

Blackwell Science, Inc.
Commerce Place
350 Main Street
Malden, MA 02148
(Telephone orders: 800-215-1000 or 781-388-8250;
Fax orders: 781-388-8270)

Canada

Login Brothers Book Company
324 Saulteaux Crescent
Winnipeg, Manitoba, R3J 3T2
(Telephone orders: 204-224-4068)

Australia

Blackwell Science, Pty, Ltd.
54 University Street
Carlton, Victoria 3053
(Telephone orders: 03-9347-0300;
Fax orders: 03-9349-3016)

Outside North America and Australia

Blackwell Science, Ltd.
c/o Marston Book Services, Ltd.
P.O. Box 269
Abingdon
Oxon, OX14 4YN
England
(Telephone orders: 44-01235-465500;
Fax orders: 44-01235-465555)

All rights reserved. Except as permitted under the Copyright Act of 1976, no part of this book may be reproduced in any form or by any electronic or mechanical means, including information storage and retrieval system, without written permission of the publisher.

Printed in the United States of America
99 00 01 02 5 4 3 2 1

Table of Contents

Preface

Quick Look: Metabolism is intended to help medical students prepare for examinations, particularly the United States Medical Licensing Examination (USMLE) Step 1. The study of human metabolism integrates biochemical pathways with themes traditionally covered in physiology, cell structure, nutrition, and histology. The two questions most frequently asked by medical students are: "What do I need to know?" and "What is the significance of this information?" Hopefully, *Quick Look: Metabolism* will provide answers to these questions, not only for the immediate task of passing an examination, but also for the long-range goal of providing a conceptual framework that will be helpful in understanding problems presented by future patients. This book emphasizes the function and underlying principles of metabolic pathways, their cellular and organ distribution, how they are regulated and coordinated with one another, and the clinical significance of the pathways.

Quick Look: Metabolism addresses 74 themes that are fundamental to the understanding of metabolism. Each theme has comprehensive illustrations on one page and concise text on the facing page. The text begins with a brief overview, is followed by thumb-nail sketches of key concepts, and ends with a discussion of clinical significance. The themes are grouped into six context-related parts and each part ends with a series of questions and answers that are accompanied by explanations.

Carole J. Coffee

Abbreviations

ACAT	acylcholesterol-acyltransferase		COMT	catechol-O-methyltransferase
ACTH	adrenocorticotropic hormone		CoQ	coenzyme Q
ACP	acyl carrier protein		CPA	carboxypeptidase A
ADP	adenosine diphosphate		CPB	carboxypeptidase B
Ala	alanine		CPS	carbamoyl phosphate synthetase
ALA	aminolevulinic acid		CRE	cAMP regulatory element
ALT	alanine aminotransferase		CREB	cAMP regulatory element binding protein
AMI	acute myocardial infarct		CRF	corticotropin releasing factor
AMP	adenosine monophosphate		CT	carnitine transporter
ANF	atrial natriuretic factor		CTP	cytidine triphosphate
APRT	adenine phosphoribosyltransferase		Cys	cysteine
Asn	asparagine		DAG	diacylglycerol
α_1-AT	α_1-antitrypsin		dATP	deoxyadenosine triphosphate
ATP	adenosine triphosphate		DG	diglyceride
AZT	azidothymidine		DH	dehydrogenase
BCAA	branched chain amino acid		DHAP	dihydroxyacetone phosphate
BCKA	branched chain keto acid		DHB	dihydrobiopterin
BEE	basal energy expenditure		DHEA	dehydroepiandrosterone
BMR	basal metabolic rate		DIT	diiodotyrosine
1,3BPG	1,3-bisphosphoglycerate		dTMP	deoxythymidine monophosphate
2,3BPG	2,3-bisphosphoglycerate		DNA	deoxyribonucleic acid
cAMP	cyclic adenosine monophosphate		dNDP	deoxynucleoside diphosphate
CAT	carnitine acyltransferase		DOPA	dihydroxyphenylalanine
CCK	choleocystokinin		DNP	dinitrophenol
CCK-PZ	choleocystokinin pancreozymin		E^o	standard reduction potential
CDP	cytidine diphosphate		ER	endoplasmic reticulum
CE	cholesterol ester		FA	fatty acid
CETP	cholesterol ester transfer protein		FAD	flavin adenine dinucleotide
CGD	chronic granulocytic disease		FADH	reduced flavin adenine dinucleotide
cGMP	cyclic guanosine monophosphate		FBPase-1	fructose bisphosphatase-1
CK	creatine kinase		FBPase-2	fructose bisphosphatase-2
CM	chylomicron		FeS	iron sulfur center
CMP	cytidine monophosphate		FH	familial hypercholesterolemia
CMR	chylomicron remnant		FIGLU	formiminoglutamate
CNS	central nervous system		F6P	fructose-6-phosphate
CNZ	condensing enzyme		$F1,6P_2$	fructose-1,6-bisphosphate
CoA	coenzyme A		$F2,6P_2$	fructose-2,6-bisphosphate

Fuc	fucose	K_{eq}	equilibrium constant
ΔG	free energy change	K_m	Michaelis constant
ΔG°	standard free energy change	LCAD	long chain acyldehydrogenase
ΔG^{*}	activation energy	LCAT	lecithin-cholesterol acyltransferase
G_i	inhibitory GTP binding protein	LDH	lactate dehydrogenase
G_s	stimulatory GTP binding protein	LDL	low density lipoprotein
GABA	γ-aminobutyrate	Leu	leucine
GAG	glycosaminoglycan	LH	luteinizing hormone
Gal	galactose	LHON	Leber's hereditary optic neuropathy
GalNAc	N-acetylgalactosamine	LpL	lipoprotein lipase
GDP	guanosine diphosphate	LT	leukotriene
GK	glucokinase	Man	mannose
GlcNAc	N-acetylglucosamine	MAO	monoamine oxidase
Gln	glutamine	Mb	myoglobin
GLUT	glucose transporter	MCAD	medium chain acyldehydrogenase
GMP	guanosine monophosphate	MELAS	mitochondrial encephalomyopathy, lactic acidosis, stroke-like episodes
G1P	glucose-1-phosphate		
G3P	glyceraldehyde-3-phosphate	MEOS	microsomal ethanol oxidizing system
G6P	glucose-6-phosphate	MERRF	myoclonic epilepsy and ragged-red fibers
G6Pase	glucose-6-phosphatase	Met	methionine
G6PD	glucose-6-phosphate dehydrogenase	MG	monoglyceride
GSH	reduced glutathione	MI	myocardial infarct
GSSG	oxidized glutathione	MIT	monoiodotyrosine
GTP	guanosine triphosphate	mRNA	messenger RNA
H^+	proton	MSUD	maple syrup urine disease
H_2	hydrogen gas	mtDNA	mitochondrial DNA
Hb	hemoglobin	NAD^+	nicotinamide adenine dinucleotide
HCl	hydrochloric acid	NADH	reduced nicotinamide adenine dinucleotide
HCO_3^-	bicarbonate	$NADP^+$	nicotinamide adenine dinucleotide phosphate
H_2CO_3	carbonic acid	NADPH	reduced nicotinamide adenine dinucleotide phosphate
HDL	high density lipoprotein		
HGPRT	hypoxanthine-guanine phosphoribosyltransferase	NAG	N-acetylglutamate
5-HI	5-hydroxyindolacetate	NANA	N-acetylneuraminic acid
5-HTP	5-hydroxytryptophan	NDP	nucleoside diphosphate
5-HT	5-hydroxytryptamine	NH_3	ammonia
HMG-CoA	hydroxymethylglutarate coenzyme A	NH_4^+	ammonium ion
HOCl	hypochlorous acid	NO	nitric oxide
H_2O_2	hydrogen peroxide	NOS	nitric oxide synthase
HPETE	5-hydroperoxyeicosatetraenoic acid	OAA	oxaloacetate
HSD	hydroxysteroid dehydrogenase	O_2^-	superoxide
IDL	intermediate density lipoprotein	OMP	orotidine monophosphate
Ile	isoleucine	OPRT	orotate phosphoribosyltransferase
IMM	inner mitochondrial membrane	OTC	ornithine transcarbamoylase
IMP	inosine monophosphate	PABA	p-aminobenzoic acid
INF	interferon	PAF	platelet activating factor
IP_3	inositol triphosphate	PAPS	phosphoadenosinephosphosulfate

PBG	porphobilinogen	rRNA	ribosomal RNA
PEP	phosphoenolpyruvate	tRNA	transfer RNA
PEPCK	phosphoenolpyruvate carboxykinase	SAM	S-adenosylmethionine
PFK-1	phosphofructose kinase-1	SCAD	short chain acyldehydrogenase
PFK-2	phosphofructose kinase-2	SCID	severe combined immunodeficiency
PG	prostaglandin	SER	smooth endoplasmic reticulum
2PG	2-phosphoglycerate	Ser	serine
3PG	3-phosphoglycerate	SGLUT	sodium-dependent glucose transporter
6-PG	6-phosphogluconate	SGOT	serum glutamate-oxaloacetate transaminase
6-PGD	6-phosphogluconate dehydrogenase	SGPT	serum glutamate-pyruvate transaminase
PLP	pyridoxal phosphate	T	absolute temperature
PNMT	phenylalanine-N-methyltransferase	T_3	triiodothyronine
pO_2	partial pressure of oxygen	T_4	tetraiodothyronine
pCO_2	partial pressure of carbon dioxide	TCA	tricarboxylic acid cycle
PDH	pyruvate dehydrogenase	TG	triglyceride
pH	negative log of hydrogen ion concentration	THB	tetrahydrobiopterin
P_i	inorganic phosphate	Thr	threonine
pK_a	negative log of dissociation constant	TNF	tumor necrosis factor
PKA	protein kinase A	TPP	thiamine pyrophosphate
PKU	phenylketonuria	TX	thromboxane
PP_i	pyrophosphate	UDP	uridine diphosphate
PRPP	phosphoribosylpyrophosphate	UMP	uridine monophosphate
PTH	parathyroid hormone	UTP	uridine triphosphate
R	gas constant	Val	valine
RBC	red blood cell	$\dot{V}_{max}$	maximum velocity
RDA	recommended daily allowance	VLDL	very low density lipoprotein
RER	rough endoplasmic reticulum	VMA	vanillylmandelic acid
RNA	ribonucleic acid		

PART I
Fundamentals of Metabolism

Cellular Organelles and Their Metabolic Functions

1

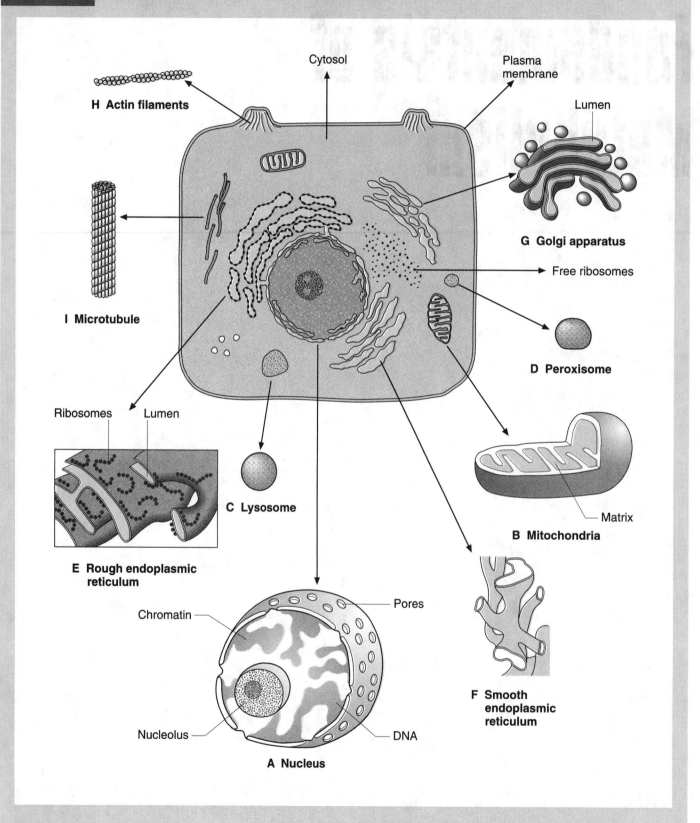

H Actin filaments

Cytosol

Plasma membrane

Lumen

G Golgi apparatus

Free ribosomes

I Microtubule

D Peroxisome

Ribosomes   Lumen

C Lysosome

Matrix

B Mitochondria

E Rough endoplasmic reticulum

Pores

Chromatin

F Smooth endoplasmic reticulum

Nucleolus

DNA

A Nucleus

OVERVIEW

The cell is the fundamental unit of metabolism. The periphery of the cell is defined by the plasma membrane that separates the contents of the cell from the external environment. Eukaryotic cells have an internal membrane system that organizes the cell into several subcellular compartments, each with discrete metabolic functions. The extensive compartmentation gives cells the ability to fine-tune the regulation of metabolism by partitioning different metabolic pathways between cellular compartments.

Nucleus

The nucleus (**Part A**) is the largest of the organelles. It is separated from the cytosol by the **nuclear envelope**, which consists of two membranes that contain **numerous pores**, allowing macromolecules to move in and out of the nucleus. The major metabolic function of the nucleus is the synthesis of DNA and RNA. Eukaryotic DNA is present as **chromatin**, a complex of DNA and histones. The **nucleolus** is a region within the nucleus where rRNA is synthesized and ribosomes are assembled.

Mitochondria

Mitochondria (**Part B**) are cigar-shaped structures; each has a smooth outer membrane and an inner membrane that is tightly folded into projections known as cristae. The inner mitochondrial membrane is highly impermeable and contains numerous transport and shuttle systems for moving metabolites in and out of the mitochondrial matrix. The major functions of mitochondria are the oxidation of metabolic fuels and the synthesis of ATP. The enzymes for oxidizing fatty acids, pyruvate, and many amino acids are found in the **matrix**. The electron transport chain and ATP synthase are located in the inner mitochondrial membrane. Unlike other organelles, mitochondria contain their own DNA as well as the enzymes that synthesize DNA, RNA, and protein.

Lysosomes

Lysosomes (**Part C**) are vesicles surrounded by a single membrane; they constitute the major degradative compartment of the cell. More than 50 different **acid hydrolases** that degrade nucleic acids, proteins, glycolipids, and proteoglycans are found in the lysosomes. A unique feature of the lysosomal membrane is the presence of an **ATP-dependent H$^+$ pump** that transports H$^+$ from the cytosol into the lysosomal lumen in exchange for sodium, thereby maintaining the low pH required for optimal activity of the lysosomal degradative enzymes.

Peroxisomes

The liver and kidney are rich in peroxisomes (**Part D**), which specialize in oxidative reactions that produce hydrogen peroxide as a by-product. Peroxisomes are rich in **catalase**, which degrades hydrogen peroxide. Metabolic reactions that occur in peroxisomes include the oxidation of amino acids, very long chain fatty acids, branched chain fatty acids, and ethanol. Synthesis of plasmalogens and bile acids also occurs in peroxisomes.

Endoplasmic Reticulum

Flattened sheets, stacks, and tubular networks of membrane are found throughout the cytoplasm of eukaryotic cells. The endoplasmic reticulum membrane is continuous with the nuclear membrane. The major metabolic function of the endoplasmic reticulum is the **synthesis and transport of lipids and membrane proteins**. The **rough endoplasmic reticulum (Part E)** appears as flat sheets with ribosomes attached to the outer surface. Lysosomal enzymes and proteins destined for secretion or incorporation into the endoplasmic reticulum membrane, Golgi membrane, and plasma membrane are synthesized by the rough endoplasmic reticulum. In contrast, mitochondrial proteins, nuclear proteins, peroxisomal proteins, and proteins destined to reside in the cytosol are synthesized by polyribosomes in the cytosol. The **smooth endoplasmic reticulum (Part F)** is more tubular in structure and contains no ribosomes. It plays a central role in lipid synthesis and in a variety of cytochrome P-450-dependent detoxification reactions.

Golgi Apparatus

The Golgi apparatus (**Part G**) consists of stacks of flat membrane sacs that are continuous with the endoplasmic reticulum. It is responsible for **sorting** and **targeting** proteins to specific destinations. **Glycosylation** and **sulfation** reactions occur in the Golgi apparatus.

Cytoskeleton

The cytoskeleton is an organized network of protein filaments found inside cells but not surrounded by membranes. **Actin filaments (Part H)** and **microtubules (Part I)** give cells their shape and mobility, whereas **intermediate filaments** are rope-like networks that provide mechanical strength.

Cytosol

The cytosol contains many of the substrates and enzymes involved in **carbohydrate metabolism, fatty acid synthesis, nucleotide synthesis, and protein synthesis**.

Clinical Significance

More than 35 inherited diseases have been associated with defects in lysosomal enzymes, resulting in a family of lysosomal storage diseases. These include **Gaucher** disease and **Tay Sachs** disease. Defects in mitochondrial function have been associated with **ammonia toxicity, viral infections**, and **cirrhosis of the liver**. Defects in peroxisomal function are responsible for **Zellweger syndrome** and **adrenoleukodystrophy**. A defect in the Golgi targeting mechanism that directs enzymes to lysosomes results in **I-cell disease**. Numerous other defects that occur within particular subcellular organelles will be introduced in other sections.

For more information see Coffee C, *Metabolism*. Fence Creek, pp 2–7.

2 Biologic Buffers and Acid-Base Equilibrium

Overview. Homeostasis requires tight control of acid-base balance to maintain the characteristic pH of specific biological fluids and cellular compartments

Fluid/Compartment	pH
Blood plasma	7.4
Interstitial fluid	7.4
Intracellular fluids	
Cytosol (liver)	6.9
Lysosomes	5.0
Gastric juice	1.5–3.0
Urine	5.0–8.0

A Some Important Weak Acids (HA) and Their Conjugate Bases (A⁻)

Acid	pK_a	Conjugate Base
Acetoacetic acid	3.6	Acetoacetate
Lactic acid	3.9	Lactate
β-Hydroxybutyric acid	4.7	β-Hydroxybutyrate
Acetic acid	4.7	Acetate
Ammonium ion	9.3	Ammonia

B Predictions from the Henderson-Hasselbach Equation

pH	% HA	% A⁻
$pK_a - 2$	99	1
$pK_a - 1$	90	10
pK_a	50	50
$pK_a + 1$	10	90
$pK_a + 2$	1	99

C Titration Curve of a Weak Acid ($pK_a = 7.0$)

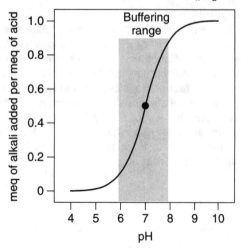

D Important Physiological Buffering Systems

Buffering System	pK_a
HCO_3^-/CO_2	6.1
Phosphate	
Inorganic phosphate	6.8
Organic phosphate esters	6.5–7.5
Proteins	
Histidine side chains	5.6–7.0

The pH of body fluids and subcellular compartments is maintained at a constant and characteristic value by a number of biologic buffers. Buffers consist of a weak acid and its conjugate base that are in equilibrium with one another. The weak acid donates protons and its conjugate base accepts protons from the surrounding medium. The most important biologic buffers are bicarbonate, phosphate, and proteins.

Properties of Weak Acids

Weak acids, in contrast to strong acids, are not completely dissociated under the conditions found in biologic systems. The undissociated acid (HA) is known as the **conjugate acid**; the dissociated form (A⁻) is the **conjugate base (Part A)**. The equilibrium between the conjugate acid and base is described by the following equation:

$$HA \rightleftharpoons H^+ + A^-$$

The equilibrium constant for this reaction is known as K_a, the dissociation constant for the conjugate acid. It is defined as follows:

$$K_a = \frac{[H^+][A^-]}{[HA]}$$

The Henderson-Hasselbach Equation

The relationship between pH and the concentrations of the conjugate acid and conjugate base is described by the following equation, where $pH = -\log[H^+]$ and $pK_a = -\log K_a$.

$$pH = pK_a + \log \frac{[A^-]}{[HA]}$$

According to this equation, the **pK_a of any weak acid can be defined as the pH where the concentration of A⁻ is equal to the concentration of HA.** If the pK_a for a weak acid is known, the Henderson-Hasselbach equation can be used to calculate the amounts of HA and A⁻ at any pH. The logarithmic nature of the equation predicts that small changes in pH can result in large changes in the relative concentrations of A⁻ and HA (**Part B**).

Buffering Properties of Weak Acids

Buffers are solutions that resist a change in pH when acid or base is added. The titration curve for a weak acid (**Part C**) shows that when equal increments of base are added unequal changes in pH occur. The smallest changes in pH are observed when the initial pH of the solution is closest to the pK_a of the weak acid. Therefore, the buffering power of a weak acid and conjugate base is most effective in a pH range within 1.0 pH unit above or below the pK_a.

Important Physiologic Buffers

The major buffer in extracellular fluids is the bicarbonate system, whereas proteins, inorganic phosphate, and organic phosphate esters are the major intracellular buffers (**Part D**).

The **bicarbonate buffering system** maintains the pH of blood and interstitial fluid near 7.4. The equilibria involved in this system are described by the equation below:

$$CO_2 + H_2O \rightleftharpoons H_2CO_3 \rightleftharpoons H^+ + HCO_3^-$$

Carbonic acid (H_2CO_3) is a weak acid with a pK_a of 6.1. Although the pK_a of H_2CO_3 is 1.3 pH units below the normal pH of plasma, its effectiveness as a buffer lies in the ability of the lungs and kidneys to regulate the concentrations of dissolved CO_2 and HCO_3^-, respectively. This buffering system is frequently referred to as the HCO_3^-/CO_2 system because the concentration of H_2CO_3 is insignificant relative to the concentration of dissolved CO_2 in the blood. The concentration of dissolved CO_2 is usually expressed as the partial pressure of the dissolved gas (P_{CO_2}).

Protein buffering systems rely primarily on the histidine content of proteins. The pK_a of the histidine side chains ranges from 5.6 to 7.0 depending on its microenvironment. Hemoglobin, which is present in very high concentrations in the red blood cell and has multiple histidine side chains, plays a major role in maintaining a constant pH inside the red blood cell.

The **phosphate buffering system** consists of $H_2PO_4^-$, a weak acid with a pK_a of 6.8, and its conjugate base HPO_4^{2-}. There are also many organic phosphates in cells that have pK_a values between 6.5 and 7.5. Phosphate buffers are very important in red blood cells and kidney tubules, which contain high concentrations of phosphates.

Clinical Significance

Disturbances in acid-base balance can lead to acidosis (plasma pH less than 7.35) or alkalosis (plasma pH greater than 7.45). Acidosis can result from either hypoventilation (**respiratory acidosis**) or from overproduction of H⁺ or overexcretion of HCO_3^- (**metabolic acidosis**). Alkalosis can result from either hyperventilation (**respiratory alkalosis**) or from overexcretion of H⁺ or ingestion of a variety of alkalis (**metabolic alkalosis**). The body usually compensates for changes in pH by adjusting the rate of CO_2 loss by the lungs or the rate of HCO_3^- filtration by the kidneys. A summary of the primary and compensatory changes in acidosis and alkalosis is shown in the following table:

ABNORMALITIES IN ACID-BASE BALANCE*

	pH	Primary Change	Compensatory Response
Respiratory acidosis	Decrease	P_{CO_2} increase	HCO_3^- increase
Respiratory alkalosis	Increase	P_{CO_2} decrease	HCO_3^- decrease
Metabolic acidosis	Decrease	HCO_3^- decrease	P_{CO_2} decrease
Metabolic alkalosis	Increase	HCO_3^- increase	P_{CO_2} increase

*Normal values: pH = 7.4; P_{CO_2} = 40 mm Hg; HCO_3^- = 24 mM.

For more information see Coffee C, *Metabolism*. Fence Creek, pp 8–10.

3 Protein Structure

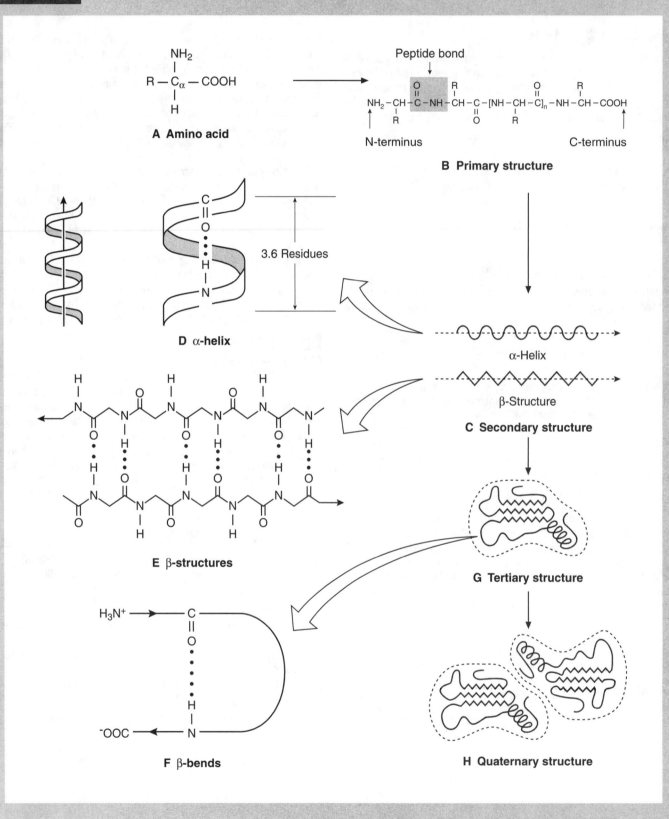

A Amino acid

Peptide bond

N-terminus

C-terminus

B Primary structure

3.6 Residues

D α-helix

α-Helix

β-Structure

C Secondary structure

E β-structures

F β-bends

G Tertiary structure

H Quaternary structure

OVERVIEW

Proteins are responsible for almost all functions that occur in the body. Each protein has a unique three-dimensional structure that is ideally suited to its physiologic function. Proteins are composed of linear polymers of amino acids held together by peptide bonds. Each protein has a unique sequence of amino acids that dictates its three-dimensional structure and biologic function.

Building Blocks of Proteins

Proteins are synthesized from 20 **amino acids**. All of the amino acids except proline have an α-carbon atom (**Part A**) to which is attached a carboxyl group, an amino group, a hydrogen atom, and a side chain group (R group). Differences in the R groups distinguish the amino acids from one another. Proteins contain two major classes of amino acids. **Hydrophilic amino acids** have side chains containing either charged groups (aspartate, glutamate, lysine, arginine, histidine) or oxygen, nitrogen, or sulfur atoms that can form a hydrogen bond with water (serine, threonine, cysteine, asparagine, glutamine). The side chains of hydrophilic amino acids are usually found on the surface of proteins where they interact favorably with the aqueous environment. **Hydrophobic amino acids** have either aliphatic side chains (alanine, valine, isoleucine, leucine, proline, methionine) or aromatic side chains (phenylalanine, tyrosine, tryptophan). The hydrophobic side chains are usually protected from water by being buried in the interior of the protein.

Primary Structure

The primary structure is defined as the **polypeptide backbone**, which is made up of a unique **sequence of amino acids** joined by **peptide bonds** (**Part B**). The carboxyl group of one amino acid reacts with the amino group of the next amino acid to form a peptide bond. The atoms in the peptide bond (C, O, N, H) lie in a plane, thereby limiting the rotations that can occur in the polypeptide backbone.

Secondary Structure

The formation of **hydrogen bonds** between the carbonyl oxygen ($\supset$C=O) of one peptide bond and the amide hydrogen (—NH) of another peptide bond gives rise to repeating patterns of secondary structure (**Part C**). The most common types of secondary structure found in proteins are α-helices, β-structures, and β-bends. α-Helices (**Part D**) are stabilized by **intrachain hydrogen bonds** that are formed between the carbonyl oxygen of one amino acid and the amide hydrogen of the amino acid located four residues ahead of it in the linear sequence. β-Structures (**Part E**), sometimes called β-sheets or β-barrels, are stabilized by **interchain hydrogen bonds** between carbonyl oxygen and amide hydrogen atoms that are located on different polypeptide chains (or different parts of the same chain that is folded back on itself). A third type of secondary structure is the β-bend (**Part F**) which reverses the direction of the polypeptide chain in globular proteins. β-Bends are stabilized by hydrogen bonds between the first and the fourth amino acid residue in the bend.

Tertiary Structure

The tertiary structure (**Part G**) describes the overall three-dimensional structure of a protein. It is stabilized by a large number of **noncova**lent interactions between side chains of amino acids that are often far apart in the linear sequence but close together when the polypeptide chain folds into a compact three-dimensional structure. Stabilizing forces include **ionic interactions** between charged side chains, **hydrophobic interactions** between aromatic or aliphatic side chains, and **hydrogen bonds** between side chains containing hydroxyl, sulfhydryl, amino, carboxyl, or imidazole groups. Some proteins also contain covalent **disulfide bonds** that are formed between cysteine side chains.

Motifs and Domains

The tertiary structure of proteins usually consists of several functional segments of structure. Motifs are **small functional sequences** of amino acids. For example, the serine residue in the sequence -Arg-Arg-X-**Ser**-Y- (where X is any amino acid and Y is a hydrophobic amino acid) is found in proteins that are phosphorylated by protein kinase A. Domains are **larger functional sequences** of amino acids that have a unique three-dimensional shape. They often contain more than 100 amino acids, and the sequence is encoded by an exon in the DNA. For example, many proteins that bind ATP or GTP contain a domain known as the **nucleotide fold**.

Quaternary Structure

Proteins that consist of more than one subunit (polypeptide chain) have quaternary structure (**Part H**). The subunits are held together by the same types of noncovalent interactions that stabilize tertiary structure.

Fibrous and Globular Proteins

Fibrous proteins are **asymmetrical** in shape and usually serve as **structural proteins** (collagen, myosin, tropomyosin, fibrin, keratin). Secondary structure is the highest order of structure in many fibrous proteins. Globular proteins are **tightly folded** into compact structures and perform **dynamic functions** (enzymes, transport proteins, hormones).

Simple and Complex Proteins

Simple proteins contain only amino acids, whereas complex proteins contain additional components such as carbohydrate (glycoproteins), lipid (lipoproteins), or metals (metalloproteins).

Clinical Significance

More than 1500 human diseases can be traced to the production of abnormal proteins. In about a third of these cases, the change of a single amino acid residue leads to disease.

For more information see Coffee C, *Metabolism*. Fence Creek, pp 15–17.

Collagen: The Major Connective Tissue Protein

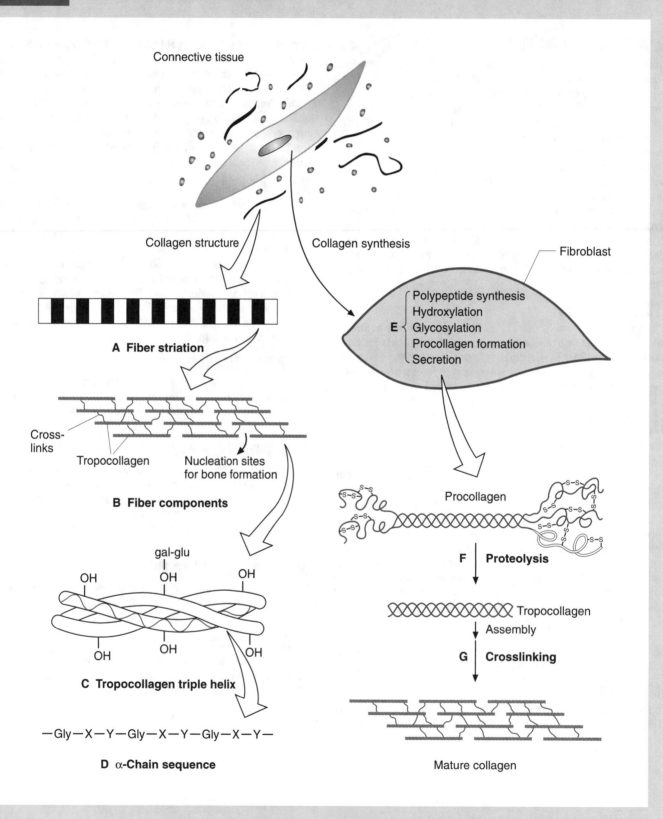

Connective tissue

Collagen structure

Collagen synthesis

Fibroblast

E
- Polypeptide synthesis
- Hydroxylation
- Glycosylation
- Procollagen formation
- Secretion

A Fiber striation

Cross-links

Tropocollagen

Nucleation sites for bone formation

B Fiber components

Procollagen

F Proteolysis

Tropocollagen

Assembly

G Crosslinking

gal-glu

OH   OH   OH

OH   OH   OH

C Tropocollagen triple helix

—Gly—X—Y—Gly—X—Y—Gly—X—Y—

D α-Chain sequence

Mature collagen

OVERVIEW

Connective tissue holds cells together, provides support for the organs, and serves as a vehicle for delivery of nutrients to cells. It consists of insoluble fibrous proteins that are embedded in an extracellular matrix of proteoglycans. Collagen, the most abundant protein in connective tissue, is synthesized by fibroblasts and other cells in the extracellular matrix. Collagen constitutes about 30% of the total protein in the body. It is made up of three peptide chains, known as α-chains, that are wound around one another in a rope-like structure. More than 20 different α-chains have been identified. Different types of collagen have different combinations of α-chains. For a particular type of collagen, the α-chains may either be identical or nonidentical. There are four major types of collagen. **Type I** is found primarily in **bone** and skin, **type II** in **cartilage, type III** in **arterial walls**, and **type IV** in **basement membranes**. Type IV collagen, unlike the other major types, is assembled in sheets rather than fibers. The most abundant collagen is type I, making up about 90% of the collagen in the body.

Collagen Structure

Collagen fibers are made up of **tropocollagen** molecules that are aligned in a parallel fashion. The ends of adjacent tropocollagen molecules are staggered, resulting in the characteristic **striation pattern** seen in electron micrographs.(**Part A**) The spaces between the end of one tropocollagen and the beginning of another act as **nucleation sites** where calcium phosphate is deposited during bone formation (**Part B**). Tropocollagen molecules are held together by **covalent crosslinking**, which gives collagen its high tensile strength, rigidity, and insolubility. Tropocollagen consists of **three peptide chains** that are wrapped around each other to form a rope-like **triple helix** (**Part C**). Distinguishing features of collagen are the high content of glycine and proline and the presence of hydroxyproline and hydroxylysine. The amino acid sequence of the α-chains (**Part D**) is characterized by a **repeating tripeptide sequence of Gly-X-Y**, where X is often proline and Y is often hydroxyproline.

Collagen Synthesis

Synthesis begins inside the cell and is completed after procollagen is secreted from the fibroblast. The synthetic pathway involves extensive posttranslational modifications including hydroxylation, glycosylation, proteolysis, and crosslinking.

Intracellular Steps (Part E)

The peptides found in collagen are synthesized as precursors known as **pro-α-collagen** chains. During synthesis, some of the proline and lysine side chains become hydroxylated. The **hydroxylation** reactions are catalyzed by **prolyl** and **lysyl hydroxylases**, enzymes that require O_2, Fe^{2+}, vitamin C, and α-ketoglutarate for activity. Following hydroxylation, **glycosylation** of some of the hydroxylysine side chains occurs by the sequential addition of galactose and glucose. The extent of glycosylation varies with different types of collagen. Type IV collagen is the most heavily glycosylated. The last step that occurs within the cell is **assembly of procollagen** from three pro-α-chains. Procollagen has a dumbbell-type shape with a long triple helix flanked by globular regions at each end. Every third amino acid residue in the triple helix passes through the center of the rope-like structure. Glycine is the only amino acid with a side chain small enough to fit into the crowded interior of the triple helix, thereby explaining the requirement for glycine at every third position. The globular peptides at the ends prevent premature assembly of procollagen and help align the three chains as they come together to form the triple helix. The triple helix is stabilized by hydroxyproline.

Extracellular Steps

The globular peptides are removed from the amino (N) and carboxyl (C) ends of procollagen by **proteolysis (Part F)**, producing tropocollagen. These reactions are catalyzed by N- and C-procollagen peptidases. Tropocollagen molecules assemble spontaneously into collagen fibers. The final step in collagen synthesis is **crosslinking**, which gives the fiber rigidity and high tensile strength (**Part G**). Crosslinking is initiated by **lysyl oxidase**, an extracellular enzyme that requires O_2, copper, and pyridoxal phosphate for activity. This enzyme acts near the gaps between tropocollagen molecules, where some of the lysine side chains are oxidized to the aldehyde derivative, **allysine**. Allysine then reacts spontaneously with either hydroxylysine, unmodified lysine, or other allysine side chains to form covalent crosslinks.

Clinical Significance

Abnormalities in collagen synthesis can result from mutations in the genes for pro-α-collagen chains or mutations in genes that encode enzymes involved in the post-translational modification of collagen. Abnormalities in collagen synthesis can also result from a nutritional deficiency in either vitamin C or copper.

DISEASES RESULTING FROM ABNORMALITIES IN COLLAGEN SYNTHESIS

Disease	Inheritance[a]	Cause	Symptoms
Osteogenesis imperfecta	AD (most forms)	Mutations in type I collagen genes	Brittle bones, blue sclerae, cardiac insufficiency, deafness
Ehlers-Danlos syndrome			
Type IV	AD	Mutations in type III collagen genes	Arterial and intestinal ruptures
Type V	XR	Lysyl oxidase deficiency[b]	Extensible skin, hypermobile joints
Type VI	AR	Lysyl hydroxylase deficiency	Extensible skin, hypermobile joints
Type VII	AD	N-procollagen peptidase deficiency	Hypermobile joints, hip dislocation
Spondyloepiphyseal dysplasia	AD	Mutations in type II collagen genes	Short-limb dwarfism
Scurvy	—	Vitamin C deficiency	Bleeding gums, hemorrhage, poor wound healing

[a] Abbreviations: AD, autosomal dominant; AR, autosomal recessive XR, X-linked recessive.
[b] Similar symptoms can result from a deficiency in copper.

5 Plasma Proteins

A Separation of plasma proteins by electrophoresis

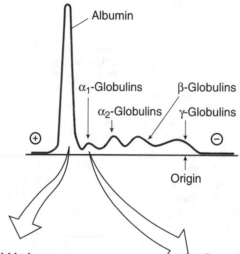

Albumin

α_1-Globulins

α_2-Globulins

β-Globulins

γ-Globulins

$\oplus$ $\ominus$

Origin

B Albumin helps regulate fluid balance between plasma and the interstitial fluid

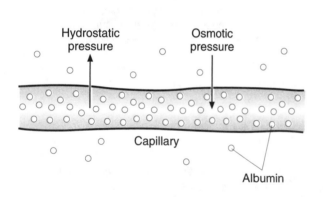

Hydrostatic pressure

Osmotic pressure

Capillary

Albumin

C α_1-Antitrypsin protects lung tissue by blocking the action of elastase

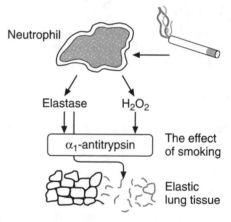

Neutrophil

Elastase

H_2O_2

α_1-antitrypsin

The effect of smoking

Elastic lung tissue

D The use of plasma electrophoretic profiles in diagnosis of disease

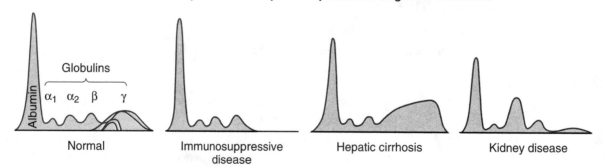

Globulins

Albumin α_1 α_2 β γ

Normal

Immunosuppressive disease

Hepatic cirrhosis

Kidney disease

Blood plasma contains hundreds of different proteins, most of which are synthesized as complex glycoproteins by the liver. They include transport proteins, enzyme inhibitors, clotting factors, and immunoglobulins. They can be separated into five major classes by **electrophoresis** at pH 8.6, a pH where most of these proteins have a net negative charge. When placed in an electric field, they move toward the positive electrode at a rate that is dependent on the charge:shape ratio. With the exception of albumin, each peak contains many different proteins (**Part A**).

Albumin

The albumin peak contains a single protein comprising 55% of the total plasma proteins. Because of its abundance and relatively low molecular weight, it makes a large contribution to the osmotic pressure of the blood, a factor accounting for the importance of albumin in **regulating fluid balance between the blood and the interstitial fluid** (**Part B**). The opposing forces that act to move fluid across the capillary wall are **hydrostatic pressure** and **colloid osmotic pressure**, also known as oncotic pressure. Hydrostatic pressure tends to push fluid out of the capillary, while colloid osmotic pressure favors the movement of fluid into the blood. The albumin concentration is much higher in the blood than in the interstitial fluid, thereby providing an osmotic pressure gradient that results in movement of water into the plasma. Factors that result in decreased plasma albumin, such as protein-calorie malnutrition, may also result in edema. Albumin also functions as a **nonspecific transport protein**, having sites that bind many kinds of hydrophobic molecules including fatty acids, bilirubin, bile acids, steroids, and a number of drugs. Additionally, albumin binds more than 50% of the total calcium in the plasma.

The α_1-Globulins

The major α_1-globulin is α_1**-antitrypsin** (α_1-AT) accounting for 70% to 90% of the total protein in this fraction. It functions as an **inhibitor of elastase**, an enzyme released from neutrophils in lung tissue, thereby preventing loss of lung function (**Part C**). Elastase degrades elastin, the major connective tissue protein that gives lungs their elasticity. A genetic deficiency in α_1-AT leads to **pulmonary emphysema**. Cigarette smoke contributes to obstructive lung disease by two mechanisms: 1) it stimulates the neutrophil to release hydrogen peroxide (H_2O_2), which oxidizes a specific methionine side chain in α_1-AT, rendering it inactive; and 2) it stimulates neutrophils to release elastase. Some cases of α_1-AT deficiency are also associated with **hepatic cirrhosis**, resulting from the accumulation of a mutant form of α_1-AT in liver that cannot be secreted.

The α_2-Globulins

Included in the α_2-globulins are ceruloplasmin and haptoglobulin. **Ceruloplasmin** is a copper transport protein, and its deficiency results in **Wilsons disease**, a copper storage disease in which copper deposits are responsible for the Kaiser-Fleischer rings seen in the eyes of affected patients. Another function of ceruloplasmin is to oxidize iron to the Fe^{3+} state so that it can bind to transferrin, accounting for the observation that copper deficiency is associated with some cases of anemia.

Haptoglobulin prevents the loss of heme iron by binding to free hemoglobin that has been released by intravascular hemolysis. The haptoglobulin–hemoglobin complex is too large to be filtered by the kidneys, whereas free hemoglobin is small enough to pass through the glomerulus and enter the tubules. The level of haptoglobulin in plasma may vary significantly. During bouts of hemolytic anemia, haptoglobulin may be depleted because the hemoglobin–haptoglobulin complex turns over much more rapidly than free haptoglobulin.

The β-Globulins

Quantitatively, the most important β-globulin is **transferrin**, constituting about 60% of the β-globulin fraction. Transferrin plays a key role in iron metabolism by **transporting Fe^{3+}** to the liver, bone marrow, and other organs. The transferrin–Fe^{3+} complex binds to **transferrin receptors** and is taken up by receptor-mediated endocytosis. Following release of Fe^{3+} inside the cell, transferrin remains bound to the receptor and returns to the plasma membrane, where it reenters the plasma and picks up more Fe^{3+}. The plasma level of **transferrin is increased during periods of iron-deficiency anemia and pregnancy** and **decreased in protein-calorie malnutrition**. The half-life of transferrin is about 8 days, making it an excellent marker for the diagnosis of protein malnutrition.

The γ-Globulins

The major types of γ-globulin found in plasma are IgG, IgM, and IgD, with IgG constituting about 70% of the plasma immunoglobulins. The first immunoglobulin made in response to a new antigen is IgM, whereas the major immunoglobulin made after repeated exposure to an antigen is IgG. Since IgG can cross the placenta, it confers immunity against infection in utero and during the neonatal period. The largest immunoglobulin is IgM, having a pentameric structure made up of five immunoglobulin monomers joined together by disulfide bonds and a joining protein, known as the J piece. Both IgG and IgM can activate the complement cascade. IgD constitutes about 1% of the plasma immunoglobulins, and its function is unclear.

Clinical Significance

Variations in the electrophoretic pattern of plasma proteins are commonly used in the diagnosis of disease. Examples of altered profiles associated with specific clinical conditions are shown in **Part D** of the figure. **Immunosuppressive disease** shows decreased or undetectable levels of γ-globulins; **hepatic cirrhosis** shows a broad increase in the γ-globulins and a marked decrease in albumin; **kidney disease** shows selective loss of albumin and other small proteins but retention of high molecular weight proteins, particularly in the α_2-globulin and β-globulin fractions.

For more information see Coffee C, *Metabolism*. Fence Creek, pp 26–29.

6 Membrane Structure and Transport Properties

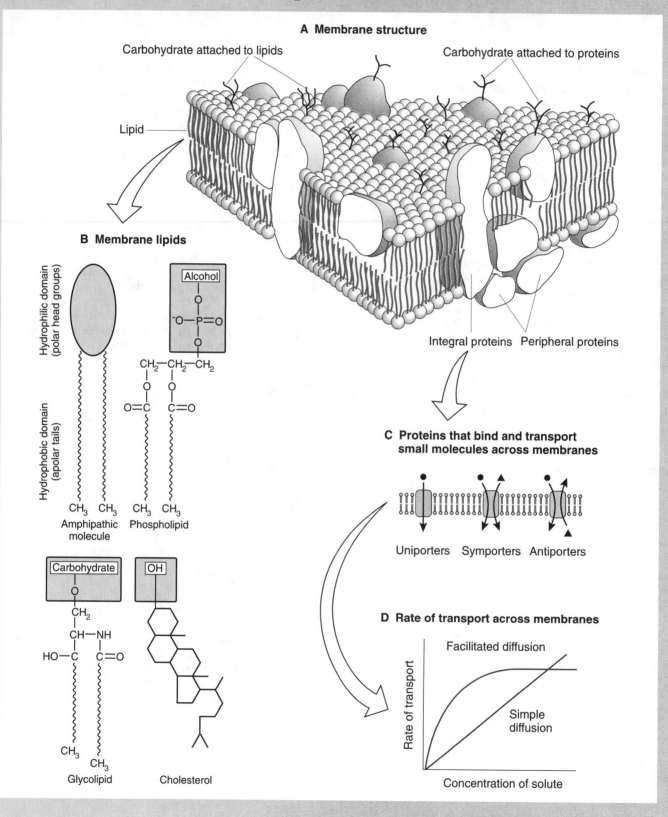

A Membrane structure

Carbohydrate attached to lipids

Carbohydrate attached to proteins

Lipid

Integral proteins   Peripheral proteins

B Membrane lipids

Hydrophilic domain (polar head groups)

Hydrophobic domain (apolar tails)

Alcohol

CH_2—CH_2—CH_2

CH_3 CH_3
Amphipathic molecule

CH_3 CH_3
Phospholipid

Carbohydrate

CH_2

CH—NH

HO—C   C=O

CH_3

CH_3
Glycolipid

OH

Cholesterol

C Proteins that bind and transport small molecules across membranes

Uniporters   Symporters   Antiporters

D Rate of transport across membranes

Facilitated diffusion

Simple diffusion

Rate of transport

Concentration of solute

OVERVIEW

Biologic membranes are bilayers that are assembled from a mixture of lipids and proteins (**Part A**). The lipids provide the structural framework, while the proteins perform the dynamic functions associated with the membrane. The relative proportion of lipid to protein varies with different membranes. In general, the more dynamic functions associated with the membrane, the greater the proportion of protein.

Membrane Lipids

The lipids that are found in membranes are amphipathic molecules, having one end that is hydrophobic and another that is hydrophilic (**Part B**). **Phospholipids** are the universal building blocks of membranes, constituting between 50% and 60% of the total membrane lipid. The four major phospholipids are phosphatidylcholine, phosphatidylethanolamine, phosphatidylserine, and phosphatidylinositol. **Cholesterol** is a major component of the plasma membrane but is found in small amounts, if any, in membranes of subcellular organelles. **Glycolipids** constitute less that 10% of the total membrane lipids and are found almost exclusively in the plasma membrane. The carbohydrate portion of both glycolipids and glycoproteins is always on the outer surface of the plasma membrane.

Membrane Proteins

The proteins found in membranes are classified into two major groups based on the ease with which they can be released from the lipid bilayer. **Integral membrane proteins** are usually transmembrane proteins that span the lipid bilayer one or more times. The sequence of amino acids spanning the bilayer is usually a segment of α-helix consisting of about 20 amino acids, most of which are hydrophobic. The removal of these proteins from the bilayer usually requires detergents. **Peripheral membrane proteins** are located near the surface of the membrane and can often be removed by altering the pH or ionic strength of the solution.

Transport Properties of Membranes

Membranes serve as **selective permeability barriers** that limit the exchange of materials between the inside and outside of cells or between intracellular compartments. Water, gases, ethanol, and urea can pass directly through the bilayer by simple diffusion, but the transport of almost all other molecules such as monosaccharides, amino acids, or ions requires the assistance of a specific integral membrane protein.

Properties of Transport Proteins

Proteins that transport small molecules across membranes bind to a specific molecule on one side of the membrane and release it on the other side (**Part C**). Proteins that carry a single solute from one side of the membrane to the other are known as **uniporters**. Other proteins function as **cotransporters**, in which two different solutes are transported simultaneously. If the two solutes move in the same direction, the carrier proteins are known as **symporters**, whereas if they move in opposite directions, they are known as **antiporters**.

Passive Transport

The movement of molecules across the membrane from a region of higher concentration to a region of lower concentration is defined as passive transport. Passive transport by **simple diffusion** describes the movement of molecules directly through the bilayer without the assistance of a carrier protein. The rate of simple diffusion is directly proportional to the concentration gradient across the membrane (**Part D**). Passive transport by **facilitated diffusion** requires an integral membrane protein that is specific for the molecule being transported. The rate of facilitated transport shows saturation kinetics and is limited by the number of carrier proteins in the membrane. The transport of glucose from the blood into cells is facilitated by a family of **transport proteins** known as the GLUT family.

Active Transport

The movement of molecules across a membrane from a region of low concentration to a region of high concentration requires both a carrier protein and a source of energy. In some cases, the energy is supplied by direct **ATP hydrolysis**. For example, the transport of Na^+ out of the cell in exchange for K^+ entering the cell is mediated by **Na^+/K^+-ATPase** acting as an antiporter. In other cases, the energy is supplied by an **ion gradient**. For example, the Na^+-dependent uptake of glucose from the intestinal lumen is mediated by **SGLUT**, a symporter that simultaneously transports Na^+ and glucose into the intestinal cell. The energy for transporting glucose uphill against a concentration gradient is provided by the movement of Na^+ down a concentration gradient.

Clinical Significance

The process of transport across membranes is essential for maintaining homeostasis. For example, the ability to lower blood glucose levels after eating is mediated by insulin. One of the effects of insulin is to increase the number of glucose transporters in the plasma membrane of muscle tissue and adipose tissue, thereby increasing the uptake of glucose by these tissues. Defective transport proteins result in several diseases. **Cystinuria**, the most common defect in amino acid metabolism, results from a genetic defect in the protein that transports cystine across the luminal membrane of both intestinal and kidney cells. Several transport proteins are targets for commonly used drugs. The **cardiac glycosides** are a family of drugs that exert their effect by binding to the plasma membrane Na^+/K^+-ATPase. The cellular **uptake of some chemotherapeutic drugs** involves carrier proteins in the plasma membrane.

For more information see Coffee C, *Metabolism*. Fence Creek, pp 2–5.

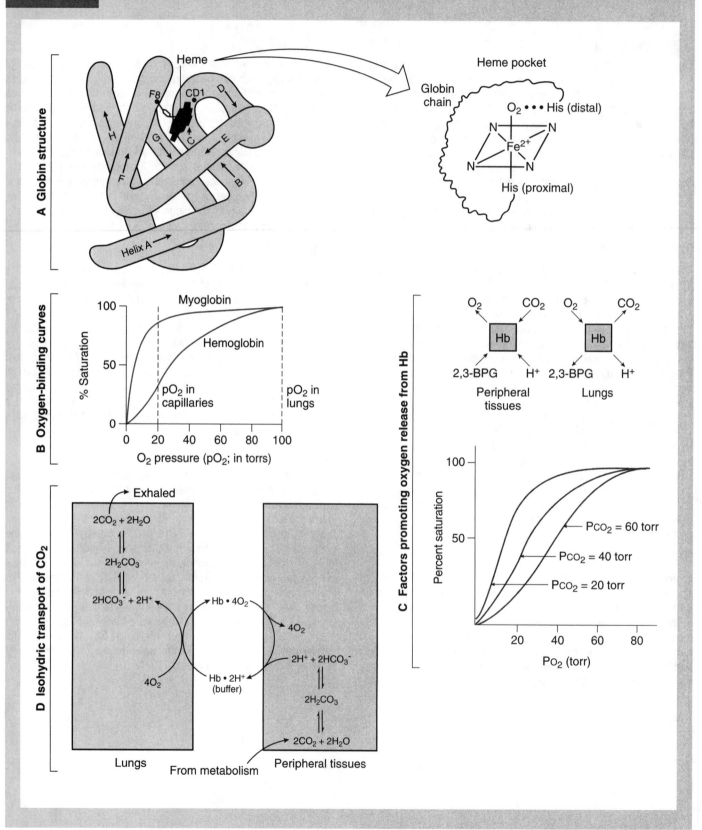

A Globin structure

Heme

F8 CD1 D

H G C E

F B

Helix A

Heme pocket

Globin chain

O_2 ••• His (distal)

N   N

Fe^{2+}

N   N

His (proximal)

B Oxygen-binding curves

Myoglobin

Hemoglobin

% Saturation

pO_2 in capillaries

pO_2 in lungs

O_2 pressure (pO_2; in torrs)

C Factors promoting oxygen release from Hb

O_2 CO_2 O_2 CO_2

Hb   Hb

2,3-BPG H^+ 2,3-BPG H^+

Peripheral tissues   Lungs

Percent saturation

$P_{CO_2} = 60$ torr

$P_{CO_2} = 40$ torr

$P_{CO_2} = 20$ torr

P_{O_2} (torr)

D Isohydric transport of CO_2

Exhaled

$2CO_2 + 2H_2O$

$2H_2CO_3$

$2HCO_3^- + 2H^+$

$Hb \cdot 4O_2$

$4O_2$

$2H^+ + 2HCO_3^-$

$4O_2$ $Hb \cdot 2H^+$ (buffer)

$2H_2CO_3$

$2CO_2 + 2H_2O$

Lungs   Peripheral tissues

From metabolism

OVERVIEW

Hemoglobin (Hb) plays an important role in the transport of O_2 and CO_2, as well as in the maintenance of blood pH. Normal adult hemoglobin (HbA) is a tetramer with an $\alpha_2\beta_2$ subunit composition. The genes for the α- and β-globin subunits are located on chromosomes 16 and 11, respectively. Each subunit contains heme, the cofactor for binding O_2. The binding and release of O_2 occur in the lung and tissue capillaries, respectively. The partial pressure of CO_2 (Pco_2) and the concentration of 2,3-bisphosphoglycerate (2,3-BPG) in the red blood cells strongly influence the release of O_2 from Hb. Fetal hemoglobin (HbF), with a subunit structure of $\alpha_2\gamma_2$, has a higher affinity for O_2 than HbA. Diseases resulting from abnormalities in Hb structure and synthesis are among the most common known genetic diseases.

Key Structural Features of Globin Subunits

The tertiary structure of all globin chains is essentially identical, including that of myoglobin (Mb), the O_2 storage protein in muscle. Globin chains consist of eight α-helical segments that are folded to form a V-shaped pocket for binding heme (**Part A**). The **heme-binding pocket** is lined with hydrophobic amino acid side chains that exclude water, thereby protecting the heme iron from oxidation. Heme iron must be in the Fe^{2+} state to bind O_2. Only two hydrophilic amino acid side chains are found in the heme pocket: the **proximal histidine** that acts as a ligand for binding Fe^{2+} to heme, and the **distal histidine** that stabilizes oxyHb by forming a hydrogen bond with O_2.

Oxygen-Binding Properties of Hemoglobin and Myoglobin

The curve describing the binding of O_2 to Mb is **hyperbolic**, while that for Hb is **sigmoidal**, a difference that reflects the subunit structure of the two proteins (**Part B**). Mb is a monomer having a single binding site for O_2, while Hb is a tetramer having four O_2-binding sites. The sigmoidal curve for Hb indicates **positive cooperativity** between the O_2-binding sites. As blood passes through the lungs, binding of O_2 to the first site facilitates binding to the other sites. Similarly, as blood flows through the tissue bed, release of O_2 from the first site facilitates release from other sites. Mb has a higher affinity for O_2 than Hb. The partial pressure of O_2 required for half-saturation (P_{50}) is 3 to 5 torr for Mb and 25 to 30 torr for Hb.

Effect of CO_2, H^+, and 2,3-BPG on O_2 Release from Hemoglobin

An increase in Pco_2 results in the release of O_2 from Hb, a phenomenon known as the **Bohr effect**. As the Pco_2 increases, the O_2 saturation curve for Hb is shifted to the right (**Part C**). The same effect is produced by an increase in H^+ or a decrease in pH. Metabolically active tissues produce CO_2, which diffuses into the red blood cells where it is converted to $H_2CO_3^-$ by **carbonic anhydrase**. H_2CO_3 is a weak acid, having a pK_a of 6.1, and at physiologic pH it dissociates to H^+ and HCO_3^-, as shown below:

$$CO_2 + H_2O \rightleftharpoons H_2CO_3 \rightleftharpoons HCO_3^- + H^+$$

The ability of H^+ to promote O_2 release from Hb is due to the fact that **oxyHb is a stronger acid than deoxyHb**, as shown in the following equation where H^+ is released from ionizable amino acid side chains of oxyHb. Clearly, an increase in H^+ (or CO_2) pushes this reaction in the reverse direction, releasing O_2:

$$H\text{-}Hb + O_2 \rightleftharpoons [H\text{-}HbO_2] \rightleftharpoons HbO_2 + H^+$$

The effect of 2,3-BPG on the O_2 saturation curve is qualitatively similar to that of CO_2 and H^+ (**Part C**, upper portion). The binding of 2,3-BPG promotes release of O_2. The binding site for 2,3-BPG is between the two β-subunits of deoxy HbA and the two γ-subunits of deoxy HbF. It does not bind to oxyHb. The affinity of HbA for 2,3-BPG is higher than that of HbF.

Role of Hemoglobin in CO_2 Transport

Hb participates in the **isohydric transport** of CO_2 by acting as a buffer that absorbs H^+ (**Part D**). About 75% of the CO_2 is transported as HCO_3^- in the plasma. DeoxyHb absorbs H^+ produced by the dissociation of H_2CO_3, thereby shifting the equilibrium toward the formation of more HCO_3^- (see equation above). In the capillaries of peripheral tissues, the Pco_2 is high and the formation of H_2CO_3 is favored. In the capillaries of lungs, the Pco_2 is low and the breakdown of H_2CO_3 to CO_2 and H_2O is favored. An additional 15% to 20% of the CO_2 is transported as **carbamoyl-Hb**, a covalent adduct formed between CO_2 and the amino terminus of the globin chains. This reaction (shown below) is reversible, allowing CO_2 to be released in the lungs:

$$CO_2 + NH_2\text{-}Hb \rightleftharpoons {}^-O\text{-}\overset{\displaystyle O}{\overset{\displaystyle \|}{C}}\text{-}NH\text{-}Hb$$

Clinical Significance

Diseases involving Hb are classified into two broad categories, resulting from abnormalities in Hb: hemoglobinopathies and thalassemias. The most well characterized hemoglobinopathy is **sickle cell anemia**, resulting from a single amino acid substitution in the β-chain. Glutamate at position $\beta6$ in HbA is replaced by valine at $\beta6$ in sickle cell hemoglobin (HbS). This substitution markedly **decreases the solubility of deoxyHbS**. In the capillaries where deoxyHbS predominates, polymers of HbS form that distort the shape of the red blood cells. These "sickle-shaped" cells are fragile and have a short lifespan. The extent of sickling is increased by any condition that promotes release of O_2 from HbS.

The thalassemias are a group of syndromes resulting from an imbalance in the synthesis of α- and β-chains. In α-**thalassemia**, α-chain synthesis is impaired. **Hydrops fetalis** is an α-thalassemia resulting from total absence of α-chains. Bart's Hb (γ_4) is formed in utero and HbH (β_4) is formed postnatally. Both Bart's Hb and HbH have a high affinity for O_2 and are unable to release adequate O_2 to tissues. β-Thalassemias result from an absence or decreased production of β-chains. β-**Thalassemia major** occurs in individuals with mutations in both alleles of the β gene. It is characterized by severe anemia that has to be treated by transfusions throughout life. β-**Thalassemia minor** occurs in carriers having only one mutant allele. The β-thalassemias are characterized by elevated levels of HbF ($\alpha_2\gamma_2$) and HbA_2 ($\alpha_2\Delta_2$).

For more information see Coffee C, *Metabolism*. Fence Creek, pp 49–60.

8 General Properties of Enzymes

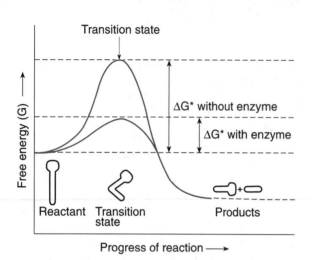

A Energy changes during reactions

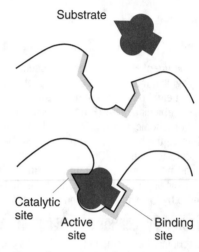

Substrate

Catalytic site

Active site

Binding site

B Formation of enzyme-substrate complex

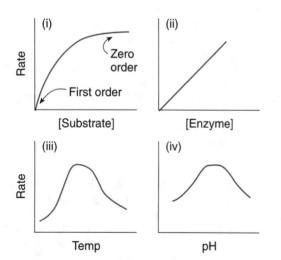

C Factors affecting rate of enzyme-catalyzed reactions

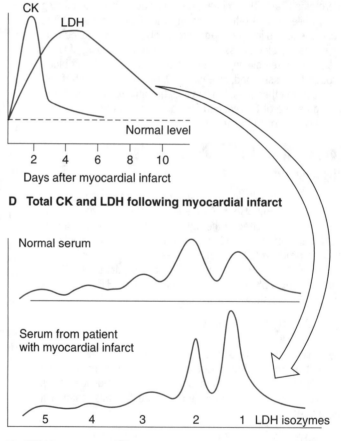

CK

LDH

Normal level

Days after myocardial infarct

D Total CK and LDH following myocardial infarct

Normal serum

Serum from patient with myocardial infarct

5   4   3   2   1 LDH isozymes

E LDH isozyme profiles

OVERVIEW

Enzymes are biocatalysts that increase the rate of chemical reactions without altering the equilibrium of the reaction. All chemical reactions proceed through a high-energy barrier known as the transition state. An enzyme lowers the energy of the transition state, thereby increasing the rate at which the reaction occurs. In enzyme-catalyzed reactions the substrate binds to a specialized region of the enzyme known as the active site, where it is transformed into product and released, leaving the enzyme unchanged. Enzymes are highly specific for the reaction they catalyze, and they have much greater catalytic power than other catalysts.

Energy Changes During a Chemical Reaction

During the course of a chemical reaction, intermediates are formed that have structures resembling both the reactant and product. The intermediate with the highest energy state is defined as the **transition state (Part A)**. The difference in the energy content of the reactant and the transition state is defined as the **activation energy** (ΔG^*) of the reaction. The magnitude of ΔG^* is inversely proportional to the rate of the reaction. Enzymes stabilize the transition state, thereby **decreasing the ΔG^*** and **increasing the rate** of the reaction. The equilibrium of the reaction is unchanged because enzymes increase the rate of the forward and reverse reactions equally.

Formation of Enzyme–Substrate Complex

The first step in an enzyme-catalyzed reaction is the formation of an enzyme–substrate complex (**Part B**). The substrate binds to the **active site**, a specialized region on the enzyme created by the side chains of several amino acids. The amino acids can be widely separated in the linear sequence, but the enzyme is folded in such a way that the side chains are in close proximity at the active site. The active site has regions responsible for binding the substrate and separate regions that catalyze the reaction. The side chains in the active site can be classified into two functional groups. **Binding residues** interact with the substrate through multiple noncovalent interactions, and **catalytic residues** create a superactive microenvironment that enhances the rate at which substrate is converted to product.

The high degree of **specificity** of enzymes for their substrates has been explained by two models of interaction between the enzyme and substrate. In the **template (lock-and-key) model**, the active site is a rigid structure that is complementary to the structure of the substrate. In the **induced-fit (hand-in-glove) model**, the active site is more flexible and substrate binding induces a conformational change in the enzyme, leading to an active site structure that is complementary to the substrate.

The **catalytic power** of enzymes is attributed to the side chains in the catalytic site, which are usually positioned near the bonds that are being made or broken during the reaction. Some catalytic residues, such as histidine, aspartic acid, glutamic acid, and lysine, act as conjugate acids and conjugate bases by donating and accepting protons during a catalytic cycle. Other amino acids such as serine, cysteine, and histidine have nucleophilic groups in their side chains that can assist in the cleavage of covalent bonds.

Factors Affecting the Rate of Enzyme-Catalyzed Reactions

The rate (velocity) of an enzyme-catalyzed reaction varies with the **substrate concentration (Part C, i)**. At very low substrate concen-

trations a first-order reaction is observed, with the rate being directly proportional to the substrate concentration. When the concentration of substrate is sufficiently high so that all of the active sites are occupied, a zero-order reaction occurs, with the rate being independent of substrate concentration. The rate of an enzyme-catalyzed reaction is directly proportional to the **concentration of enzyme**, provided the substrate concentration is high enough for all of the enzyme to exist as the enzyme-substrate complex (**Part C, ii**). The rates of most reactions increase approximately twofold with an increase in **temperature** of 10°C. For enzyme-catalyzed reactions, however, there is an optimal temperature beyond which the enzyme begins to denature (**Part C, iii**). The rate of enzyme-catalyzed reactions varies with **pH (Part C, iv)**. The optimal rate usually occurs between pH 5 and 9. The shape of the curve reflects different ionization states for specific amino acid side chains in the active site.

Isozymes

Isozymes are enzymes that catalyze the same reaction but have different chemical, physical, and kinetic properties. Isozymes frequently have organ-specific localization, a property that has been exploited for diagnostic purposes. For example, the diagnosis of acute myocardial infarct (AMI) routinely analyzes the total serum creatine kinase (CK) and lactate dehydrogenase (LDH), and the isozyme patterns of each. Following cardiac tissue damage, the total activity of both CK and LDH in the serum increases, with the release of CK occurring considerably earlier than that of LDH (**Part D**). Since these enzymes are also present in other tissues, analyses of isozyme patterns are needed to determine the origin of the activity. The change in the CK profile that is specific for cardiac tissue is an increase in the CK-MB isozyme, which is synthesized only in cardiac tissue. The change in the isozyme pattern for LDH associated with AMI is in the ratio of LDH_1/LDH_2 isozymes (**Part E**). Normally, the serum concentration of LDH_2 is greater than LDH_1, but after an AMI the LDH_1 is the predominant isozyme.

Clinical Significance

The principles of enzymology are important in both the diagnosis and the treatment of disease. Many inborn errors of metabolism result from a deficiency in a single enzyme. Decreased enzyme activity can result either from a structural change in the enzyme itself or from decreased synthesis of the enzyme.

For more information see Coffee C, *Metabolism*. Fence Creek, pp 33–44.

9 Enzyme Kinetics

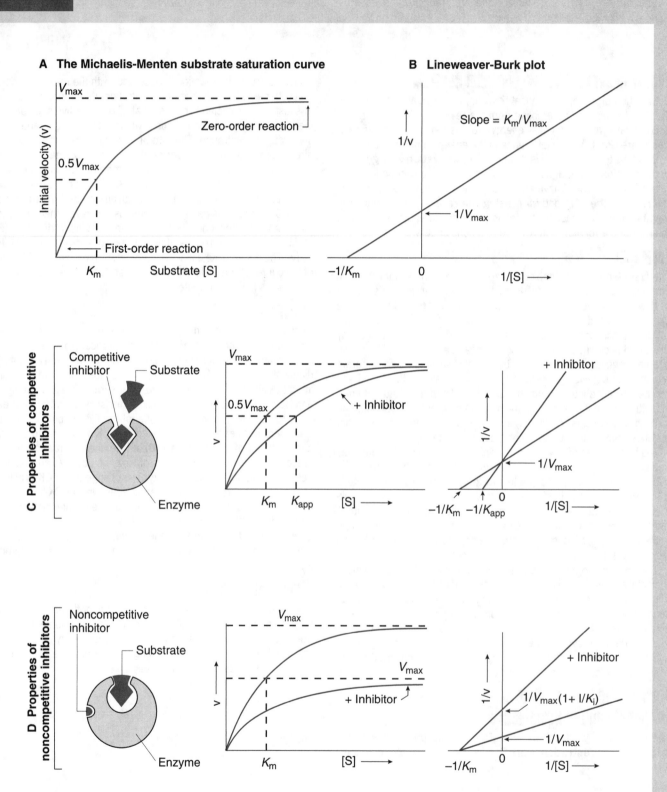

A The Michaelis-Menten substrate saturation curve

V_{max}

Initial velocity (v)

Zero-order reaction

$0.5 V_{max}$

First-order reaction

K_m — Substrate [S]

B Lineweaver-Burk plot

Slope = K_m/V_{max}

1/v

$1/V_{max}$

$-1/K_m$ — 0 — 1/[S] →

C Properties of competitive inhibitors

Competitive inhibitor

Substrate

Enzyme

V_{max}

$0.5 V_{max}$

v

+ Inhibitor

K_m K_{app} [S] →

+ Inhibitor

1/v

$1/V_{max}$

$-1/K_m$ $-1/K_{app}$ 0 1/[S] →

D Properties of noncompetitive inhibitors

Noncompetitive inhibitor

Substrate

Enzyme

V_{max}

v

V_{max}

+ Inhibitor

K_m [S] →

+ Inhibitor

1/v

$1/V_{max}(1 + I/K_i)$

$1/V_{max}$

$-1/K_m$ 0 1/[S] →

A useful model for quantitating the catalytic activity of enzymes is the Michaelis-Menten equation. This equation describes the relationship between the initial velocity of an enzyme-catalyzed reaction and the substrate concentration. The Michaelis-Menten equation defines two kinetic parameters, K_m and V_{max}, which are related to intrinsic properties of the enzyme. Lineweaver-Burk plots are commonly used to determine the values for K_m and V_{max}. The therapeutic action of many drugs is based on the principles of enzyme inhibition. Inhibitors bind to enzymes and decrease the catalytic activity by altering either the K_m or the V_{max}.

The Michaelis-Menten Equation

The relationship between the rate of an enzyme-catalyzed reaction and the substrate concentration is shown in **Part A**. This curve is described by the following equation:

$$v = \frac{V_{max}\,[S]}{K_m + [S]}$$

The V_{max} is defined as the velocity observed when all of the binding sites on the enzyme are filled with substrate; it is an index of the catalytic efficiency of an enzyme. It is directly proportional to the enzyme concentration and is sensitive to changes in pH and temperature. The units for V_{max} are rate units. The K_m (Michaelis constant) can be defined as the substrate concentration required to achieve half-maximum velocity, and is therefore an index of the affinity of the enzyme for its substrate. A low K_m corresponds to a high affinity and vice-versa. The units for K_m are concentration units. Values for V_{max} and K_m can be extrapolated from the substrate saturation curve (**Part A**). Values obtained by this method, however, are subject to considerable error.

Lineweaver-Burk Plots

Lineweaver-Burk plots are commonly used to obtain values for K_m and V_{max} (**Part B**). The following equation for this double reciprocal plot is obtained by inverting the Michaelis-Menten equation:

$$\frac{1}{V} = \frac{1}{V_{max}} + \frac{K_m}{V_{max}} \times \frac{1}{[S]}$$

The relationship between $1/V$ and $1/[S]$ describes a straight line having a slope equal to K_m/V_{max}. The point at which the line crosses the x-axis is equal to $-1/K_m$, and the point at which the line crosses the y-axis is equal to $1/V_{max}$. Therefore, values for K_m and V_{max} can be calculated directly from the numerical values of the x and y intercepts, respectively.

Enzyme Inhibitors

Inhibitors can produce either reversible or irreversible effects on the catalytic activity of an enzyme. Compounds that are reversible inhibitors can be classified into two major categories: competitive and noncompetitive inhibitors. The effects of these inhibitors on the kinetic parameters of a reaction can be readily seen by examining either the substrate saturation curve or Lineweaver-Burk plots. **Competitive inhibitors** are structural analogs of the substrate and compete with the substrate for the same binding site on the enzyme (**Part C**). The effects of a competitive inhibitor can be reversed by increasing the substrate to a concentration sufficiently high to occupy all the binding sites. Competitive inhibitors increase the apparent K_m (K_{app}) but have no effect on the V_{max}. Competitive inhibitors are readily identified by Lineweaver-Burk plots, where the lines for the inhibited and uninhibited reactions intersect on the y-axis. **Noncompetitive inhibitors** are not structurally related to the substrate and bind to a site that is independent of the substrate-binding site (**Part D**). The effect of a noncompetitive inhibitor cannot be reversed by increasing the concentration of substrate. Noncompetitive inhibitors decrease the V_{max} but have no effect on the K_m. Noncompetitive inhibitors are readily identified by Lineweaver-Burk plots, where the lines for the inhibited and uninhibited reactions intersect on the x-axis. Both competitive and noncompetitive inhibitors increase the slope of the line in the Lineweaver-Burk plot relative to that observed in the absence of inhibitor.

Irreversible inhibitors react covalently with an amino acid side chain on the enzyme, forming a stable complex that is permanently inactivated. Some irreversible inhibitors are known as **mechanism-based inhibitors**. These inhibitors are structurally related to the substrate and bind to the active site. After binding they inactivate the enzyme by reacting with some amino acid side chain in the active site. Mechanism-based inhibitors are also known as **suicide substrates**. The kinetic effect of an irreversible inhibitor is similar to that of a noncompetitive inhibitor, resulting in a decrease in V_{max} but having no effect on the K_m. An irreversible inhibitor has the same kinetic effect as decreasing the amount of enzyme.

Clinical Significance

Many drugs exert their effects by inhibiting specific enzymes. Most inhibitors that are used therapeutically are either competitive inhibitors or irreversible mechanism-based inhibitors. Most of the drug development in modern pharmacology is based on the principles of enzyme inhibition and enzyme kinetics. Some commonly used drugs that exert their effects by inhibiting enzymes are listed in the following table.

Drug	Therapeutic Use	Target Enzyme	Type of Inhibitor
Mevinolin	Hypercholesterolemia	HMG-CoA reductase	Competitive
5-Fluorouracil	Cancer	Thymidylate synthase	Suicide
Methotrexate	Cancer	Dihydrofolate reductase	Competitive
Allopurinol	Gout	Xanthine oxidase	Suicide
Aspirin	Anti-inflammatory	Cyclooxygenase	Suicide
Captopril	High blood pressure	Angiotensin-converting enzyme	Competitive

For more information see Coffee C, *Metabolism*. Fence Creek, pp 33–44.

10 Regulation of Enzyme Activity

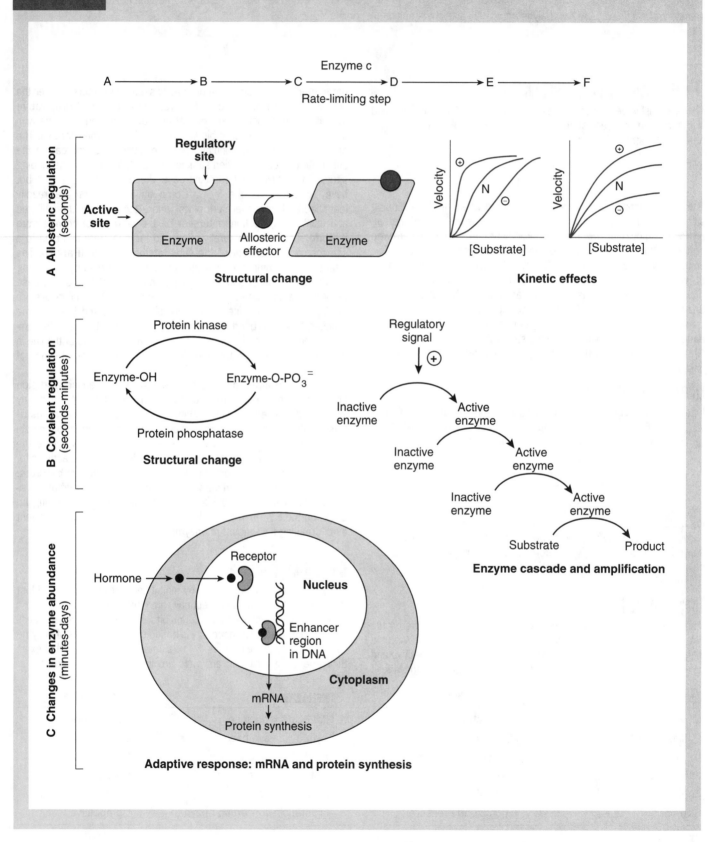

Enzyme c

A ———→ B ———→ C ———→ D ———→ E ———→ F

Rate-limiting step

A Allosteric regulation (seconds)

Regulatory site

Active site

Enzyme

Allosteric effector

Enzyme

Structural change

Velocity

[Substrate]

⊕   N   ⊖

Velocity

[Substrate]

⊕   N   ⊖

Kinetic effects

B Covalent regulation (seconds-minutes)

Protein kinase

Enzyme-OH   Enzyme-O-PO$_3^=$

Protein phosphatase

Structural change

Regulatory signal

⊕

Inactive enzyme → Active enzyme

Inactive enzyme → Active enzyme

Inactive enzyme → Active enzyme

Substrate → Product

Enzyme cascade and amplification

C Changes in enzyme abundance (minutes-days)

Hormone →

Receptor

Nucleus

Enhancer region in DNA

Cytoplasm

mRNA

Protein synthesis

Adaptive response: mRNA and protein synthesis

OVERVIEW

A variety of mechanisms exist within cells that allow metabolism to proceed in an orderly and balanced fashion. Imposed on the intracellular mechanisms are hormonal mechanisms that coordinate the metabolic activities between different cells and tissues. Each metabolic pathway has at least one key regulatory enzyme, usually the enzyme that catalyzes the rate-limiting step in the pathway. Secondary sites of regulation in metabolic pathways are frequently enzymes that catalyze irreversible reactions or reactions that create branch points in pathways. There are three major mechanisms for regulating the activity of enzymes: 1) allosteric interactions, 2) covalent modification, and 3) changes in enzyme abundance. The time required for an enzyme to respond to each of these mechanisms differs, ranging from minutes to days. A particular enzyme may be regulated by all three mechanisms.

Allosteric Regulation

The most rapid type of regulation occurs when a small molecule, having little structural resemblance to the substrate, binds to a regulatory site on the enzyme, resulting in a conformational change that alters the K_m for the substrate and/or the V_{max} of the reaction (**Part A**). The regulatory site is known as the **allosteric site** and the molecules that bind to these sites are **allosteric effectors**. Most allosteric enzymes are multisubunit enzymes having **sigmoidal substrate saturation curves** that cannot be described by Michaelis-Menten kinetics. **Positive effectors** (allosteric activators) decrease the K_m or increase the V_{max}, whereas **negative effectors** (allosteric inhibitors) increase the K_m or decrease the V_{max}. In many cases, an effector can alter both the K_m and V_m. The types of molecules that act as allosteric effectors are usually end products of pathways (heme, cholesterol, and purine and pyrimidine nucleotides) or molecules that serve as indicators of the energy state of the cell (ATP, ADP, AMP). The accumulation of ATP indicates a high-energy state, whereas the accumulation of ADP or AMP indicates a low-energy state. Many catabolic pathways (glycolysis, tricarboxylic acid cycle) lead to ATP synthesis, and regulatory enzymes in these pathways are inhibited by ATP and activated by ADP or AMP. Conversely, anabolic pathways usually require energy and are activated by ATP and inhibited by ADP or AMP. The accumulation of acetyl CoA and citrate also indicate a high-energy state in the cell.

Covalent Regulation

Covalent regulation may be reversible or irreversible (**Part B**). The most common type of reversible covalent regulation in metabolism is phosphorylation and dephosphorylation, reactions catalyzed by a family of **protein kinases** and **protein phosphatases**, respectively. Protein kinases transfer a phosphate group from ATP to the hydroxyl group of a specific serine, threonine, or tyrosine residue in the target enzyme. The residue that is phosphorylated is surrounded by a specific amino acid sequence, known as the **consensus sequence**. Each protein kinase recognizes a different consensus sequence. The addition or removal of phosphate groups produces a change in both the conformation of the enzyme and its kinetic properties. The K_m or V_{max} and, in some cases, the affinity for an allosteric effector are altered. Each protein kinase is activated by a specific **second messenger molecule** (cAMP, cGMP, DAG, Ca^{2+}). The concentration of second messengers in the cell is regulated, in turn, by hormones that bind to the surface of cells.

The most common type of irreversible covalent regulation is **limited proteolysis**, a mechanism used to convert inactive precursors to active enzymes. Limited proteolysis is involved in activating enzymes responsible for many important processes, including collagen assembly, blood clotting, complement activation, and protein digestion. Both phosphorylation and limited proteolysis are used to establish **enzyme cascades**. Cascades are generated when one molecule of enzyme activates many molecules of another enzyme, thereby providing a mechanism for **amplification** of small regulatory signals. The amplification potential is increased by increasing the number of enzymes in the cascade.

Changes in Enzyme Abundance

The rate at which a particular reaction occurs is dependent on the amount of enzyme present in the cell. Although most enzymes are present at a constant level throughout the life of the cell, regulatory enzymes can vary significantly in concentration, depending on the needs of the cell. An adaptive response resulting in an increase in the amount of enzyme involves both mRNA and protein synthesis, and is subject to hormonal regulation (**Part C**). The rate of mRNA synthesis is controlled by a group of proteins known as **transcriptional factors**, some of which are hormone receptors. Steroid and thyroid hormones regulate transcription by binding directly to the transcriptional factor, whereas other hormones such as glucagon can regulate transcription by stimulating the phosphorylation of specific transcriptional factors. Activated transcriptional factors bind to regulatory sequences in DNA known as **enhancers** or **silencers**, resulting in either an increase or a decrease in the rate of mRNA synthesis, respectively. Following transcription, mRNA is translocated to the cytosol where it directs the synthesis of a specific enzyme. A period of time extending from hours to days may pass between the initiating signal and the actual change in enzyme concentration.

Clinical Significance

Homeostasis can be defined as the maintenance of a constant cellular environment. This is a remarkable feat, considering that each cell obtains nutrients from the surrounding interstitial fluid, metabolizes the nutrients by dozens of different pathways, and releases its waste products into the same fluid. The ability of the cell to maintain a narrow concentration range for each of the thousands of metabolites is achieved primarily by a few key regulatory enzymes that are able to respond to small changes that occur both in the cell and in the fluid surrounding the cell. Loss of the regulatory properties of an enzyme is frequently associated with disease.

For more information see Coffee C, *Metabolism*. Fence Creek, pp 112–120.

11 Transduction of Hormonal Signals Across Membranes

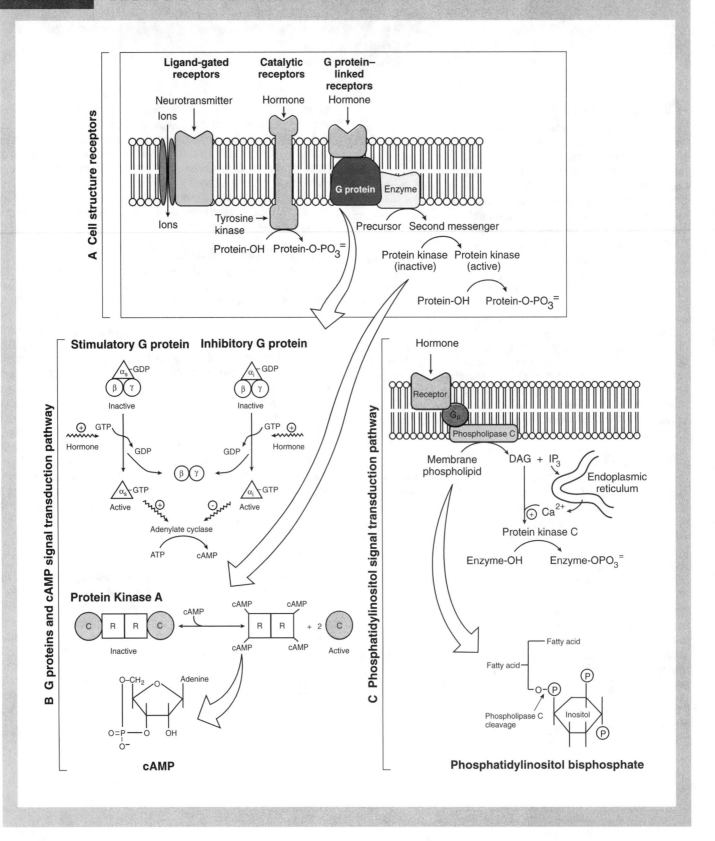

A Cell structure receptors

Ligand-gated receptors

Neurotransmitter

Ions

Ions

Catalytic receptors

Hormone

Tyrosine kinase

Protein-OH → Protein-O-PO$_3^=$

G protein–linked receptors

Hormone

G protein

Enzyme

Precursor → Second messenger

Protein kinase (inactive) → Protein kinase (active)

Protein-OH → Protein-O-PO$_3^=$

B G proteins and cAMP signal transduction pathway

Stimulatory G protein

α_s-GDP
β γ
Inactive

$+$ GTP
Hormone
GDP

α_s-GTP
Active
$+$

Inhibitory G protein

α_i-GDP
β γ
Inactive

GTP $+$
Hormone
GDP

β γ

α_i-GTP
Active
$-$

Adenylate cyclase

ATP → cAMP

Protein Kinase A

C R R C
Inactive

cAMP

cAMP cAMP
R R
cAMP cAMP

$+$ 2 C
Active

O-CH$_2$ Adenine
O=P-O OH
O$^-$

cAMP

C Phosphatidylinositol signal transduction pathway

Hormone

Receptor

G$_p$

Phospholipase C

Membrane phospholipid

DAG + IP$_3$

Endoplasmic reticulum

$+$ Ca^{2+}

Protein kinase C

Enzyme-OH → Enzyme-OPO$_3^=$

Fatty acid

Fatty acid

O P

P

Phospholipase C cleavage

Inositol

P

Phosphatidylinositol bisphosphate

OVERVIEW

The metabolic activities of different cells and organs are coordinated by hormones that are synthesized in endocrine glands and released into the circulation. The hormones act as chemical signals or **primary messengers** that produce a characteristic response in other tissues, known as target tissues. The **target tissues** that respond to a particular hormone have **receptors** that bind the hormone with a high degree of specificity. **Lipid-soluble hormones** such as steroid hormones and thyroid hormones can cross the plasma membrane and enter the cell where they bind to their receptors. Peptide hormones, catecholamines, and neurotransmitters are water-soluble molecules that cannot cross the plasma membrane, and they transmit their signal to the inside of cells by binding to **cell-surface receptors**. The hormone–receptor complex stimulates the production of an intracellular molecule known as a **second messenger**.

Cell-Surface Receptors

There are three major classes of cell-surface receptors that differ from one another in their mechanism of signal transduction across the plasma membrane (**Part A**). **Ligand-gated receptors** have an ion channel that spans the plasma membrane and a ligand-binding domain on the extracellular surface of the membrane that binds to a specific ligand, usually a neurotransmitter. The binding of a ligand results in a conformational change in the receptor that renders the ion channel selectively permeable to one or more ions. The direction that a particular ion moves is determined by the concentration gradient of that ion across the membrane. **Catalytic receptors** span the plasma membrane, having an extracellular domain that binds a hormone or growth factor and a cytosolic domain that has intrinsic enzyme activity. The most well-characterized catalytic receptors are those that bind insulin, growth factors, and atrial natriuretic factor (ANF). Binding of insulin or growth factors to their respective receptors activates tyrosine kinase activity, which is associated with an intracellular domain of the receptor. The active tyrosine kinase catalyzes the phosphorylation of a number of proteins that propagate the signal along various pathways in the cell. The ANF receptor has intrinsic guanylate cyclase activity. The binding of ANF to its receptor stimulates the conversion of GTP to cGMP, the second messenger for ANF. **G protein–linked receptors** are a family of homologous membrane proteins. These receptors have an extracellular domain that binds a specific hormone (glucagon, epinephrine, adrenocorticotropic hormone, parathyroid hormone, etc.) and a domain within the membrane that binds to a G protein. All G protein–linked receptors are structurally similar in that they span the membrane seven times. The G proteins provide a communication link between the hormone receptor and an enzyme that synthesizes second-messenger molecules, such as cAMP and diacylglycerol (DAG). Each type of second messenger activates a specific protein kinase that catalyzes the phosphorylation of a subset of cellular proteins, resulting in a change in their biologic activity.

G Proteins and the cAMP Signal Transduction Pathway

The G proteins (**Part B**) are trimers consisting of α-, β-, and γ-subunits. Two types of G proteins are involved in the **cAMP signal transduction pathway**, G_s and G_i. Adenylate cyclase, the enzyme that synthesizes cAMP, is stimulated by G_s and inhibited by G_i. The G proteins differ only in their α-subunits (α_s and α_i, respectively). The α-subunits bind a guanine nucleotide, either GTP or GDP, and have intrinsic GTPase activity that slowly hydrolyzes GTP to GDP. The cell contains both inactive and active forms of G proteins. The inactive form, the $\alpha\beta\gamma$ trimer, binds GDP, whereas the active form is the free α-subunit, which binds GTP. Binding of a hormone to its receptor results in the displacement of GDP by GTP, followed by the dissociation of the complex, releasing the active α-subunit. The active α_s- and α_i-subunits can associate with **adenylate cyclase**, and either increase or decrease the rate at which ATP is converted to cAMP. The α-subunits retain their ability to interact with adenylate cyclase only as long as GTP is bound. When GTP is hydrolyzed to GDP, the inactive $\alpha\beta\gamma$ trimer is reformed.

The only known function of cAMP in mammalian cells is to activate **protein kinase A**. Protein kinase A contains separate regulatory (R) and catalytic (C) subunits. The presence of the regulatory subunits inhibits the activity of the C subunits. The binding of cAMP to the R subunits results in the release of active C subunits, which phosphorylate specific serine residues in several cellular proteins, thereby altering their biologic activity. cAMP is degraded by **cAMP phosphodiesterase**, an enzyme that is activated by insulin and inhibited by caffeine.

The Phosphatidylinositol Signal Transduction Pathway

Hormones that use the phosphatidylinositol signal transduction pathway (**Part C**) activate a different G protein (G_p) which, in turn, activates **phospholipase C**. This enzyme cleaves a specific membrane phospholipid, phosphatidylinositol bisphosphate, generating two second messengers, DAG and inositol triphosphate (IP_3). DAG activates **protein kinase C**, while IP_3 binds to receptors on the smooth endoplasmic reticulum, resulting in the release of Ca^{2+}. The increase in cytosolic Ca^{2+} activates several **Ca^{2+}-calmodulin-dependent protein kinases** found in the cell. Both protein kinase C and Ca^{2+}-calmodulin-dependent protein kinases catalyze the phosphorylation several enzymes in the cell. IP_3 and DAG can be used to resynthesize phosphatidylinositol, but only after the three phosphate groups have been removed from IP_3, producing inositol. **Lithium**, a drug used to treat manic depression, inhibits one or more of the phosphatases involved in converting IP_3 to inositol.

Clinical Significance

Cellular transformation leading to cancer is closely linked to abnormalities in signal transduction pathways. **Oncogenes** that are expressed during malignant transformation of cells are mutant genes that code for abnormal components of signal transduction pathways. The abnormal proteins stimulate uncontrolled cellular growth and differentiation. The proteins encoded by oncogenes include abnormal forms of growth factors, growth factor receptors, hormone receptors, G proteins, protein kinases, and transcriptional factors.

Several bacterial toxins establish disease by modifying the structure and function of G proteins. These toxins catalyze the **ADP-ribosylation** of the α-subunits. **Cholera toxin** modifies the α_s-subunit, resulting in loss of GTPase activity. The inability to hydrolyze GTP to GDP locks the α_s-subunit into a permanently active form that persistently stimulates adenylate cyclase. **Pertussis toxin** modifies the α_i-subunit, resulting in the inability of the $\alpha\beta\gamma$ trimer to dissociate, a change that prevents adenylate cyclase from being inhibited. Both toxins lead to very high levels of cellular cAMP.

For more information see Coffee C, *Metabolism*. Fence Creek, pp 120–125.

12 Nutritional Basis of Metabolism: Macronutrients

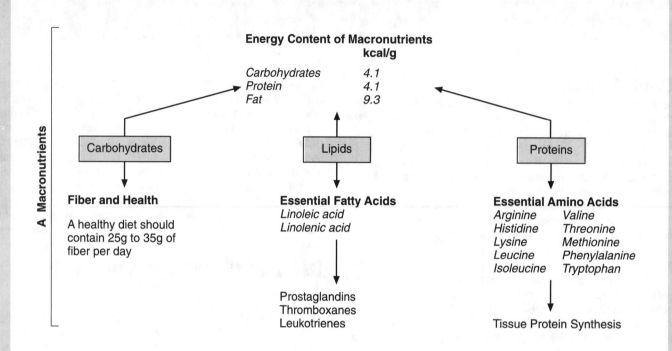

A Macronutrients

Energy Content of Macronutrients
kcal/g

Carbohydrates	*4.1*
Protein	*4.1*
Fat	*9.3*

Carbohydrates

Lipids

Proteins

Fiber and Health

A healthy diet should contain 25g to 35g of fiber per day

Essential Fatty Acids
Linoleic acid
Linolenic acid

Prostaglandins
Thromboxanes
Leukotrienes

Essential Amino Acids

Arginine	*Valine*
Histidine	*Threonine*
Lysine	*Methionine*
Leucine	*Phenylalanine*
Isoleucine	*Tryptophan*

Tissue Protein Synthesis

B Defining a healthy diet

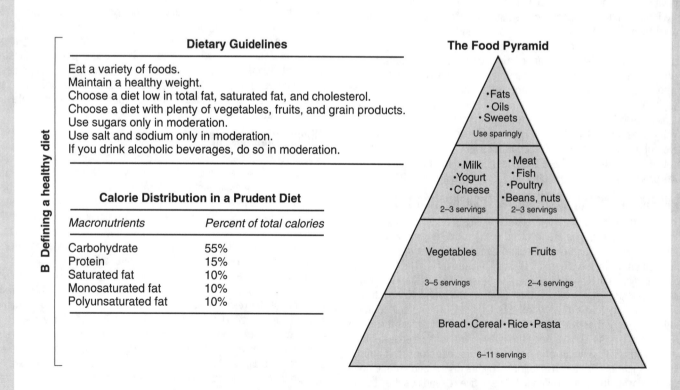

Dietary Guidelines

Eat a variety of foods.
Maintain a healthy weight.
Choose a diet low in total fat, saturated fat, and cholesterol.
Choose a diet with plenty of vegetables, fruits, and grain products.
Use sugars only in moderation.
Use salt and sodium only in moderation.
If you drink alcoholic beverages, do so in moderation.

Calorie Distribution in a Prudent Diet

Macronutrients	*Percent of total calories*
Carbohydrate	55%
Protein	15%
Saturated fat	10%
Monosaturated fat	10%
Polyunsaturated fat	10%

The Food Pyramid

- Fats
- Oils
- Sweets
Use sparingly

- Milk
- Yogurt
- Cheese
2–3 servings

- Meat
- Fish
- Poultry
- Beans, nuts
2–3 servings

Vegetables
3–5 servings

Fruits
2–4 servings

Bread • Cereal • Rice • Pasta
6–11 servings

Nutrition is the study of dietary requirements necessary to maintain good health. The human body needs a variety of nutrients for growth, reproduction, maintenance of organ structure, and repair of damaged tissues. The three major types of nutrients are macronutrients, vitamins, and minerals. Nutrients are described as essential if they cannot be synthesized by the body in sufficient amounts.

Macronutrients and Energy

Energy for the body is provided by the macronutrients: carbohydrates, lipids, and proteins (**Part A**). Lipids are highly reduced and anhydrous, containing more than twice the energy found in carbohydrates and proteins. The energy needed each day to maintain normal functions when the body is at rest is known as the **basal metabolic rate (BMR)**. The BMR depends on weight, height, and sex. Men have a higher BMR than women, a reflection of the fact that women have a higher proportion of body fat. The metabolic activity of fat is very low compared with other tissues such as liver, muscle, and kidneys. The approximate BMR can be predicted as follows:

Men $\quad$ BMR = 1.0 kcal/hr/kg body weight
Women + D $\quad$ BMR = 0.9 kcal/hr/kg body weight

Additional energy is needed for physical activity and for the digestion, absorption, and distribution of nutrients. The energy required for physical activity is known as the **energy expenditure of activity (EEA)** and varies widely among individuals depending on the type of exercise involved in work and recreation. The amount of energy needed to digest, absorb, and distribute nutrients varies with the type of nutrient, being highest for protein and lowest for fat. It is approximately 10% of the sum of the BMR and EEA. In addition to providing energy, each macronutrient has specialized functions, as described below.

Carbohydrate

There are two types of dietary carbohydrate: **available carbohydrate**, which is used for energy, and **nonavailable carbohydrate**, which supplies dietary **fiber**. Fiber is not degraded by the digestive enzymes and does not serve as a source of energy. It is, however, a significant component of the diet. In general, fiber increases stool bulk and decreases the time that waste stays in the gastrointestinal tract. Fiber from different sources has different physiologic effects. The presence of fiber in the diet has been correlated with a decreased incidence of cardiovascular disease and colon cancer, although too much fiber may lower the absorption of essential minerals.

Lipid

The two essential functions of dietary lipid are to provide a vehicle for the **absorption of fat-soluble vitamins** and to supply the body with **essential fatty acids**. The two essential fatty acids in humans are linoleic acid (an ω-6 fatty acid) and linolenic acid (an ω-3 fatty acid). Both linoleic and linolenic acids have 18 carbons and are polyunsaturated, having two and three double bonds, respectively. Humans are unable to insert double bonds into either the ω-6 or the ω-3 position of fatty acids. The essential fatty acids are the **precursors of prostaglandins, thromboxanes, and leukotrienes**. The substitution of polyunsaturated fatty acids for some of the saturated fatty acids in the diet has been shown to be effective in lowering serum cholesterol levels. Plants generally have a high proportion of polyunsaturated fatty acids, while animal tissues have a high proportion of saturated fatty acids.

Protein

The major function of dietary protein is to supply the body with **essential amino acids**. Ten of the 20 amino acids found in proteins cannot be synthesized by newborns in amounts sufficient to support growth. These amino acids include the basic amino acids (arginine, histidine, lysine), the branched-chain amino acids (valine, leucine, isoleucine, threonine), two of the three aromatic amino acids (phenylalanine and tryptophan), and one of the sulfur-containing amino acids (methionine). The ability to synthesize arginine and histidine is acquired in early childhood, but the other eight amino acids remain essential throughout life.

Recommendations for a Healthy Diet

The key features of a healthy diet are balance, variety, and moderation (**Part B**). **Dietary guidelines** for promoting health and reducing the risk of chronic diseases have been developed by government agencies. The **calorie distribution in a prudent diet** should have no more than 30% of the total calories coming from fat, with only 10% of the fat being saturated. Extensive tables of nutrient standards have been published listing the **recommended daily allowance (RDA)** for well-characterized nutrients. The RDA is an estimate of the amount of a particular nutrient required to meet the needs of 95% of the population in the United States. It is an overestimate that provides a margin of safety for most healthy people. A number of food guides have been developed that provide practical information on how to implement sound nutrient standards. For example, the **food pyramid** is a graphic representation of a good diet. The food group at the bottom of the pyramid should be consumed most frequently, while the group at the top should be consumed sparingly. A range of servings is suggested for each food group. The lower number of servings is appropriate for individuals requiring 1600 kcal/day, while the higher number is for individuals requiring 2500 kcal/day.

Clinical Significance

Inadequate intake of macronutrients results in a wide range of clinical disorders. The two extreme forms of malnutrition are **marasmus** and **kwashiorkor**. In marasmus, there is a deficiency in both energy and protein intake, whereas in kwashiorkor, only protein intake is inadequate. These diseases also involve deficiencies in vitamins and minerals. The clinical features of marasmus and kwashiorkor are summarized below:

Symptom	Marasmus	Kwashiorkor
Edema	Absent	Present
Hepatomegaly	Absent	Present
Muscle wasting	Severe	Absent or mild
Body fat	Absent	Diminished
Serum albumin	Moderately diminished	Severely diminished
Insulin levels	Low	Normal
Cortisol levels	High	Normal

For more information see Coffee C, *Metabolism*. Fence Creek, pp 63–67.

13 Nutritional Basis of Metabolism: Micronutrients

A Micronutrients

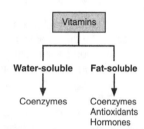

Vitamins
- Water-soluble → Coenzymes
- Fat-soluble → Coenzymes, Antioxidants, Hormones

Minerals
- Major minerals → Structural role, Electrolytes, Enzyme cofactors
- Trace elements → Structural roles, Regulatory roles, Enzyme cofactors

B Water-soluble vitamins

Vitamin	Physiologic function	Deficiency symptoms
Vitamin C	Reduction of iron and hydroxylation reactions (collagen, catecholamine, carnitine synthesis)	Scurvy
Niacin	Oxidation-reduction reactions (carbohydrate, lipid metabolism)	Pellagra
Riboflavin	Oxidation-reduction reactions (carbohydrate, lipid, amino acid metabolism)	Ariboflavinosis
Thiamine	Oxidative decarboxylation and transketolation reactions (carbohydrate, branched-chain amino acid metabolism)	Beriberi
Pantothenic acid	Acyl group transfer reactions (terminal oxidation of all fuels, lipid metabolism)	Adrenal insufficiency[a]
Pyridoxine	Transamination and decarboxylation reactions (amino acid metabolism)	Irritability, convulsions, and confusion
Biotin	Carboxylation reactions (gluconeogenesis, fatty acid synthesis, branched-chain amino acid metabolism)	Alopecia and dermatitis
Folic acid	One-carbon transfer reactions (purine and pyrimidine synthesis, amino acid interconversions)	Megaloblastic anemia
Cobalamin	Methylation and isomerization reactions (amino acid metabolism)	Pernicious anemia and neurologic effects

[a]Observed only in experimental animals

C Fat-soluble vitamins

Vitamin	Physiologic function	Deficiency symptoms
Vitamin A	Vision, reproduction, maintenance, and differentiation of epithelial tissue	Night blindness and hyperkeratosis
Vitamin D	Calcium and phosphate metabolism and maintenance of skeletal integrity	Rickets (children) and osteomalacia (adults)
Vitamin E	Antioxidant	Lipid peroxidation and hemolytic anemia
Vitamin K	Carboxylation of clotting factors	Hemorrhage and bruising

D Major minerals

Major mineral	Physiologic function	Deficiency symptoms
Calcium	Calcification of bone, blood clotting, and regulation of nerve, muscle, and hormone function	Tetany, muscle cramps, convulsions, bone fractures, and loss of height and bone mass
Phosphorus	Constituent of bones, teeth, nucleic acids, and ATP; required for energy metabolism	Growth retardation, skeletal deformities, muscle weakness, diminished phagocytic function, and increased hemolysis of RBCs
Magnesium	Cofactor for many enzymes; essential for ATP metabolism, muscle contraction, membrane transport, and nerve transmission	Muscle spasms, tetany, seizures, and deficiency secondary to malabsorption, diarrhea
Sodium	Principal extracellular cation; essential for regulation of plasma volume, acid-base balance, nerve and muscle function; sodium (Na^+), potassium (K^+)-ATPase	Fluid volume depletion and deficiency secondary to vomiting, diarrhea, diuretic abuse, or adrenal insufficiency
Potassium	Principal intracellular cation; nerve and muscle function; Na^+, K^+-ATPase	Muscle weakness, paralysis, and mental confusion; deficiency usually associated with alkalosis
Chloride	Principal extracellular anion; component of gastric fluid; bicarbonate transport in RBCs	Deficiency secondary to vomiting and diarrhea
Sulfur	Connective tissue proteoglycans; bile acid conjugation; detoxification reactions	Unknown

E Trace elements

Trace element	Physiologic function	Deficiency symptoms
Chromium	Potentiates the effect of insulin	Impaired glucose metabolism
Cobalt	Constituent of vitamin B_{12}	Macrocytic anemia
Copper	Iron absorption and mobilization; oxidative enzymes	Microcytic anemia, depigmentation of skin and hair, connective tissue and skeletal abnormalities
Fluoride	Component of calcified tissues; teeth and bone strength	Dental caries
Iodine	Constituent of thyroid hormones	Cretinism (children) and goiter (adults)
Iron	Oxygen transport and storage; oxidative reactions; electron transport chain	Pallor, fatigue, and microcytic anemia
Manganese	Cofactor for enzymes of glycoprotein and proteoglycan synthesis	Not well defined
Molybdenum	Cofactor for xanthine oxidase, sulfite oxidase, and aldehyde oxidase	Unknown
Selenium	Cofactor for glutathione peroxidase; protects cells against membrane peroxidation	Cardiomyopathy
Zinc	Growth, sexual maturation, fertility, and immune function; cofactor for enzymes in DNA, RNA, and protein synthesis	Hypogonadism, growth failure, impaired wound healing, defects in taste and smell, and loss of appetite

OVERVIEW

The micronutrients consist of vitamins and minerals, which perform a variety of functions in the human body (**Part A**). **Vitamins** are converted to coenzymes, small organic molecules that are required by specific enzymes for catalytic activity. The required amount of a vitamin depends on the sex, age, body weight, diet, and physiologic status. The best source of vitamins for a healthy person is a well-balanced diet. There are, however, several normal conditions that warrant specific vitamin supplements. For example, vegetarians are particularly susceptible to vitamin B_{12} deficiency; both folate and vitamin B_{12} are required in higher amounts during pregnancy and lactation; and women taking oral contraceptives require increased levels of vitamin B_6. Vitamins are classified into two major groups, water soluble and fat soluble. **Minerals** are inorganic elements that have vital structural and functional roles in the human body. They are classified into two major groups, the major minerals that are required in amounts greater than 100 mg/day and the trace elements that are required in amounts less than 100 mg/day. The mineral requirements are usually met by a diet that is adequate in dairy products, whole-grain cereals, legumes, and leafy green vegetables. Deficiency diseases have been reported for most of the vitamins and some of the minerals. Symptoms of toxicity result from excessive intake of some of the vitamins.

Water-Soluble Vitamins

The nine water-soluble vitamins play important roles in metabolism (**Part B**). They are required in pathways that use carbohydrates, lipids, and proteins as a source of energy and in pathways that generate building blocks for macromolecule synthesis. These vitamins are the precursors for the coenzymes that are required in many types of metabolic reactions, including hydroxylation, oxidation-reduction, carboxylation, decarboxylation, acyl transfer, amino transfer, and one-carbon transfer reactions. The enzymes that catalyze these reactions have no activity in the absence of their coenzymes. The water-soluble vitamins are readily absorbed from the intestine and transported to tissues where they are converted to coenzymes. The absorption of most of the water-soluble vitamins is mediated by carrier proteins that cotransport Na^+. An exception is vitamin B_{12}, which requires **intrinsic factor**, a protein secreted by the stomach. The water-soluble vitamins can be excreted by the kidneys, and with the exception of vitamin B_{12}, are not stored in significant amounts in the body.

Fat-Soluble Vitamins

The four fat-soluble vitamins have diverse biologic functions (**Part C**). They act as coenzymes (vitamins A and K), as antioxidants (vitamins A and E), and as hormones that regulate DNA transcription (vitamins A and D). The fat-soluble vitamins are present in foods from both plant and animal sources, and they are absorbed from the intestine along with the other dietary lipids. Malabsorption syndromes are frequently accompanied by deficiencies in one or more of the fat-soluble vitamins. Large quantities of these vitamins can be stored in the liver and adipose tissue. **Toxicity syndromes** are associated with excessive intake of vitamins A and D. Vitamin A exists in three active forms, retinol, retinal, and retinoic acid. **Retinal** is the cofactor for rhodopsin, which serves as the light receptor in the visual process. **Retinol** and **retinoic acid** are required for normal reproduction and for growth and differentiation of epithelial cells. These forms of vitamin A bind to nuclear receptors and regulate the transcription of specific genes in DNA. Vitamin D plays a crucial role in calcium and phosphate metabolism. The dietary form of vitamin D is inactive, but is converted to its active form, **1,25-dihydroxycholecalciferol**, by sequential hydroxylation reactions that occur in the liver and kidney. The mechanism by which vitamin D regulates calcium and phosphate metabolism involves binding to nuclear receptors and regulating the rate of gene transcription. Vitamin E belongs to a family of compounds known as tocopherols. These compounds have a protective effect on membrane integrity by acting as antioxidants. The most powerful form of vitamin E is **α-tocopherol**. Vitamin K is essential for normal blood clotting. It serves as a cofactor for **γ-glutamate carboxylase**, the liver enzyme that catalyzes the carboxylation of glutamate side chains in several of the clotting factors, including factors II, VII, IX, and X. The carboxylation of these clotting factors allows Ca^{2+} to bind to them and anchor them to the surface of platelets.

Major Minerals

The major minerals are the components of body fluids and the inorganic matrix of bone (**Part D**). About 99% of the calcium in the body is found in the bones and teeth where it exists as **calcium phosphate** (hydroxyapatite) crystals. **Magnesium** is required for normal muscle and nerve function, and it is essential for the metabolism of ATP. It is required as a cofactor for more than 300 different enzymes. **Sodium and potassium** are the principal minerals in the extracellular and intracellular fluids, respectively.

Trace Elements

The trace elements are required for a number of highly specific processes (**Part E**). Some of the trace elements such as fluoride have **structural roles** in the body. Others have regulatory roles (chromium) or function as **cofactors for enzymes**. Iron, copper, and zinc are cofactors for many enzymes, whereas selenium, molybdenum, and iodine are required by only one, or at most a few enzymes.

Clinical Significance

The importance of vitamins and minerals in normal metabolism is underscored by the large number of diseases resulting from a deficiency in one or more of these nutrients. Vitamin deficiencies can result from inadequate intake or impaired absorption, or the deficiency may be induced secondary to treatment of other clinical conditions. For patients that must be fed intravenously for long periods of time, care must be taken to avoid vitamin and mineral deficiencies. The administration of isoniazid to treat tuberculosis or penicillamine to treat copper-storage disease can result in vitamin B_6 deficiency unless excess vitamin is provided. Treatment of infections with broad spectrum antibiotics for a prolonged period of time will diminish the bacterial flora in the gut, and consequently may result in vitamin K and biotin deficiency.

For more information see Coffee C, *Metabolism*. Fence Creek, pp 67–75.

Questions 1–20

Directions: For each of the following questions, choose the **one best** answer.

1. Which of the following conditions would be expected in a patient with chronic obstructive pulmonary disease (COPD)?

(A) Metabolic acidosis

(B) Respiratory acidosis

(C) Metabolic alkalosis

(D) Respiratory alkalosis

(E) None of the above

2. The pK_a for lactic acid is 3.9. According to the Henderson-Hasselbach equation, the [lactate]/[lactic acid] ratio in a normal person with a plasma pH of 7.6 would be approximately:

(A) 10

(B) 70

(C) 1000

(D) 3200

(E) 10,000

3. Alzheimer's disease is characterized by the accumulation of amyloid plaques in the brain. The major protein in the plaques is a protease-resistant protein that is rich in β-structure. Which of the following bonds or interactions stabilize the β-structure in this protein?

(A) Electrostatic interactions between amino acid side chains

(B) Hydrogen bonds between amino acid side chains

(C) Hydrophobic interactions between amino-acid side chains

(D) Hydrogen bonds between components of the peptide bonds

(E) Disulfide bonds between cysteine side chains

4. The side chains of the following pairs of amino acids would most likely be found in the interior of a globular protein?

(A) Lysine and glutamate

(B) Glycine and serine

(C) Leucine and phenylalanine

(D) Asparagine and valine

(E) Histidine and tryptophan

Questions 5 and 6 are based on the following clinical case:

A woman came to the hospital because of a retinal detachment, she had a previous history of multiple joint dislocations and was easily bruised. Analysis of collagen that was isolated from fibroblasts showed normal hydroxylation but a low degree of crosslinking.

5. Based on the information provided, the most likely diagnosis for this patient is:

(A) Osteogenesis imperfecta

(B) Ehlers-Danlos syndrome

(C) Scurvy

(D) Marfan syndrome

(E) Spondyloepiphyseal dysplasia

6. The symptoms described for this patient are most consistent with a deficiency in which of the following enzymes?

(A) Prolyl hydroxylase

(B) Lysyl hydroxylase

(C) N-Procollagen peptidase

(D) Lysyl oxidase

(E) None of the above

7. The transport system that maintains Na^+ and K^+ gradients across the plasma membrane:

(A) Transports Na^+ into the cell in exchange for K^+

(B) Requires energy that is supplied by ATP hydrolysis

(C) Is an example of passive transport

(D) Is an example of a symporter

(E) None of the above

8. Integral plasma membrane proteins:

(A) Can be released from the membrane by altering the ionic strength

(B) Contain α-helical segments of about 20 amino acids that span the membrane

(C) Always have their N-terminus on the extracellular side of the membrane

(D) Frequently have carbohydrate attached to the cytosolic domain

(E) Are stabilized by covalent interactions with the lipid bilayer

9. Which of the following conditions facilitates the release of oxygen from hemoglobin?

(A) An increase in pH

(B) A decrease in 2,3-bisphosphoglycerate concentration

(C) An increase in P_{CO_2}

(D) A decrease in H^+ concentration

(E) An increase in carbon monoxide concentration

10. In a patient with sickle cell disease, all of the following conditions would promote sickling of red cells **except:**

(A) Metabolic acidosis

(B) Oxidation of heme iron

(C) Decreased pO_2

(D) Decreased rate of respiration

(E) Decreased 2,3-bisphosphoglycerate concentration

11. Enzymes:

(A) Decrease the free energy change (ΔG) of a reaction

(B) Increase the activation energy (ΔG^*) of a reaction

(C) Increase the rate of the forward and reverse reactions equally

(D) Increase the equilibrium constant (K_{eq}) of a reaction

(E) None of the above

12. Which of the following serum enzyme profiles for creatine kinase (CK) and lactate dehydrogenase (LDH) is most useful in the diagnosis of acute myocardial infarct?

(A) An increase in the total serum CK

(B) An increase in the LDH_2/LDH_1 isozyme ratio

(C) An increase in the total serum LDH

(D) An increase in the MB isozyme of CK

(E) An increase in the MM isozyme of CK

13. The K_m of an enzyme:

(A) Is equal to the intercept on the 1/[S] axis of a Lineweaver-Burk plot

(B) Is a function of enzyme concentration

(C) Is an index of the affinity of the enzyme for its substrate

(D) Is decreased by a noncompetitive inhibitor

(E) Is equal to the substrate concentration that results in the maximum velocity

14. Aspirin is a nonsteroidal anti-inflammatory drug that inhibits cyclooxygenase irreversibly. Which of the following effects would aspirin have on the kinetic properties of cyclooxygenase?

(A) The K_m for arachidonic acid is increased

(B) The V_{max} of the reaction is decreased

(C) The K_m for arachidonic acid is decreased

(D) The K_m for arachidonic acid is increased and the V_{max} is decreased

(E) None of the above

15. Which of the following characteristics best describes an allosteric enzyme?

(A) The substrate affinity is increased by an allosteric activator

(B) The substrate saturation curve is usually hyperbolic

(C) The allosteric site binds both substrate and allosteric effectors

(D) The substrate saturation curve is shifted to the right by an allosteric activator

(E) None of the above

16. Steroid hormones increase the activity of an enzyme by:

(A) Activating protein kinases

(B) Activating protein phosphatases

(C) Increasing the concentration of second messenger molecules

(D) Increasing the amount of enzyme present

(E) Decreasing the rate of gene transcription

17. Which of the following statements about cAMP is most accurate?

(A) The synthesis is inhibited by hormones that activate G_s proteins

(B) The degradation is stimulated by insulin

(C) The concentration is decreased by pertussis toxin

(D) It activates protein kinase C

(E) It is a second messenger for insulin

18. G_s, proteins that participate in signal transduction pathways:

(A) Are heterodimers

(B) Have GTPase activity associated with the β-subunit

(C) Are ADP-ribosylated by cholera toxin

(D) Are active when GDP is bound to the α-subunit

(E) Have intrinsic tyrosine kinase activity

19. The calories needed by a 50-kg woman to maintain the normal resting body functions for 24 hours is approximately:

(A) 500 kcalories

(B) 1100 kcalories

(C) 1400 kcalories

(D) 1600 kcalories

(E) 2000 kcalories

20. Which of the following symptoms is seen in patients with marasmus but not in patients with kwashiorkor?

(A) Hepatomegaly

(B) Depigmentation

(C) Elevated cortisol

(D) Edema

(E) None of the above

Directions: The groups of questions below consist of lettered choices followed by several numbered items. For each numbered item, select the most appropriate lettered option. Each lettered option may be used once, more than once, or not at all.

Questions 21–22
For each metabolic function listed below, select the subcellular compartment where it occurs.

(A) Mitochondria

(B) Cytosol

(C) Lysosomes

(D) Endoplasmic reticulum

21. Carbohydrate metabolism

22. Detoxification of drugs

Questions 23–24
For each clinical condition listed below, select the most closely related plasma protein.

(A) Albumin

(B) α_1-Antitrypsin

(C) Haptoglobulin

(D) Transferrin

(E) Ceruloplasmin

23. Wilson's disease

24. Pulmonary emphysema

Questions 25–26
For each clinical condition listed below, select the vitamin most likely to be deficient.

(A) Niacin

(B) Folic acid

(C) Vitamin E

(D) Vitamin K

25. Hemolytic anemia

26. Pellagra

Questions 27–28
For each clinical condition listed below, select the mineral most likely to be deficient.

(A) Selenium

(B) Iodine

(C) Chromium

(D) Iron

27. Microcytic anemia

28. Gucose intolerance

PART I: ANSWERS AND EXPLANATIONS

1. The answer is B.

The rate of respiration is reduced in patients with COPD, resulting in decreased expiration of CO_2. The increase in P_{CO_2} shifts the following equilibria to the right, resulting in an increase in $[H^+]$ and a decrease in the plasma pH.

$$CO_2 + H_2O \rightleftharpoons H_2CO_3 \rightleftharpoons H^+ + HCO_3^-$$

2. The answer is D.

The Henderson-Hasselbach equation for the ionization of lactic acid at pH 7.6 is shown below.

$$7.6 = 3.9 + \log \frac{[\text{lactate}]}{[\text{lactic acid}]}$$

The pK_a of and weak acid is defined as the pH where the concentration of the conjugate base is equal to that of the conjugate acid. Therefore, at pH 3.9 (the pK_a for lactic acid), the concentration of lactate is equal to the concentration of lactic acid. The logarithmic nature of the Henderson-Hasselbach equation predicts that a change of 1 pH unit results in approximately a 10-fold change in the [conjugate base]/[conjugate acid] ratio. As the pH increases, the ratio increases, and as the pH decreases the ratio decreases. Rearrangement of the above equation shows that: log [lactate]/lactic acid] = 7.6 − 3.9 = 3.7. Therefore, at pH 7.6, which is 3.7 pH units above the pK_a, the [lactate]/[lactic acid] ratio will be between 10^3 and 10^4. The only answer that falls within this range is D.

3. The answer is D.

The primary, secondary, tertiary, and quaternary structures of proteins are characterized by the types of bonds and interactions that stabilize that particular level of structure. The two major types of secondary structure found in proteins are α-helix and β-structures. Both types are stabilized by hydrogen bonds that are formed between the amide-hydrogen atom of one peptide bond and the carbonyl-oxygen atom of another. In contrast, the primary structure is stabilized by amide (peptide) bonds; the tertiary and quaternary structures are stabilized by various types of bonds and interactions that occur between the side chains of amino acids, including hydrogen bonds, hydrophobic interactions, electrostatic interactions, and disulfide bonds.

4. The answer is C.

Hydrophobic amino acid side chains are usually found buried in the interior globular proteins where they are protected from water and stabilized by hydrophobic interactions with each other. In contrast, hydrophilic amino acid side chains are usually found on the surface of proteins where they are stabilized by interaction with the aqueous medium. Hydrophobic amino acids have either aromatic or aliphatic side chains, while hydrophilic amino acids have side chains that are either charged or have N, O, or S atoms that can hydrogen bond with water.

5. The answer is B.

Ehlers-Danlos syndrome is a connective tissue disease that is characterized by weak collagen that leads to hypermobile joints, hyperextensible skin, poor wound healing, and easily bruised skin. Numerous other symptoms, including retinal detachment, are seen in some cases of Ehlers-Danlos syndrome. These diseases usually result from mutations that lead to deficiencies in enzymes that alter the structure of collagen by post-translational modification reactions. Osteogenesis imperfecta is a bone disease that results from an inherited defect in type I collagen. Scurvy results from vitamin C deficiency and is characterized by poorly cross-linked collagen secondary to decreased hydroxylation of lysyl side chains. Marfan syndrome is a connective tissue disease resulting from defective fibrillin, a connective tissue protein associated with elastic fibers. Spondyloepiphyseal dysplasia results from mutations in the type II collagen genes and is characterized by short-limb dwarfism.

6. The answer is D.

Lysyl oxidase catalyzes the oxidative deamination of lysyl side chains, producing allysine, an aldehyde that forms covalent crosslinks in collagen by reacting with hydroxylysine, lysine, or other allysine residues. Covalent crosslinks give the collagen fibers strength and rigidity.

7. The answer is B.

Large differences in the concentration of Na^+ and K^+ are found on different sides of the plasma membrane. The intracellular Na^+ concentration is about 10 mM and the extracellular concentration is about 145 mM; the intracellular concentration of K^+ is about 140 mM and the extracellular concentration is about 5 mM. The energy required to maintain these ion gradients is provided by the hydrolysis of ATP. Transporters that move solutes against a concentration gradient are active transport systems and require energy. The NaK-ATPase is an example of an antiporter that simultaneously transports Na^+ out of the cell and K^+ into the cell.

8. The answer is B.

Integral membrane proteins are usually transmembrane proteins that span the lipid bilayer one or more times. The segment of amino acids spanning the bilayer is usually an α-helix consisting of about 20 amino acids, most of which are hydrophobic. The protein is stabilized in the membrane by hydrophobic interactions between the amino acid side chains and the lipid bilayer. The removal of integral membrane proteins from the lipid bilayer requires detergents. The N-terminus of some integral membrane proteins is on the extracellular side, while that of others is on the cytosolic side of the plasma membrane. The carbohydrate moiety of integral membrane proteins is always found on the extracellular side of the plasma membrane.

9. The answer is C.

Any factor that decreases the percentage of oxygenated hemoglobin facilitates the release of oxygen, which can be recognized by a shift in the oxygen saturation curve to the right. Factors that facilitate O_2 release from hemoglobin are an increase in Pco_2, an increase in H^+ concentration (which corresponds to a decrease in pH), and an increase in the concentration of 2,3-bisphosphoglycerate. Carbon monoxide shifts the oxygen saturation curve of hemoglobin to the left.

10. The answer is E.

Any condition that increases the proportion of deoxy HbS relative to oxy HbS (or shifts the oxygen saturation curve to the right) will promote sickling of red cells. The only condition listed that increases the relative proportion of oxy HbS is a decrease in the concentration of 2,3-bisphosphoglycerate. All of the other conditions listed increase the relative amount of deoxy HbS.

11. The answer is C.

An enzyme increases the rate of a chemical reaction by decreasing the activation energy (also known as the transition state energy). Because the same transition state is involved in both the forward and reverse reactions the rates of these opposing reactions are increased equally. The K_{eq} can be expressed as the ratio of the rates of the forward and reverse reactions, and therefore is not altered by an enzyme.

12. The answer is D.

The total CK and LDH levels in the serum are increased following an acute myocardial infarct, but the source is not necessarily specific for cardiac tissue. However, the MB isozyme of CK is synthesized only by cardiac tissue, and an increase in the serum concentration of the MB isozyme is diagnostic of damage to cardiac tissue. The amount of LDH_1 in the serum increases following an acute myocardial infarct, and the ratio of LDH_2/LDH_1 decreases.

13. The answer is C.

The K_m is related to the affinity of the enzyme for its substrate. A high K_m indicates a low affinity and vice versa. The K_m is equal to the substrate concentration that results in half-maximum velocity, and the intercept on the 1/[S] axis of a Lineweaver-Burk plot is equal to $-1/K_m$. The K_m is independent of the enzyme concentration. The K_m is increased by a competitive inhibitor but is unchanged by a noncompetitive inhibitor.

14. The answer is B.

Aspirin is an irreversible inhibitor of cyclooxygenase. It effectively decreases the concentration of active enzyme, thereby lowering the V_{max}. The effect of an irreversible inhibitor is kinetically indistinguishable from that of a noncompetitive inhibitor. Both types of inhibitors decrease the V_{max} and have no effect on the K_m.

15. The answer is A.

Allosteric activators either increase the affinity (decrease the K_m) of the enzyme for its substrate or increase the V_{max} of the reaction. Allosteric enzymes usually have sigmoidal substrate saturation curves, a property that reflects cooperative interaction between substrate binding sites. Allosteric effectors that alter the K_m shift the substrate saturation curve to the left (activators) or to the right (inhibitors). Activators and inhibitors that alter the V_{max} shift the plateau of the curve up and down, respectively. The allosteric site on an enzyme is separate and distinct from the active site, and in some cases can even be located on a separate regulatory subunit.

16. The answer is D.

Steroid hormones increase the activity of an enzyme by increasing the amount of enzyme present in the cell. The mechanism by which this occurs involves an increase in the rate at which the gene for the enzyme is expressed. In contrast, peptide hormones exert their effect by increasing and decreasing the cellular level of second messenger molecules, which in turn alter the activity of protein kinases and protein phosphatases.

17. The answer is B.

The binding of insulin to liver and adipose results in the activation of cAMP phosphodiesterase, the enzyme that hydrolyzes cAMP to 5'-AMP. The synthesis of cAMP is stimulated by hormones that activate G_s proteins. cAMP is the second messenger for many peptide hormones including glucagon, parathyroid hormone, and luteinizing hormone. The primary target for cAMP is protein kinase A, which is inactive in the absence of cAMP.

18. The answer is C.

G proteins are located in the plasma membrane where they transmit information between hormone receptors and the enzymes that synthesize second messengers. G_s proteins increase the rate of second messenger synthesis, whereas G_i proteins decrease the rate of second messenger synthesis. The G proteins are heterotrimers consisting of α-, β-, and γ-subunits. The α-subunit binds both GTP and GDP and has intrinsic GTPase activity. The G proteins are active only when GTP is bound. Cholera toxin catalyzes the ADP-ribosylation of the α-subunit of G_s, resulting in inactivation of the GTPase activity.

19. The answer is B.

The BMR is defined as the calories needed to maintain normal functions when the body is at rest. The BMR depends on weight, height, and sex. The BMR for a woman can be approximated from the equation: BMR = 0.9 kcal/kg/hr. For men this equation is BMR = 1.0 kcal/kg/hr. In these equations, kcal are often used interchangeably with Calories (spelled with a capital "c").

20. The answer is C.

Cortisol levels are normal in patients with kwashiorkor but high in patients with marasmus. Hepatomegaly, edema, and depigmentation of skin and hair are symptoms present in kwashiorkor but absent in marasmus.

Questions 21–22. The answers are 21-B, 22-D.
The major pathways of carbohydrate metabolism, including glycolysis, the pentose phosphate pathway, glycogen synthesis, and degradation occur in the cytosol. Many drugs are hydrophobic compounds that are relatively insoluble and are toxic if allowed to accumulate. They are detoxified by the action of enzymes located in the smooth endoplasmic reticulum of the liver. The detoxification reactions include cytochrome P_{450}-dependent hydroxylation followed by conjugation with a compound that renders the drug soluble enough to be excreted.

Questions 23–24. The answers are 23-E, 24-B.
A deficiency in ceruloplasmin results in Wilson's disease, a copper storage disease in which copper accumulates in high concentrations in the liver, brain, and eye. A deficiency in α_1-antitrypsin results in pulmonary emphysema. The function of α_1-antitrypsin is to prevent the degradation of elastin, the major connective tissue protein in lung. Elastase is irreversibly inhibited by α_1-antitrypsin.

Questions 25–26. The answers are 25-C, 26-A.
A deficiency in vitamin E leads to lipid peroxidation, resulting in lysis of red blood cells and hemolytic anemia. Pellagra, seen in patients with niacin deficiency, is characterized by dermatitis, diarrhea, and dementia.

Questions 27–28. The answers are 27-D, 28-C.
Microcytic anemia can result from either an iron or copper deficiency and is characterized by small, pale red blood cells. Chromium is required for insulin to function properly. A deficiency in either insulin or chromium can result in impaired ability to remove glucose from the circulation.

PART II
Bioenergetics

14 Thermodynamic Principles of Metabolism

A Free-energy change of reactions

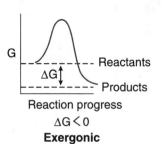

G ----- Reactants

ΔG

G ----- Products

Reaction progress
$\Delta G < 0$
Exergonic

G ----- Products

ΔG

G ----- Reactants

Reaction progress
$\Delta G > 0$
Endergonic

$$\Delta G = G_{products} - G_{reactants}$$

$$\Delta G^o = -RT\ln K_{eq}$$

For reaction:

$A \rightleftharpoons B$ $K_{eq} > 1$ and $\Delta G^o < 0$

$A \rightleftharpoons B$ $K_{eq} = 1$ and $\Delta G^o = 0$

$A \rightleftharpoons B$ $K_{eq} < 1$ and $\Delta G^o > 0$

$$\Delta G = \Delta G^o + RT\ln \frac{[B]}{[A]}$$

B Role of ATP in energy metabolism

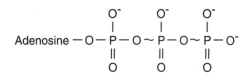

$$\text{Adenosine} - O - \underset{\underset{O}{\overset{\overset{O^-}{|}}{\|}}}{P} - O \sim \underset{\underset{O}{\overset{\overset{O^-}{|}}{\|}}}{P} - O \sim \underset{\underset{O}{\overset{\overset{O^-}{|}}{\|}}}{P} - O^-$$

Adenosine triphosphate (ATP)

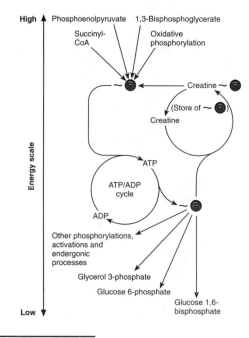

C High energy carriers in metabolism

Group	High-energy carrier	Reaction or pathway
Phosphate	Adenosine triphosphate	Kinase reactions
Sugars	Uridine diphosphate sugar	Glycogen synthesis
Acetate	Acetyl~CoA	Fatty acid synthesis
Fatty acids	Acyl~CoA	Triglyceride synythesis
Amino acids	Aminoacyl adenylate	Protein synthesis
Carboxyl	Carboxy~biotin	Carboxylation reactions
Methyl	*S*-adenosylmethionine	Methylation reactions
Sulfate	Phosphoadenosinephosphosulfate	Sulfation reactions

OVERVIEW

The concepts underlying metabolism are based on thermodynamic principles of chemical reactions. Chemical reactions either consume or release energy, depending on the relative energy content of the reactants and products. Reactions that release energy are exergonic, while those that require energy are endergonic. ATP is the principal carrier of energy in metabolism. Energy released in exergonic reactions is used to synthesize ATP and the energy contained in high-energy bonds of ATP can be used to drive reactions that require energy. The concepts of free-energy change, high-energy bonds, and coupled reactions are central themes in metabolism.

Free-Energy Change of Reactions

The free-energy change (ΔG) of a reaction is the portion of the total energy change that is available for doing work (**Part A**). For any reaction, ΔG is equal to the difference in the free energy (G) of the products and the reactants. Reactions are classified into two major groups, based on whether ΔG has a positive or negative value. Reactions having a ΔG < 0 are **exergonic** reactions and proceed spontaneously from a higher to a lower energy state. Reactions having a ΔG > 0 are **endergonic** reactions, and energy must be supplied for the reaction to proceed from a lower to a higher energy state. Thus, the **sign of ΔG predicts the direction of a reaction**. The ΔG is dependent only on the energy content of the reactants and the products, and it is **independent of the pathway** by which reactants are converted to products.

The change in free energy that occurs when all reactants and products are present at 1 M concentration and pH 7.0 is defined as the **standard free-energy change (ΔG°)** of a reaction. The ΔG° is related to the equilibrium constant (K_{eq}) by the following equation, where T is the absolute temperature, R is the universal gas constant, ln is the natural logarithm, and K_{eq} [B]/[A] for the reaction A $\rightarrow$ B at equilibrium.

$$\Delta G° = -RT \ln K_{eq}$$

Since metabolites are rarely, if ever, present at I M concentration in cells, it is important to note that ΔG may be larger or smaller than ΔG°, depending on the actual concentration of the reactants and products. The relationship between ΔG and ΔG° is given by the following equation:

$$\Delta G = \Delta G° + RT \ln \frac{[B]}{[A]}$$

Role of ATP in Energy Metabolism

ATP, consisting of adenosine with three phosphate groups attached, is the principal carrier of energy in living systems (**Part B**). The two terminal phosphate groups are joined to one another by **anhydride bonds**, which have a high-energy content, whereas the innermost phosphate is linked to adenosine by an ester bond, having considerably less energy. Because of the high-energy content of anhydride bonds, ATP is considered a **high-energy compound**. The ΔG° for the hydrolysis of ATP to ADP and P_i is -7.3 kcal/mol. A few compounds are found in cells that contain bonds having a higher energy level than ATP. Two of these compounds are intermediates in glycolysis (1,3-bisphosphoglycerate and phosphoenolpyruvate); and creatine phosphate (a reservoir of high-energy phosphate bonds in muscle and brain). The phosphate groups in these compounds can be transferred to ADP, resulting in ATP synthesis by **substrate-level phosphorylation**. Another high-energy compound is succinyl CoA, an intermediate

in the TCA cycle. Hydrolysis of the high-energy thioester bond in succinyl CoA is used to drive the synthesis of GTP from GDP and P_i. Other phosphate-containing compounds, such as various phosphate esters, contain considerably less energy than ATP. These compounds can be synthesized by the transfer of phosphate from ATP to the appropriate precursors such as glycerol and glucose. The energy for ATP synthesis by substrate-level phosphorylation comes from high-energy bonds in metabolites, whereas the energy for ATP synthesis by **oxidative phosphorylation** comes from a proton gradient across the inner mitochondrial membrane.

Other High-Energy Carriers of Chemical Groups in Metabolism

Many reactions in metabolism involve the transfer of some chemical group from a high-energy carrier to an acceptor (**Part C**). The bond that links the group to the carrier is a high-energy bond that is cleaved during the transfer, thereby providing the energy needed to make the reaction thermodynamically favorable.

Coupled Reaction Systems

Two reactions are coupled if the product of one reaction is the reactant in the other reaction, and such reactions are **additive**. Cells often couple an exergonic reaction, such as the hydrolysis of ATP, with endergonic reactions, thereby ensuring that the endergonic reaction will proceed in the desired direction. For example, cells synthesize glucose-6-phosphate (G6P) by using ATP as a phosphate donor. Hexokinase, the enzyme involved, couples the hydrolysis of ATP (an exergonic reaction) with the addition of phosphate to glucose (an endergonic reaction). Since coupled reactions are additive, the ΔG° for the overall reaction is the sum of the two reactions:

ATP + H_2O $\longrightarrow$ ADP + P_i		ΔG° = -7.3 kcal/mol
Glucose + P_i $\longrightarrow$ G6P + H_2O		ΔG° = $+3.3$ kcal/mol
Sum: Glucose + ATP $\longrightarrow$ G6P + H_2O		ΔG° = -4.0 kcal/mol

Clinical Significance

Many clinical abnormalities involve defects in energy metabolism. A diminished ability to synthesize ATP results in myopathy, weakness, blindness, deafness, and altered concentrations of many metabolites, both in the cell and in the blood. The wide range of effects is, in part, a reflection of the fact that ATP is a universal carrier of energy for many essential functions, including muscle contraction, active transport, maintenance of ionic gradients across membranes, transmission of neurochemical signals, and synthesis of many compounds in cells.

For more information see Coffee C, *Metabolism*. Fence Creek, pp 81–84.

15 Oxidative Metabolism

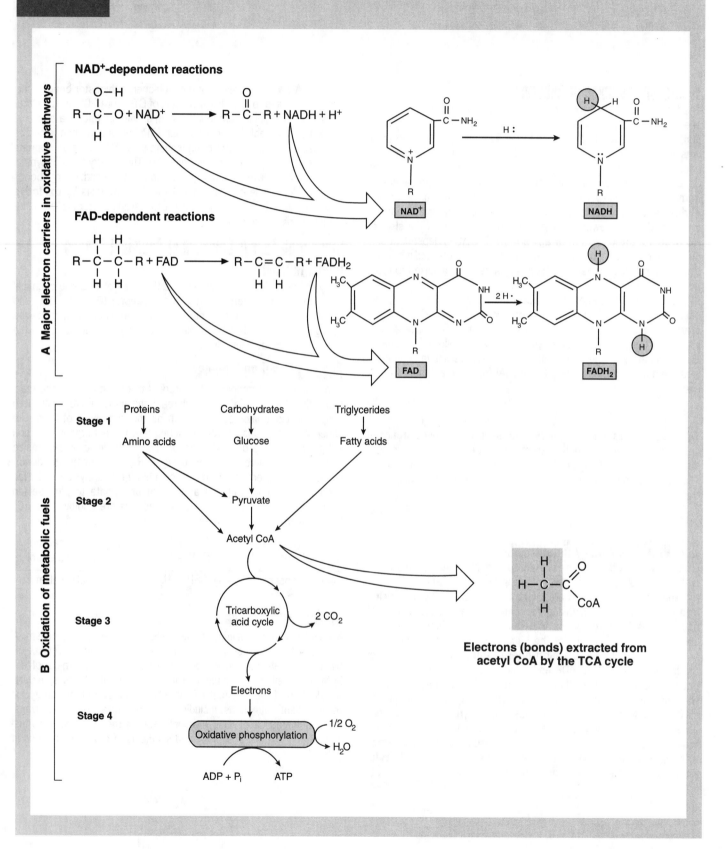

A Major electron carriers in oxidative pathways

NAD⁺-dependent reactions

$$R-\underset{\underset{H}{|}}{\overset{\overset{O-H}{|}}{C}}-O + NAD^+ \longrightarrow R-\overset{\overset{O}{\|}}{C}-R + NADH + H^+$$

NAD⁺ → H: → NADH

FAD-dependent reactions

$$R-\underset{\underset{H}{|}}{\overset{\overset{H}{|}}{C}}-\underset{\underset{H}{|}}{\overset{\overset{H}{|}}{C}}-R + FAD \longrightarrow R-\underset{\underset{H}{|}}{C}=\underset{\underset{H}{|}}{C}-R + FADH_2$$

FAD → 2 H· → FADH₂

B Oxidation of metabolic fuels

Stage 1

Proteins → Amino acids

Carbohydrates → Glucose

Triglycerides → Fatty acids

Stage 2

Pyruvate

Acetyl CoA

Stage 3

Tricarboxylic acid cycle → 2 CO₂

Electrons (bonds) extracted from acetyl CoA by the TCA cycle

Stage 4

Electrons

Oxidative phosphorylation → 1/2 O₂ → H₂O

ADP + P_i → ATP

OVERVIEW

Oxidation is defined as the loss of electrons, while reduction is defined as the gain of electrons. Every oxidation reaction is accompanied by a concomitant reduction reaction. Biologic oxidations are central to ATP synthesis in cells. Energy is extracted from food by a series of oxidation reactions, in which pairs of electrons, present in chemical bonds, are transferred through a series of electron carriers to O_2, resulting in the reduction of O_2 to H_2O. Much of the energy released in oxidative reactions is used for the synthesis of ATP. The pathways primarily responsible for the extraction of energy from food is the TCA cycle, and the pathway that uses this energy to drive ATP synthesis is oxidative phosphorylation. Both pathways occur in mitochondria. Glycolysis is the only other pathway in mammals that produces ATP. The amount of ATP produced by glycolysis is less than 10% of that produced by oxidative phosphorylation. Cells and tissues that are either deprived of O_2 or have no mitochondria are totally dependent on glycolysis for ATP synthesis.

Major Electron Carriers in Metabolism

The oxidation of metabolic fuels involves a large number of dehydrogenases that require coenzymes, either NAD$^+$ or FAD, as electron carriers (**Part A**). The vitamin precursors of NAD$^+$ and FAD are niacin and riboflavin, respectively. **NAD$^+$-dependent dehydrogenases** catalyze the transfer of a **hydride ion** (two electrons and a proton) to NAD$^+$. Most of these reactions involve the oxidation of a hydroxylated carbon atom to an aldehyde or ketone, with the concomitant reduction of NAD$^+$ to NADH. **FAD-dependent dehydrogenases** catalyze the transfer of **two hydrogen atoms** (two electrons and two protons) to FAD, resulting in the concomitant formation of FADH$_2$. The two hydrogen atoms usually come from adjacent carbon atoms, resulting in the formation of a carbon–carbon double bond.

Oxidation of Metabolic Fuels

Cells extract energy from food by the oxidation of protein, carbohydrate, and fat to CO_2 and H_2O (**Part B**). The extraction of energy from food and the use of that energy to synthesize ATP occurs in four stages. In the **first stage** macronutrients are hydrolyzed to their constituent building blocks, producing a diverse set of amino acids, sugars, and fatty acids. This is a preparatory stage and does not involve oxidation reactions. The **second stage** oxidizes these diverse compounds to a common intermediate, **acetyl CoA**, releasing only a small fraction of the total energy. Most of the energy in these compounds is conserved in acetyl CoA, where it is found in the energy-rich electron pairs that make up the carbon–hydrogen and carbon–carbon bonds of acetyl CoA. In the **third stage**, acetyl CoA is oxidized to CO_2 by the TCA cycle. Electrons are removed from acetyl CoA and transferred to NAD$^+$ and FAD, producing NADH and FADH$_2$. In the **fourth stage**, the energy present as electrons in NADH and FADH$_2$ is used to synthesize ATP by the pathway of **oxidative phosphorylation**.

Pathways in Stage 2

Most of the energy used for ATP synthesis comes from the oxidation of glucose and fatty acids. Normally, most of the amino acids derived from dietary protein are used to synthesize tissue protein, with only a small fraction being oxidized to acetyl CoA. Glucose is oxidized to pyruvate by **glycolysis**, a pathway that is located in the cytosol and produces a net of 2 mols each of pyruvate, ATP, and NADH per mol of glucose. Pyruvate is transported into the mitochondria where it is oxidized by **pyruvate dehydrogenase**. The oxidation of each mol of pyruvate results in 1 mol each of acetyl CoA, CO_2, and NADH. Fatty acids are oxidized to acetyl CoA in mitochondria by the pathway of β-oxidation. The amount of acetyl CoA produced depends on the length of the fatty acid. If the fatty acid is palmitic acid having 16 carbons, then 8 mols of acetyl CoA, 7 mols of NADH, and 7 mols of FADH$_2$ are produced. Most of the original energy in glucose and fatty acids is conserved in acetyl CoA, although some of the energy has been extracted and transferred to NADH and FADH$_2$.

The TCA Cycle

The role of the TCA cycle in energy metabolism is to oxidize acetyl CoA to two molecules of CO_2 and to transfer the electrons in the three C–H bonds and one C–C bond to electron carriers. Each turn of the cycle involves the entry of acetyl CoA and the production of 2 mols of CO_2, 3 mols of NADH, 1 mol of FADH$_2$, and 1 mol of GTP, which is energetically equivalent to ATP.

Oxidative Phosphorylation

The energy conserved in NADH and FADH$_2$ is used to synthesize ATP in the pathway of oxidative phosphorylation. The electrons in NADH and FADH$_2$ are removed and used to reduce O_2 to H_2O. The electrons move from NADH and FADH$_2$ through a series of electron carriers, known as the **electron transport chain**. The terminal electron acceptor in the chain is O_2, which is reduced to H_2O. The oxidation of NADH and FADH$_2$ by the electron transport chain is an exergonic reaction, releasing energy, which is coupled with the formation of ATP, an endergonic reaction catalyzed by **ATP synthase**. The energy released by the oxidation of 1 mol of NADH will support the synthesis of approximately 3 mols of ATP, whereas the oxidation of 1 mol of FADH$_2$ supports the synthesis of approximately 2 mols of ATP. The complete oxidation of glucose to CO_2 and H_2O results in the synthesis of 36 to 38 mols of ATP, while the complete oxidation of palmitic acid results in the synthesis of 129 mols of ATP.

Clinical Significance

The clinical significance of oxidative metabolism can be appreciated by considering what happens during acute myocardial infarction. Cardiac tissue has a higher demand for ATP than most tissues. Most of the ATP is used for contraction and for maintaining ion gradients across the plasma membrane. Cardiac tissue also has a high density of mitochondria that synthesize ATP by oxidative phosphorylation. Blockage of the coronary artery prevents blood from delivering O_2 and metabolic fuels, resulting in diminished ATP synthesis and cell death.

For more information see Coffee C, *Metabolism*. Fence Creek, pp 81–88.

16 Mitochondrial Compartments

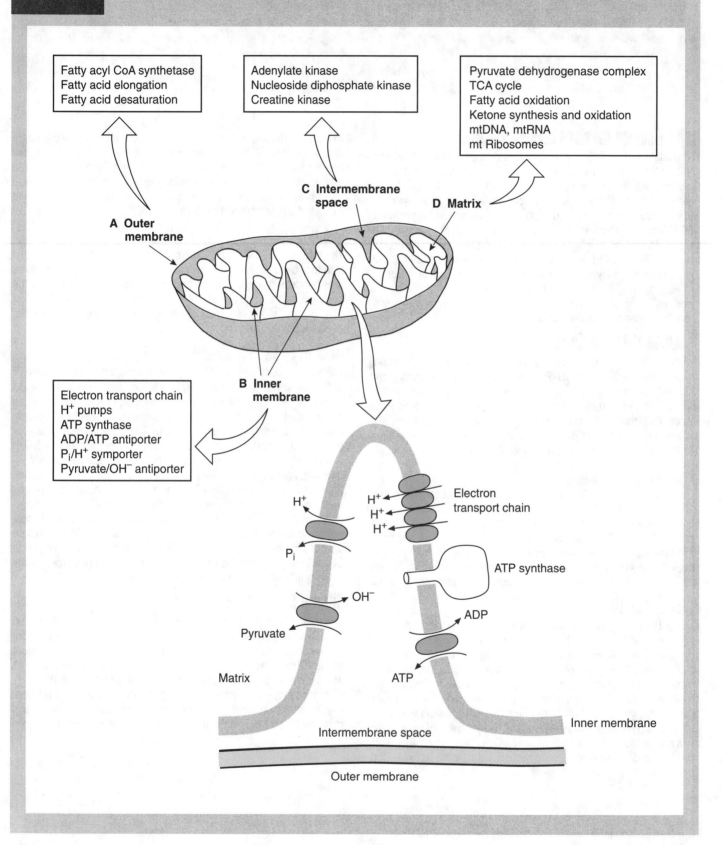

Fatty acyl CoA synthetase
Fatty acid elongation
Fatty acid desaturation

Adenylate kinase
Nucleoside diphosphate kinase
Creatine kinase

Pyruvate dehydrogenase complex
TCA cycle
Fatty acid oxidation
Ketone synthesis and oxidation
mtDNA, mtRNA
mt Ribosomes

C Intermembrane space

D Matrix

A Outer membrane

B Inner membrane

Electron transport chain
H^+ pumps
ATP synthase
ADP/ATP antiporter
P_i/H^+ symporter
Pyruvate/OH^- antiporter

H^+

P_i

OH^-

Pyruvate

Matrix

H^+
H^+
H^+

Electron transport chain

ATP synthase

ADP

ATP

Intermembrane space

Inner membrane

Outer membrane

OVERVIEW

The mitochondrion is the energy-producing organelle in animal cells. It is the compartment where most of the oxidations that produce NADH and FADH$_2$ occur. The number of mitochondria per cell varies with different tissues. The greater the energy needs of the cell, the greater the number of mitochondria. The mitochondrion consists of an outer membrane and an inner membrane that divide the mitochondrion into two compartments. The intermembrane space is located between the outer and inner membrane, and the matrix is enclosed within the inner membrane. Mitochondria also contain multiple copies of circular double-stranded DNA (mtDNA), mitochondrial-specific RNAs, and ribosomes.

Outer Membrane

The outer mitochondrial membrane (**Part A**) is composed of approximately 50% protein and 50% lipid. Its composition is similar to that of the endoplasmic reticulum. It is smooth in appearance, and has relatively few enzymatic and transport functions. The major protein in the outer membrane is **porin**, which aggregates to form large pores that allow most molecules having a mass of less than 10 kD to pass freely from the cytosol into the intermembrane space. The outer membrane can be solubilized by the detergent digitonin, leaving the inner membrane and the enclosed matrix intact.

Inner Membrane

The inner mitochondrial membrane (**Part B**) has a higher proportion of protein than other mammalian membranes, containing about 80% protein and 20% lipid. It is more complex, in both structure and function, than the outer membrane. The inner membrane is tightly folded into a series of **cristae**, thereby greatly increasing the surface area and the functional capacity of the membrane. The inner membrane, in contrast to the outer membrane, is highly **impermeable** to most molecules. The movement of small molecules across the inner membrane requires either specific **transport proteins** or **shuttle systems**. All of the enzymes in the **electron transport chain**, as well as the mitochondrial **ATP synthase**, are located in the inner membrane. Some of the components of the electron transport chain also act as **H$^+$ pumps,** transporting H$^+$ from the matrix to the intermembrane space. Most of the transport proteins, also known as **translocases**, that move molecules across the inner membrane are either antiporters or symporters. For example, the **ATP/ADP translocase** is an antiporter that transports ATP out of the matrix in exchange for ADP; the **P$_i$ translocase** is a symporter that cotransports P$_i$ and H$^+$ into the matrix; and **pyruvate translocase** is an antiporter that transports pyruvate into the matrix in exchange for OH$^-$.

Intermembrane Space

The space between the outer and inner membranes (**Part C**) contains a family of enzymes that exchange high-energy phosphate bonds between various nucleoside mono-, di-, and triphosphates. These enzymes include adenylate kinase, creatine kinase, and nucleoside diphosphate kinase. **Adenylate kinase**, an enzyme found in very high concentration in muscle, helps maintain a relatively constant concentration of ATP during strenuous exercise by converting two molecules of ADP to ATP and AMP.

$$\text{2 ADP} \xrightleftharpoons{\text{\textbf{Adenylate kinase}}} \text{AMP + ATP}$$

Creatine kinase performs a function similar to that of adenylate kinase. Creatine phosphate serves as a reservoir of high-energy phosphate bonds in muscle and brain. Creatine kinase catalyzes the transfer of phosphate from creatine phosphate to ADP, forming ATP. When ATP is high, the reverse reaction occurs.

$$\text{Creatine phosphate + ADP} \xrightleftharpoons{\text{\textbf{Creatine kinase}}} \text{Creatine + ATP}$$

Nucleoside diphosphate kinase catalyzes the interconversion of nucleoside di- and triphosphates. The enzyme has broad specificity for both the phosphate donor and the acceptor. For example, one molecule of GTP is formed during each turn of the tricarboxylic acid cycle. Nucleoside diphosphate kinase transfers the terminal phosphate of GTP to ADP, forming ATP.

$$\text{GTP + ADP} \xrightleftharpoons{\text{\textbf{Nucleoside diphosphate kinase}}} \text{ATP + GDP}$$

Matrix

A large number of enzymes are found in the mitochondrial matrix (**Part D**), including enzymes involved in pyruvate oxidation, fatty acid oxidation, and the TCA cycle. Many of these enzymes are NAD$^+$-dependent and FAD-dependent dehydrogenases that catalyze reactions, resulting in NADH and FADH$_2$. The NADH and FADH$_2$ are oxidized back to NAD$^+$ and FAD by the electron transport chain that is housed in the surrounding inner membrane. The matrix also contains multiple copies of mitochondrial DNA (mtDNA), together with ribosomes, tRNA, and the enzymes needed to transcribe mtDNA and synthesize the proteins encoded by mtDNA. The number of proteins encoded by mtDNA is relatively small compared to nuclear DNA, and all are a part of the pathway of oxidative phosphorylation. Most of the proteins in mitochondria are encoded by nuclear DNA.

Clinical Significance

An increasing number of congenital defects are being attributed to mutations in mtDNA. Several human diseases can be traced back to point mutations in mtDNA genes that code for proteins or tRNAs. Patients with these diseases have multiple phenotypes, including weakness, myopathy, inability to tolerate exercise, cardiomyopathies, and encephalopathies. The tissues that are most affected are skeletal muscle, heart, brain, and nerve. These tissues have a high energy requirement. Disorders resulting from mutations in mtDNA always show a maternal inheritance pattern.

For more information see Coffee C, *Metabolism*. Fence Creek, pp 86–96.

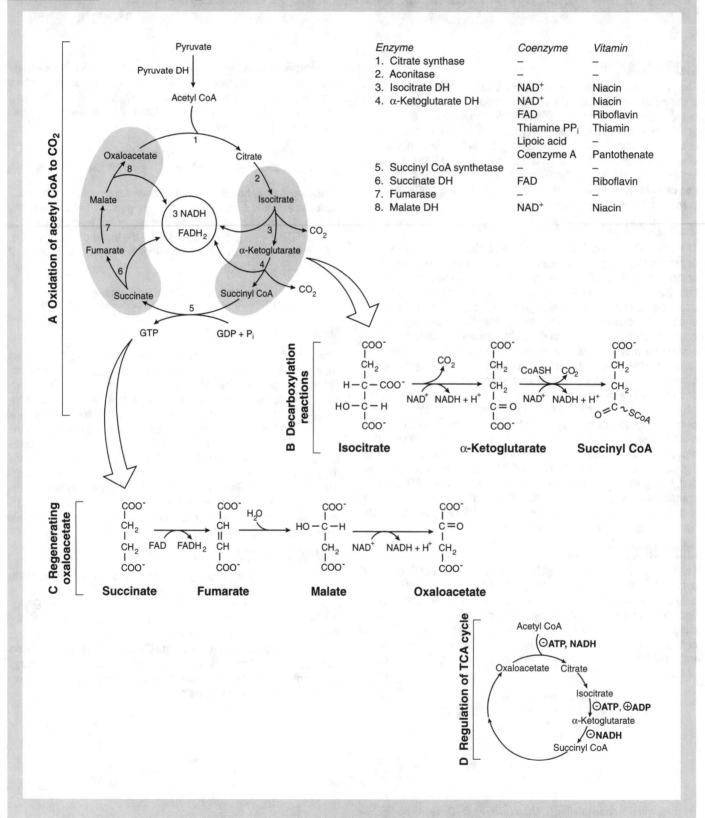

Enzyme	Coenzyme	Vitamin
1. Citrate synthase	–	–
2. Aconitase	–	–
3. Isocitrate DH	NAD^+	Niacin
4. α-Ketoglutarate DH	NAD^+	Niacin
	FAD	Riboflavin
	Thiamine PP_i	Thiamin
	Lipoic acid	–
	Coenzyme A	Pantothenate
5. Succinyl CoA synthetase	–	–
6. Succinate DH	FAD	Riboflavin
7. Fumarase	–	–
8. Malate DH	NAD^+	Niacin

A Oxidation of acetyl CoA to CO_2

B Decarboxylation reactions

Isocitrate α-Ketoglutarate   Succinyl CoA

C Regenerating oxaloacetate

Succinate   Fumarate   Malate   Oxaloacetate

D Regulation of TCA cycle

OVERVIEW

The tricarboxylic acid (TCA) cycle, also known as the citric acid cycle or the Krebs cycle, consists of eight coupled reactions, starting and ending with oxaloacetate. Five coenzymes are required for operation of the cycle: NAD^+, FAD, thiamine pyrophosphate, lipoic acid, and coenzyme A (CoA). The catabolic function of the cycle is to oxidize acetyl CoA to CO_2. Approximately 90% of the energy present in acetyl CoA is conserved in the products: NADH, $FADH_2$, and GTP. The rate at which the TCA cycle operates is dependent on both the energy state of the cell and the availability of O_2. Three enzymes in the cycle are targets of regulation: isocitrate dehydrogenase, α-ketoglutarate dehydrogenase, and citrate synthase.

Oxidation of Acetyl CoA to CO_2

The overall reaction catalyzed by the TCA cycle is shown below:

$$Acetyl\ C_0A + 3NAD^+ + FAD + GDP + P_i + 2H_2O \longrightarrow$$
$$2CO_2 + 3NADH + 3FADH_2 + GTP + 2H^+ + CoA$$

The first reaction in the cycle (**Part A**) is catalyzed by **citrate synthase**. Acetyl CoA, a C_2 compound, enters the cycle by condensing with oxaloacetate, a C_4 intermediate, producing citrate. The conversion of citrate to its isomer, isocitrate, sets the stage for the decarboxylation reactions that follow.

Decarboxylation Reactions

Isocitrate is converted to succinyl CoA by two sequential **oxidative decarboxylation** reactions (**Part B**). The first reaction results in α-ketoglutarate, followed by succinyl CoA in the second reaction. The enzymes involved are **isocitrate dehydrogenase** and **α-ketoglutarate dehydrogenase**, respectively. In each reaction, CO_2 is released and electrons are transferred to NAD^+, producing NADH. The two carbon atoms released as CO_2 are not the same two atoms that entered the cycle as acetyl CoA. However, there is no *net* contribution of carbon to the cycle; for every two carbons that enter as acetyl CoA, two atoms leave as CO_2.

Regeneration of Oxaloacetate

The function of the remaining reactions in the cycle is to regenerate oxaloacetate (**Part C**), extracting as much energy as possible in the process. Succinyl CoA contains a **high-energy thioester linkage** that is hydrolyzed, releasing succinate. The energy released is coupled to **GTP synthesis by substrate-level phosphorylation**. In the next reaction, catalyzed by succinate dehydrogenase, succinate is oxidized to fumarate, producing $FADH_2$. Succinate dehydrogenase is the only enzyme in the cycle that is not in the matrix; it is embedded in the inner mitochondrial membrane and is also known as complex II of the electron transport chain. Water is added across the double bond of fumarate, producing malate, which is oxidized by malate dehydrogenase, regenerating oxaloacetate and producing NADH.

Regulation of the TCA Cycle

The rate at which the TCA cycle operates is dependent on both the energy state of the cell and the availability of O_2. The primary site of regulation is **isocitrate dehydrogenase**, the rate-limiting enzyme in the cycle (**Part D**). It is allosterically inhibited by the accumulation of ATP and activated by the accumulation of ADP. Secondary sites of regulation are **α-ketoglutarate dehydrogenase** and **citrate synthase**. All three of these enzymes are inhibited by the accumulation of NADH, an indication of limited O_2 availability and a diminished ability to regenerate NAD^+, the coenzyme required for three of the dehydrogenases in the cycle. All three of the regulatory enzymes catalyze reactions that are irreversible under the conditions that exist in the cell.

Pyruvate: The Route for Terminal Oxidation of Glucose

Most of the acetyl CoA that is oxidized by the TCA cycle is derived either from fatty acid oxidation or from glycolysis. Pyruvate, the end product of aerobic glycolysis, is generated in the cytosol and must be transported into the mitochondrial matrix to be further oxidized. The **oxidative decarboxylation** of pyruvate to acetyl CoA is catalyzed by **pyruvate dehydrogenase**, and the reaction is summarized by the following equation:

$$Pyruvate + NAD^+ + CoA \longrightarrow Acetyl\ CoA + CO_2 + NADH$$

Although the above reaction appears to be simple, it is very complex, consisting of several sequential reactions. Similarly, pyruvate dehydrogenase is a complex enzyme, consisting of three different types of subunits that collectively require five different coenzymes: NAD^+, FAD, lipoic acid, thiamin pyrophosphate, and CoA. The subunit structure and coenzyme requirements of pyruvate dehydrogenase are very similar to that of two other mitochondrial enzymes, **α-ketoglutarate dehydrogenase** and **branched-chain ketoacid dehydrogenase**. All three of these enzymes catalyze oxidative decarboxylation reactions.

Clinical Significance

Inherited deficiencies in the TCA cycle enzymes are rarely seen, perhaps because they are seldom compatible with life. A few cases of fumarase deficiency, however, have been reported that are characterized by severe and progressive impairment of muscular and neurologic function. More commonly, vitamin deficiencies, particularly thiamin deficiency, can lead to diminished activity of several of the enzymes in the TCA cycle, resulting in lactic acidosis and a variety of neurologic effects.

For more information see Coffee C, *Metabolism*. Fence Creek, pp 87–90.

18 Anabolic Functions of the TCA Cycle

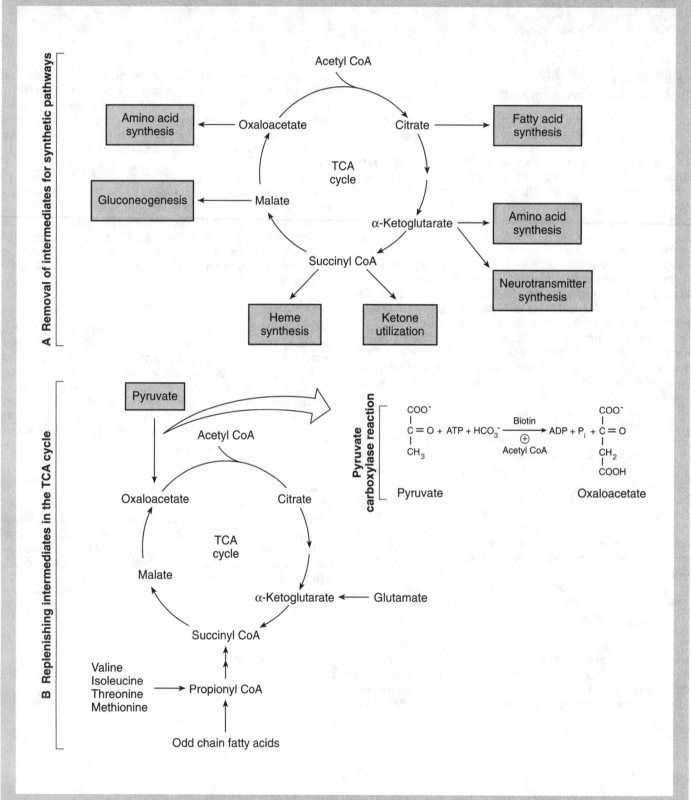

A Removal of intermediates for synthetic pathways

Acetyl CoA

Amino acid synthesis ← Oxaloacetate

Citrate → Fatty acid synthesis

TCA cycle

Gluconeogenesis ← Malate

α-Ketoglutarate → Amino acid synthesis

α-Ketoglutarate → Neurotransmitter synthesis

Succinyl CoA → Heme synthesis

Succinyl CoA → Ketone utilization

B Replenishing intermediates in the TCA cycle

Pyruvate

Acetyl CoA

Oxaloacetate

Citrate

TCA cycle

Malate

α-Ketoglutarate ← Glutamate

Succinyl CoA

Valine
Isoleucine
Threonine → Propionyl CoA
Methionine

Odd chain fatty acids

Pyruvate carboxylase reaction

$$\begin{array}{c} COO^- \\ | \\ C=O \\ | \\ CH_3 \end{array} + ATP + HCO_3^- \xrightarrow[\underset{Acetyl\ CoA}{\oplus}]{Biotin} ADP + P_i + \begin{array}{c} COO^- \\ | \\ C=O \\ | \\ CH_2 \\ | \\ COOH \end{array}$$

Pyruvate   Oxaloacetate

OVERVIEW

Several intermediates in the TCA cycle serve as substrates for biosynthetic pathways. Citrate is a source of acetyl CoA for fatty acid synthesis; malate is a source of oxaloacetate for gluconeogenesis; succinyl CoA is precursor for heme synthesis and is required for ketone utilization; and α-ketoglutarate and oxaloacetate are used for glutamate and aspartate synthesis, respectively. The removal of intermediates from the TCA cycle will decrease the rate at which the cycle operates unless the intermediates can be replenished. Reactions that replenish intermediates in the TCA cycle are known as **anaplerotic reactions**.

Removal of Intermediates for Synthetic Pathways

The liver is the main organ that uses intermediates in the TCA cycle for synthetic purposes, although most other tissues carry out one or more of the synthetic pathways (**Part A**).

Citrate: Fatty Acid Synthesis

In humans, almost all fatty acid synthesis occurs in the **liver**, following a meal. The immediate carbon precursor is acetyl CoA, which is derived from excess dietary glucose. Pyruvate is converted to acetyl CoA in mitochondria, where it condenses with oxaloacetate, producing citrate. Fatty acid synthesis, however, takes place in the cytosol. In the well-fed state, citrate accumulates in the mitochondria and is transported to the cytosol, where it is cleaved, releasing acetyl CoA that is available for fatty acid synthesis.

Malate: Gluconeogenesis

Gluconeogenesis occurs primarily in the **liver** during the fasting state. The first intermediate in the pathway is oxaloacetate, which is produced in the mitochondria. The remaining steps in gluconeogenesis occur in the cytosol. Oxaloacetate cannot be transported across the inner mitochondrial membrane, although one or more transporters exist for malate. Moreover, malate accumulates in the mitochondria during fasting and is transported into the cytosol, where it is oxidized to oxaloacetate and used for the remaining steps in gluconeogenesis. The accumulation of malate during fasting results from degradation of glucogenic amino acids whose carbon skeletons are intermediates in the TCA cycle.

Succinyl CoA: Heme Synthesis

The major tissues that synthesize heme are **bone marrow** and **liver**. The first step in the pathway of heme synthesis occurs in the mitochondria, where Δ-aminolevulenic acid synthase catalyzes the condensation of succinyl CoA and glycine, producing Δ-aminolevulenic acid. All of the atoms in heme are derived from succinyl CoA and glycine.

Succinyl CoA: Ketone Utilization

The ketone bodies, β-hydroxybutyrate and acetoacetate, can be extracted from the blood and used as fuels by most **extrahepatic tissues**. As the ketones enter the mitochondria, β-hydroxybutyrate is oxidized to acetoacetate. Acetoacetate must be converted to acetoacetyl CoA before it can be further oxidized. Acetoacetyl CoA is formed in an exchange reaction in which CoA is transferred from succinyl CoA to acetoacetate, as described in the following equation:

$$\text{Acetoacetate} + \text{Succinyl CoA} \longrightarrow \text{Acetoacetyl CoA} + \text{Succinate}$$

The absence of the enzyme catalyzing this reaction in liver accounts for the fact that the liver cannot oxidize ketones, although it is the site where they are synthesized.

α-Ketoglutarate and Oxaloacetate: Nonessential Amino Acid Synthesis

Oxaloacetate and α-ketoglutarate can be converted to aspartate and glutamate, respectively, by transamination reactions. The addition of an amide group to the side chains of glutamate and aspartate results in glutamine and asparagine, respectively. Both **transamination** and **amidation** reactions are widely distributed in tissues. The brain uses glutamate and aspartate as neurotransmitters and produces γ-aminobutyrate, another neurotransmitter by the decarboxylation of glutamate.

Replenishing Intermediates in the TCA Cycle

Although many intermediates are withdrawn from the TCA cycle, the concentrations of the intermediates remain almost constant. There are three **anaplerotic reactions** in humans that are particularly important in replenishing intermediates in the cycle (**Part B**).

Synthesis of Oxaloacetate from Pyruvate

The most important anaplerotic reaction in liver, kidney, and muscle is the carboxylation of pyruvate to oxaloacetate, which is catalyzed by **pyruvate carboxylase**. This reaction, like all carboxylation reactions, requires ATP and biotin. ATP supplies the energy for adding the carboxyl group to pyruvate, and biotin is the coenzyme that acts as a high-energy carrier of CO_2 groups. The pyruvate used in this reaction is derived from glucose and some amino acids (serine, threonine, glycine, cysteine). Acetyl CoA is an essential allosteric activatior of pyruvate carboxylase.

Synthesis of Succinyl CoA from Propionyl CoA

In tissues that do not contain pyruvate carboxylase, the conversion of propionyl CoA to succinyl CoA is an important anaplerotic pathway. Most of the propionyl CoA comes from the degradation of the branched-chain amino acids, valine and isoleucine, with smaller amounts coming from threonine, methionine, and the oxidation of odd-chain fatty acids.

Synthesis of α-Ketoglutarate from Glutamate

Transamination reactions involving glutamate as an amino donor result in α-ketoglutarate. Additionally, glutamate can be deaminated by glutamate dehydrogenase, resulting in α-ketoglutarate. Both **transaminases** and **glutamate dehydrogenase** are widely distributed in tissues.

Clinical Significance

The TCA cycle has been called the "hub of metabolism" because of its many roles in metabolism. The clinical significance of the TCA cycle can be appreciated by considering two of its anabolic functions, providing precursors for glucose and heme synthesis. Glucose is an obligatory fuel for red blood cells and the brain, yet during periods of fasting, the blood levels of glucose remain relatively constant because of gluconeogenesis. Similarly, heme is the cofactor for hemoglobin, myoglobin, and cytochromes. These proteins are responsible for transport, storage, and utilization of oxygen. Clearly, the inability to synthesize either glucose or heme would be incompatible with life.

For more information see Coffee C, *Metabolism*. Fence Creek, pp 87–88, 233–240.

Electron Transport Chain: Oxidation of NADH and FADH₂

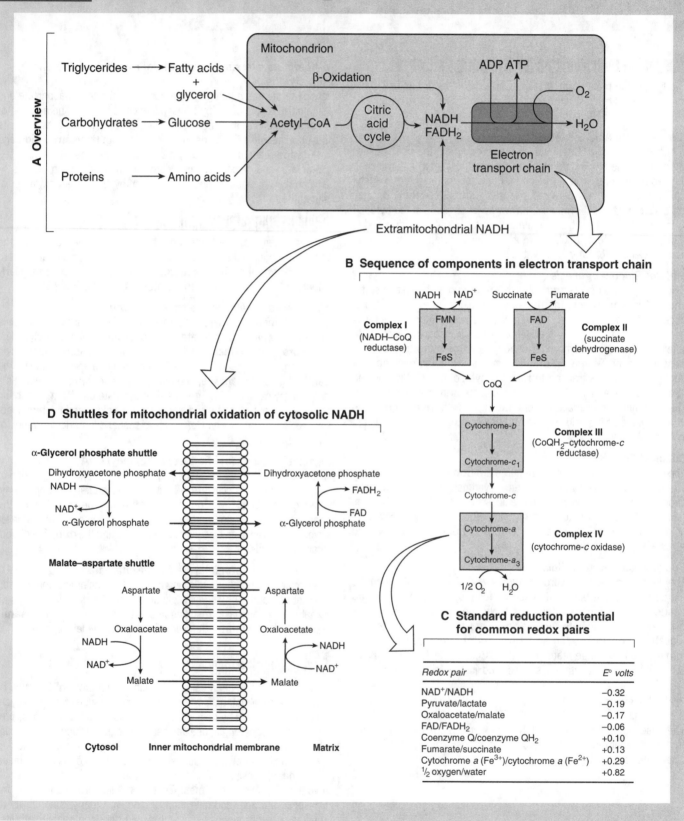

A Overview

Triglycerides → Fatty acids + glycerol

Carbohydrates → Glucose

Proteins → Amino acids

Mitochondrion

β-Oxidation

Acetyl–CoA → Citric acid cycle → NADH FADH₂ → Electron transport chain → H_2O

ADP ATP

O_2

Extramitochondrial NADH

B Sequence of components in electron transport chain

NADH   NAD⁺   Succinate   Fumarate

Complex I (NADH–CoQ reductase)
FMN → FeS

Complex II (succinate dehydrogenase)
FAD → FeS

CoQ

Complex III (CoQH₂–cytochrome-*c* reductase)
Cytochrome-*b* → Cytochrome-*c₁*

Cytochrome-*c*

Complex IV (cytochrome-*c* oxidase)
Cytochrome-*a* → Cytochrome-*a₃*

1/2 O_2 H_2O

D Shuttles for mitochondrial oxidation of cytosolic NADH

α-Glycerol phosphate shuttle

Dihydroxyacetone phosphate ← Dihydroxyacetone phosphate

NADH
NAD⁺
α-Glycerol phosphate → α-Glycerol phosphate

FADH₂
FAD

Malate–aspartate shuttle

Aspartate ← Aspartate

Oxaloacetate   Oxaloacetate
NADH   NADH
NAD⁺   NAD⁺
Malate → Malate

Cytosol   **Inner mitochondrial membrane**   **Matrix**

C Standard reduction potential for common redox pairs

Redox pair	E° volts
NAD⁺/NADH	−0.32
Pyruvate/lactate	−0.19
Oxaloacetate/malate	−0.17
FAD/FADH₂	−0.06
Coenzyme Q/coenzyme QH₂	+0.10
Fumarate/succinate	+0.13
Cytochrome *a* (Fe^{3+})/cytochrome *a* (Fe^{2+})	+0.29
½ oxygen/water	+0.82

OVERVIEW

The electron transport chain, also known as the respiratory chain, transfers electrons from NADH and $FADH_2$ to O_2, producing H_2O (**Part A**). It consists of four enzyme complexes, embedded in the inner mitochondrial membrane, and two free electron carriers, coenzyme Q (CoQ) and cytochrome c. Each electron carrier in the chain has a standard reduction potential ($E^°$) that is an index of its ability to donate electrons to some acceptor. Three of the four complexes (I, III, and IV) in the electron transport chain also function as H^+ pumps, using energy released by electron transfer to establish a proton gradient across the inner mitochondrial membrane. The inner mitochondrial membrane is impermeable to NADH; therefore, oxidation of cytosolic NADH requires shuttle systems that transfer electrons from cytosolic NADH to mitochondrial electron carriers, either NADH or $FADH_2$, which can be oxidized by the electron transport chain.

Sequence of Components in the Electron Transport Chain

The sequence of components in the electron transport chain (**Part B**) was deduced by studying the structural and functional properties of submitochondrial particles, isolated from detergent-treated mitochondria. **Complex I**, also known as NADH-CoQ reductase, accepts electrons from NADH and transfers them through flavin mononucleotide (FMN) and iron-sulfur (FeS) centers to **CoQ**. **Complex II**, also known as succinate dehydrogenase, oxidizes succinate and transfers the electrons through FAD and FeS centers to CoQ. Unlike other components of the electron transport chain, CoQ is a lipid that moves freely in the membrane, accepting electrons from FADH derived from the oxidation of several substrates. In addition to succinate dehydrogenase, fatty acyl CoA and α-glycerol phosphate dehydrogenases generate $FADH_2$, which feeds electrons into CoQ. **Complex III** accepts two electrons from CoQ and transfers them, one at a time, through cytochrome b and cytochrome c_1, to **cytochrome c**, a protein loosely associated with the inner mitochondrial membrane. CoQ occupies a pivotal point in the electron transport chain by acting as a bridge between two-electron transfer reactions (catalyzed by complexes I and II) and one-electron transfer reactions (catalyzed by complexes III and IV). **Complex IV**, also known as cytochrome oxidase, accepts electrons from cytochrome c and transfers them through cytochromes a, a_3, and copper to O_2, the terminal acceptor. The reduction of each atom of oxygen ($\frac{1}{2} O_2$) to H_2O requires two electrons.

Standard Reduction Potential and Energetics of Electron Transport

Electron transfer reactions are by definition both oxidation and reduction (redox) reactions. The loss of electrons by one compound is always accompanied by the gain of electrons by another. Every electron carrier cycles between an oxidized and a reduced form, known as a **redox pair**. Redox pairs have a **standard reduction potential** ($E^°$) expressed in volts (**Part C**). The $E^°$ for a redox pair is an index of its ability to donate electrons to some acceptor. The stronger the electron donor, the more negative the $E^°$. Electron carriers at the beginning of the electron transport chain have more negative $E^°$ values than those near the end of the chain, thereby assuring that electrons will flow spontaneously from NADH ($E^° = -0.32$ volts) or $FADH_2$ ($E^° = -0.06$ volts) to O_2 ($E^° = +0.82$ volts). The **standard free energy change** ($\Delta G^°$) for a redox reaction is related to the difference in the standard reduction potential ($\Delta E^°$) between the electron acceptor and the electron donor. The $\Delta G^°$ for a redox reaction can be calculated from the following equation, where n is the number of electrons transferred, F is a constant (23 kcal/volt), and $\Delta E^° = E^°_{electron\ acceptor} - E^°_{electron\ donor}$:

$$\Delta G^° = -nF\Delta E^°$$

Using this equation, the $\Delta G^°$ for the oxidation of NADH by O_2 is -52.6 kcal/mol, while the $\Delta G^°$ for the oxidation of $FADH_2$ by O_2 is -40.5

kcal/mol. In addition to catalyzing cyclic reduction and oxidation reactions, complexes I, III, and IV also act as H^+ pumps. The energy released by transfer of electrons through the complex is used to pump H^+ out of the mitochondrial matrix. A change of approximately one pH unit between the matrix and the surrounding medium can be measured in mitochondria that are actively oxidizing substrate.

Shuttle Systems for Mitochondrial Oxidation of Cytosolic NADH

The inner mitochondrial membrane is impermeable to NADH, and special shuttle systems carry reducing equivalents (electrons) from cytosolic NADH into the mitochondria (**Part D**). The **malate-aspartate shuttle**, found in heart, liver, and kidney mitochondria, transfers electrons from cytosolic NADH, through malate as a carrier, to mitochondrial NADH, which can be oxidized by the electron transport chain. The **α-glycerol phosphate** shuttle, found in skeletal muscle and brain mitochondria, transfers electrons from cytosolic NADH, through α-glycerol phosphate as a carrier, to mitochondrial $FADH_2$, which can be oxidized by the electron transport chain. Since electrons from $FADH_2$ bypass complex I of the electron transport chain, the energy derived from oxidation of cytosolic NADH, and ultimately the amount of ATP synthesized, varies depending on which shuttle is used.

Clinical Significance

Human mitochondrial DNA (mtDNA) contains 13 genes that encode proteins of the electron transport chain. The remaining genes code for tRNA or rRNA that are required for synthesis of proteins encoded by mtDNA. Mutations in mtDNA have been implicated in several diseases whose symptoms are summarized in the table below. Two different mutations, both single-base changes in mtDNA, have been shown to result in Leber hereditary optic neuropathy (LHON). One mutation results in a partially active complex I, while the other results in a partially active complex III. Both MERRF and MELAS result from point mutations in mtDNA genes that code for tRNAs required for synthesis of proteins encoded by mtDNA.

Disease	Clinical Features
LHON	Bilateral loss of central vision, tremor, and ataxia
MERRF disease	Abnormal eye movements, loss of hearing, ataxia, lactic acidosis, ragged-red muscle fibers, and progressive dementia
MELAS	Stroke-like episodes, abnormal motor and cognitive development, lactic acidosis, cardiomyopathy, deafness, dementia, and renal disease

LHON, Leber hereditary optic neuropathy; MERRF, myoclonic epilepsy and ragged-red fiber disease; MELAS, mitochondrial encephalomyopathy, lactic acidosis, and stroke-like episodes.

For more information see Coffee C, *Metabolism*. Fence Creek, pp 90–96.

Oxidative Phosphorylation: Mitochondrial ATP Synthesis

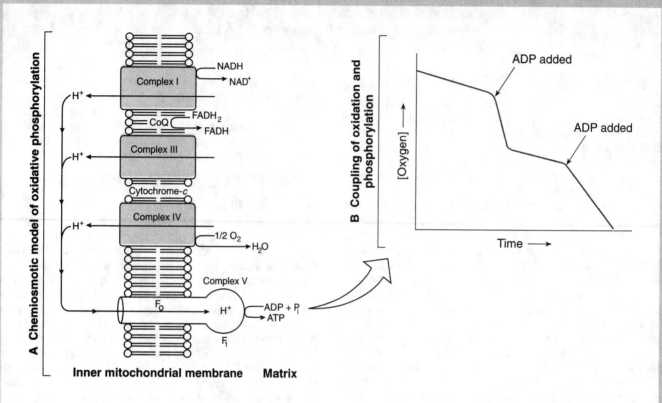

A Chemiosmotic model of oxidative phosphorylation

Complex I — NADH → NAD$^+$

H$^+$

CoQ — FADH$_2$ / FADH

Complex III

H$^+$

Cytochrome-c

Complex IV

H$^+$

1/2 O$_2$ → H$_2$O

Complex V

F$_o$

H$^+$ — ADP + P$_i$ / ATP

F$_1$

Inner mitochondrial membrane   **Matrix**

B Coupling of oxidation and phosphorylation

ADP added

ADP added

[Oxygen] →

Time →

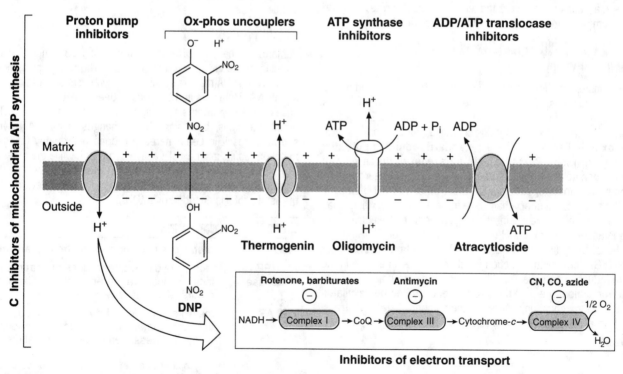

C Inhibitors of mitochondrial ATP synthesis

Proton pump inhibitors   **Ox-phos uncouplers**   **ATP synthase inhibitors**   **ADP/ATP translocase inhibitors**

O$^-$ H$^+$
NO$_2$
NO$_2$

H$^+$

ATP   ADP + P$_i$ ADP

Matrix + + + + + + + + + + + + +

Outside − − − − − − − − − − − −

H$^+$

OH
NO$_2$
NO$_2$
DNP

H$^+$
Thermogenin

H$^+$
Oligomycin

ATP
Atractyloside

Rotenone, barbiturates   **Antimycin**   **CN, CO, azide**
⊖   ⊖   ⊖
1/2 O$_2$
NADH → Complex I → CoQ → Complex III → Cytochrome-c → Complex IV
H$_2$O

Inhibitors of electron transport

OVERVIEW

The final step in converting energy contained in metabolic fuels to ATP is oxidative phosphorylation, a process that couples oxygen-consuming reactions with the phosphorylation of ADP. About 95% of the oxygen consumed by the body is used by the electron transport chain to oxidize NADH and $FADH_2$. The concomitant reduction of O_2 produces about 300 mL of H_2O per day. The energy released by the oxidation of NADH and $FADH_2$ is used for ATP synthesis, a reaction catalyzed by ATP synthase. The chemiosmotic model of oxidative phosphorylation provides a molecular explanation of how energy released by electron transfer through the respiratory chain is coupled with mitochondrial ATP synthesis.

The Chemiosmotic Model of Oxidative Phosphorylation

The chemiosmotic model (**Part A**), also known as Mitchell's hypothesis, has two basic postulates: 1) as electrons flow from NADH and $FADH_2$ through the electron transport chain, the energy released is used to create a H^+ gradient (protomotive force) across the inner mitochondrial membrane; and 2) the movement of protons back into the matrix releases energy that is used to drive the synthesis of ATP. Implicit in this model is the requirement for an intact membrane that can confer directional properties on the reactions involved. The proton gradient is established by **complexes I, III, and IV** of the electron transport chain. These complexes use energy released by electron transport to pump H^+ out of the matrix. The synthesis of ATP is catalyzed by **ATP synthase (complex V)**. ATP synthase has two major components, F_o and F_1. The F_o component spans the inner mitochondrial membrane, forming a channel through which H^+ can reenter the matrix. The F_1 component protrudes into the matrix and contains the active site where ADP and P_i are condensed, forming ATP.

Coupling of Electron Transport with ATP Synthesis

The **obligatory coupling** of electron transport with ATP synthesis can be demonstrated in isolated mitochondria that are supplied with an oxidizable substrate and O_2, but not with ADP (**Part B**). When ADP is added, the rate of O_2 consumption (a measure of electron transport) increases until the ADP is used up, when it decreases back to a basal level of respiration. If more ADP is added, the rate of oxygen consumption increases again. A quantitative index of coupling is provided by the **P/O ratio**, which is defined as the number of P_i groups incorporated into ATP per atom of oxygen consumed ($1/2\ O_2$). Substrates that are oxidized with the formation of NADH (malate, pyruvate, isocitrate) have a P/O ratio of 2.5 to 3. Substrates that are oxidized with the formation of $FADH_2$ (succinate, α-glycerol phosphate) have a P/O ratio of 1.5 to 2. The **efficiency of oxidative phosphorylation** can be calculated from the energy released when NADH is oxidized by O_2 ($\Delta G° = -52.6$ kcal/mol) and the energy required for ATP synthesis from ADP and P_i ($\Delta G° = +7.3$ kcal/mol). Assuming 3 mols of ATP are produced per mol of NADH oxidized, the efficiency would be approximately 40%. Most of the additional energy is released as heat.

Inhibitors of Mitochondrial ATP Synthesis

Several drugs and toxins inhibit oxidative phosphorylation (**Part C**). These inhibitors can be classified into four major groups. **Proton pump inhibitors**, often described as site-specific inhibitors of the electron transport chain, bind to complexes I, III, and IV and block both electron transport and H^+ pumping (**Part D**). Examples of site-specific inhibitors are cyanide and carbon monoxide, which block electron transfer from complex IV to O_2; rotenone and several barbiturates, which block the transfer of electrons from complex I to CoQ; and antimycin, which blocks the transfer of electrons from complex III to cytochrome c. **Uncouplers of oxidative phosphorylation** are compounds that abolish the H^+ gradient across the inner mitochondrial membrane, thereby inhibiting the rate of ATP synthesis. In contrast, the rate of oxidation is increased by uncouplers. The energy released by oxidation in the presence of an uncoupler is released as heat. Examples of uncouplers are dinitrophenol (DNP), aspirin, and thermogenin. DNP, a hydrophobic compound that readily crosses the membrane, carries H^+ into the matrix (**Part C**). DNP is a weak acid that is protonated at the lower pH that exists in the space between the inner and outer mitochondrial membranes. However, when DNP enters the matrix, where the pH is higher, it dissociates, releasing H^+. Similarly, aspirin uncouples oxidation and phosphorylation, and when taken in large doses, it increases the body temperature. Thermogenin, a protein found in the inner mitochondrial membrane of brown fat, abolishes the H^+ gradient by providing a path for H^+ to reenter the matrix that bypasses the F_o channel. Thermogenin plays a key role in thermogenesis, particularly in neonates. **Inhibitors that bind directly to ATP synthase** inhibit both ATP synthesis and electron transport. An example is oligomycin, an antibiotic that binds to the F_o component of ATP synthase, blocking the movement of H^+ through the F_o channel. Electron transport is inhibited because complexes I, III, and IV have difficulty pumping H^+ against a large H^+ gradient that cannot be dissipated. **Inhibitors of ADP/ATP translocase** decrease both ATP synthesis and electron transport. An example is atractyloside, which inhibits transport of ADP into the mitochondrial matrix in exchange for ATP.

Clinical Significance

The toxic and lethal effects of cyanide are due to its inhibition of complex IV (cytochrome oxidase). Cyanide binds to heme Fe^{3+} in cytochrome oxidase, blocking the transfer of electrons from complex IV to O_2. Mitochondrial ATP synthesis ceases, and death occurs unless prompt treatment is initiated. Treatment of cyanide poisoning involves diverting the cyanide away from cytochrome oxidase, followed by conversion to thiocyanide, which can be excreted in the urine. Administration of **nitrite** oxidizes the heme iron in hemoglobin to the Fe^{3+} state, forming methemoglobin, which can bind cyanide. Giving **thiosulfate** activates rhodanese, an enzyme that converts both free cyanide and methemoglobin-bound cyanide to thiocyanide, which can be excreted.

For more information see Coffee C, *Metabolism*. Fence Creek, pp 90–96.

21 Interconversion of Metabolic Fuels

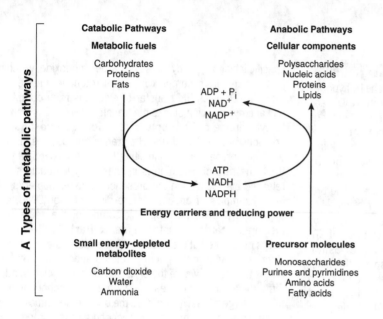

A Types of metabolic pathways

Catabolic Pathways

Metabolic fuels

Carbohydrates
Proteins
Fats

ADP + P$_i$
NAD$^+$
NADP$^+$

ATP
NADH
NADPH

Energy carriers and reducing power

Anabolic Pathways

Cellular components

Polysaccharides
Nucleic acids
Proteins
Lipids

Small energy-depleted metabolites

Carbon dioxide
Water
Ammonia

Precursor molecules

Monosaccharides
Purines and pyrimidines
Amino acids
Fatty acids

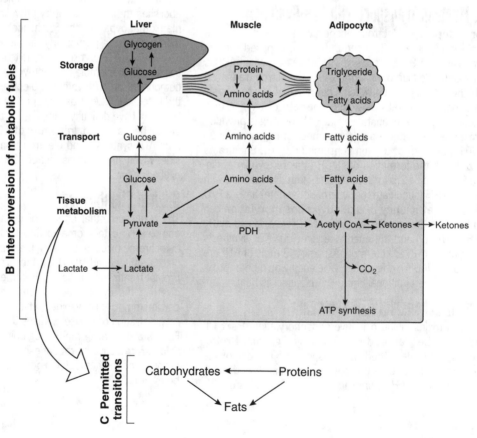

B Interconversion of metabolic fuels

| | Liver | Muscle | Adipocyte |

Storage

Glycogen
Glucose

Protein
Amino acids

Triglyceride
Fatty acids

Transport

Glucose

Amino acids

Fatty acids

Tissue metabolism

Glucose

Amino acids

Fatty acids

Pyruvate — PDH → Acetyl CoA ⇄ Ketones ← Ketones

Lactate ← → Lactate

CO$_2$

ATP synthesis

C Permitted transitions

Carbohydrates ← Proteins

Fats

OVERVIEW

Metabolic pathways are organized around two major goals that are necessary for cell maintenance and replication. The first goal of metabolism is to extract energy ATP and reducing power (NADPH) from metabolic fuels that can be used for the synthesis of more complex molecules. The second goal of metabolism is to provide a small set of precursor molecules that can be used to synthesize a diverse set of macromolecules, having both structural and functional roles in the cell. Each of the metabolic fuels has separate storage and transport forms. The pathways for glucose, amino acid, and fatty acid metabolism have a few common intermediates that permit some, but not all, of these metabolic fuels to be interconverted.

Types of Metabolic Pathways

The metabolic pathways found in cells can be divided into three major categories: catabolic, anabolic, and amphibolic (**Part A**). **Catabolic pathways** degrade large, complex molecules into smaller compounds by cleaving chemical bonds. These pathways involve oxidative processes and release energy that can be conserved as ATP, NADH, and NADPH. **Anabolic pathways** synthesize large molecules from small precursors by the formation of chemical bonds. Synthetic pathways require ATP and reducing power, usually in the form of NADPH. Catabolic and anabolic pathways are integrated by sharing ATP, NADH, and NADPH. These universal energy carriers are products of catabolic pathways and substrates for anabolic pathways. **Amphibolic pathways**, such as the TCA cycle, have both anabolic and catabolic functions.

Interconversion of Metabolic Fuels

Each metabolic fuel has a storage form, a transport or circulating form, and one or more characteristic cellular intermediates (**Part B**). The catabolic pathways for carbohydrate, lipid, and protein converge with the formation of **acetyl CoA**. The storage and transport forms for each metabolic fuel are interconvertible, although separate pathways are used to convert the storage form to the transport form, and vice versa. Separate pathways can be controlled independently, thereby preventing futile cycling of fuel. Pathways for interconverting different metabolic fuels are used to store excess dietary carbohydrate and protein as fat following a meal. During periods of fasting, these pathways are used to degrade glycogen and to convert the glucogenic amino acids to glucose. All of the transport forms, except the essential amino acids, can be synthesized in the cell. The essential amino acids must be supplied by the diet.

There are two transport forms for carbohydrate: **glucose**, which is released from glycogen stores, and **lactate**, which is derived from glucose. Lactate is formed by the NADH-dependent reduction of pyruvate and released into the blood. Lactate can be extracted from the blood by several tissues, where it is oxidized back to pyruvate. The pyruvate can be either oxidized to CO_2 and H_2O or used for gluconeogenesis.

There are two transport forms for lipids: **fatty acids**, which are released from triglyceride stores, and **ketones**, which are small water-soluble derivatives of fatty acids. Ketones are synthesized in the liver and released into the blood. They can be removed from the circulation by many tissues and either oxidized to CO_2 and H_2O or used as a substrate for membrane lipid synthesis. Ketones are formed only when an excess of acetyl CoA exists.

Permitted and Nonpermitted Transitions Between Metabolic Fuels

The pathways for degrading different metabolic fuels have some common intermediates, thereby allowing transitions between some of the metabolic fuels to occur. **Permitted transitions** are carbohydrate to fat, protein to fat, and protein to carbohydrate (**Part C**). **Nonpermitted transitions** are fat to carbohydrate, fat to protein, and carbohydrate to protein. Protein cannot be synthesized from either carbohydrate or fat because the essential amino acids must be supplied by the diet. Fat cannot be converted to carbohydrate because there is no enzyme in human tissues that can convert acetyl CoA (a C_2 compound) to pyruvate (a C_3 compound). The conversion of pyruvate to acetyl CoA, a reaction catalyzed by **pyruvate dehydrogenase (PDH)**, is an irreversible reaction under the conditions that exist in the cell.

Clinical Significance

The relationship between PDH and nonpermitted transitions of metabolic fuels has several clinical implications. The fact that PDH catalyzes an irreversible reaction in human tissues is the reason why fat (or acetyl CoA derived from fat oxidation) cannot be used as a source of carbon for net glucose synthesis. The regulatory properties of PDH are responsible for sparing of glucose and protein during fasting. The PDH reaction controls the rate at which carbohydrates and many amino acid carbon skeletons enter the TCA cycle for terminal oxidation. During fasting, the oxidation of fatty acids and ketones supply both acetyl CoA which is oxidized by the TCA cycle and NADH which is oxidized by the electron transport chain. Both acetyl CoA and NADH also inhibit PDH, thereby conserving glucose, which is an obligatory fuel for some tissues. Inhibition of PDH also inhibits the terminal oxidation of amino acids, thereby sparing protein for other functions.

For more information see Coffee C, *Metabolism*. Fence Creek, pp 101–103.

Directions: For each of the following questions, choose the **one best** answer.

1. The standard free energy change ($\Delta G°$) for the hydrolysis of phosphoenolpyruvate to pyruvate and P_i is -14.8 kcal/mol and the $\Delta G°$ for the hydrolysis of ATP to ADP and P_i is -7.3 kcal/mol. What is the $\Delta G°$ for the following reaction?

$$\text{Phosphoenolpyruvate} + \text{ADP} \longrightarrow \text{ATP} + \text{pyruvate}$$

(A) -14.8 kcal/mol

(B) $+7.3$ kcal/mol

(C) $+7.5$ kcal/mol

(D) -7.5 kcal/mol

(E) $+14.8$ kcal/mol

2. All of the following compounds participate in substrate-level phosphorylation reactions **except:**

(A) Phosphoenolpyruvate

(B) Creatine phosphate

(C) Fructose-1,6-bisphosphate

(D) Succinyl CoA

(E) 1,3-Bisphosphoglycerate

3. Which of the following properties best describes NAD^+?

(A) It accepts two hydrogen atoms from various substrates

(B) It is found in higher concentration in mitochondria than in the cytosol

(C) It is derived from the vitamin riboflavin

(D) It is readily transported across the inner mitochondrial membrane

(E) It participates in several reductive reactions in biosynthetic pathways

4. How many mols of ATP (or equivalent high-energy phosphate bonds) can be formed by the complete oxidation of acetyl CoA to CO_2 and H_2O?

(A) 12

(B) 11

(C) 5

(D) 3

(E) 1

5. The rate-limiting step in the TCA cycle is catalyzed by:

(A) Citrate synthase

(B) Isocitrate dehydrogenase

(C) α-Ketoglutarate dehydrogenase

(D) Succinate dehydrogenase

(E) Malate dehydrogenase

6. A deficiency in which of the following vitamins would impair the TCA cycle most severely?

(A) Folate

(B) Pyridoxine

(C) Biotin

(D) Thiamine

(E) Vitamin B_{12}

7. Which enzyme in the TCA cycle catalyzes a reaction whose product is used for the synthesis of heme?

(A) α-Ketoglutarate dehydrogenase

(B) Isocitrate dehydrogenase

(C) Succinate dehydrogenase

(D) Fumarase

(E) Malate dehydrogenase

8. Which of the following enzymes catalyzes an anaplerotic reaction that replenishes intermediates in the TCA cycle?

(A) Succinate dehydrogenase

(B) Citrate lyase

(C) Pyruvate carboxylase

(D) Citrate synthase

(E) Pyruvate dehydrogenase

9. The addition of rotenone to a preparation of muscle mitochondria will inhibit the oxidation of all of the following substrates **except:**

(A) Pyruvate

(B) Succinate

(C) Glutamate

(D) β-Hydroxybutyrate

(E) NADH

10. The chemiosmotic coupling hypothesis of oxidative phosphorylation proposes that:

(A) Protons are pumped from the inner membrane space into the mitochondrial matrix

(B) ADP is transported out of the mitochondrial matrix in exchange for ATP

(C) A proton gradient is established across the inner mitochondrial membrane

(D) High-energy phosphate bonds are formed in mitochondrial proteins

(E) The inner mitochondrial membrane becomes more permeable to NADH

11. Which of the following transitions among metabolic fuels is a non-permitted transition?

(A) Protein to fat

(B) Fat to carbohydrate

(C) Carbohydrate to fat

(D) Protein to carbohydrate

(E) None of the above

12. Which of the following is an amphibolic pathway?

(A) Glycolysis

(B) Gluconeogenesis

(C) Fatty acid synthesis

(D) Tricarboxylic acid cycle

(E) β-Oxidation

Directions: The groups of questions below consist of several lettered choices followed by numbered items. For each number item, select the most appropriate lettered option. Each lettered option may be used once, twice, or not at all.

Questions 13–16

For each enzyme or protein listed below, select the mitochondrial compartment where it is located.

(A) Outer mitochondrial membrane

(B) Intermembrane space

(C) Inner mitochondrial membrane

(D) Mitochondrial matrix

13. Adenylate kinase

14. Porin

15. ATP synthase

16. Succinate dehydrogenase

Questions 17–18

For each description given below, select the compound that is most closely associated.

(A) Aspirin

(B) Cyanide

(C) Oligomycin

(D) Atracycloside

17. Inhibits ATP synthesis most directly

18. Uncouples oxidation and phosphorylation

PART II: ANSWERS AND EXPLANATIONS

1. The answer is D.

The reaction shown in this question is the sum of two half-reactions. In one half-reaction, phosphoenolpyruvate is hydrolyzed to pyruvate and P_i, with a ΔG° of -14.8 kcal/mol. In the other half-reaction, ADP is condensed with P_i to form ATP. This reaction is the reverse of ATP hydrolysis and has a ΔG° of $+7.3$ kcal/mol. The sum of these two half reactions has a ΔG° that is equal to sum of the ΔG° for the two half reactions: $\Delta G^\circ = [-14.8 \text{ kcal/mol} + 7.3 \text{ kcal/mol}] = -7.5 \text{ kcal/mol}$.

2. The answer is C.

Fructose-1,6-bisphosphate does not have bonds with sufficient energy to drive the synthesis of ATP. In contrast, the large negative ΔG° for the hydrolysis of phosphate groups from phosphoenolpyruvate (-14.8 kcal/mol), creatine phosphate (-10.3 kcal/mol), and position 1 of 1,3-bisphosphoglycerate (-11.8 kcal/mol) provides more than enough energy required for synthesis of ATP ($+7.3$ kcal/mol). Similarly, the hydrolysis of the thioester bond that links CoA to succinate releases sufficient energy to drive the synthesis of GTP. The hydrolysis of succinyl CoA is coupled with the condensation of GDP and P_i to form GTP.

3. The answer is B.

NAD^+, a coenzyme derived from niacin, is used by many enzymes in oxidative reactions in catabolism. In contrast, NADPH is the major coenzyme involved in reductive reactions in biosynthetic pathways. NAD^+ accepts a hydride ion (two electrons and one proton) from substrates, resulting in the production of NADH. An additional proton is released from the substrate into solution. Most of the NAD^+ and NADH in the cell is concentrated in the mitochondria. The inner mitochondrial membrane is impermeable to both the oxidized and reduced forms of this coenzyme, and special shuttle systems are required to transfer the electrons in cytosolic NADH to electron carriers in the mitochondrial matrix.

4. The answer is A.

The oxidation of 1 mol of acetyl CoA by the TCA cycle results in 2 mols of CO_2, 1 mol of GTP (which is readily converted to ATP by nucleoside-diphosphokinase), 3 mols of NADH, and 1 mol of $FADH_2$. The oxidation of 1 mol of NADH by the electron transport chain releases enough energy to support the synthesis of 3 mols of ATP, whereas the oxidation of one mol of $FADH_2$ supports the synthesis of 2 mols of ATP.

5. The answer is B.

Isocitrate dehydrogenase is the rate-limiting enzyme and the primary site for regulation of the TCA cycle. The cycle is inhibited when the energy state of the cell is high. Isocitrate dehydrogenase is inhibited by ATP and activated by ADP. Secondary sites of regulation are citrate synthase and α-ketoglutarate dehydrogenase; both of these enzymes are inhibited by ATP.

6. The answer is D.

Thiamine pyrophosphate is one of the five coenzymes required for the oxidative decarboxylation of α-ketoglutarate, a reaction catalyzed by α-ketoglutarate dehydrogenase. None of the other vitamins listed are precursors for coenzymes that are used in the TCA cycle.

7. The answer is A.

All of the atoms in heme are derived from succinyl CoA and glycine. Succinyl CoA is formed by the oxidative decarboxylation of α-ketoglutarate, a reaction catalyzed by α-ketoglutarate dehydrogenase.

8. The answer is C.

Intermediates that are removed from the TCA cycle for use in biosynthetic pathways are replenished primarily by the action of pyruvate carboxylase, which catalyzes the carboxylation of pyruvate to oxaloacetate.

9. The answer is B.

Rotenone binds to complex I of the electron transport chain and inhibits the transfer of electrons from complex I to CoQ. Because complex I oxidizes NADH, the oxidation of NADH or any substrate that results in NADH production will be inhibited by rotenone. The oxidation of pyruvate, glutamate, and β-hydroxybutyrate all produce NADH. In contrast, the oxidation of succinate is independent of complex I. Oxidation of succinate produces $FADH_2$, which feeds electrons into the electron chain at CoQ, thereby bypassing complex I.

10. The answer is C.

The chemiosmotic coupling hypothesis proposes that the energy released by the transfer of electrons through the electron transport chain is used to pump protons from the matrix into the inner membrane space, thereby creating a proton gradient. Complexes I, III, and IV all act as proton pumps, creating the proton gradient. The movement of protons back into the matrix occurs through a proton channel in the inner mitochondrial membrane that is created by the F_o subunit of mitochondrial ATP synthase. The movement of protons through the F_o channel into the matrix releases energy that is used by the F_1 subunit of ATP synthase to drive the synthesis of ATP.

11. The answer is B.

The conversion of fat to carbohydrate is a nonpermitted transition. The synthesis of carbohydrate requires C_3 intermediates. Acetyl CoA, a C_2 compound, cannot be converted back to pyruvate or any other C_3 compound by human tissues. The reaction that converts pyruvate to acetyl CoA is an irreversible reaction, and there is no other enzyme in human tissues that will circumvent the irreversible reaction catalyzed by pyruvate dehydrogenase.

12. The answer is D.

The tricarboxylic acid cycle has both anabolic and catabolic functions, making it an amphibolic pathway. Glycolysis and β-oxidation of fatty acids are catabolic pathways, whereas gluconeogenesis and fatty acid synthesis are anabolic pathways.

Questions 13–16. The answers are 13-B, 14-A, 15-C, 16-C.

Adenylate kinase is found in the inner membrane space where it catalyzes the reversible formation of ATP and AMP from 2 mols of ADP. Porin is a protein found in the outer mitochondrial membrane, where it aggregates to form large pores that allow most molecules having a molecular of less than 10 kD to pass freely from the cytosol into the inner membrane space. Both ATP synthase (sometimes called complex V) and succinate dehydrogenase (also known as complex II) are located in the inner mitochondrial membrane. Succinate dehydrogenase is the only enzyme in the TCA cycle that is not located in the mitochondrial matrix.

Questions 17–18. The answers are 17-C, 18-A.

Oligomycin binds to the F_o subunit of ATP synthase and prevents the movement of protons through the proton channel. Aspirin uncouples oxidation and phosphorylation, accounting for the observation that aspirin overdose is accompanied by a fever.

PART III
Carbohydrate Metabolism

22

Digestion and Absorption of Carbohydrates

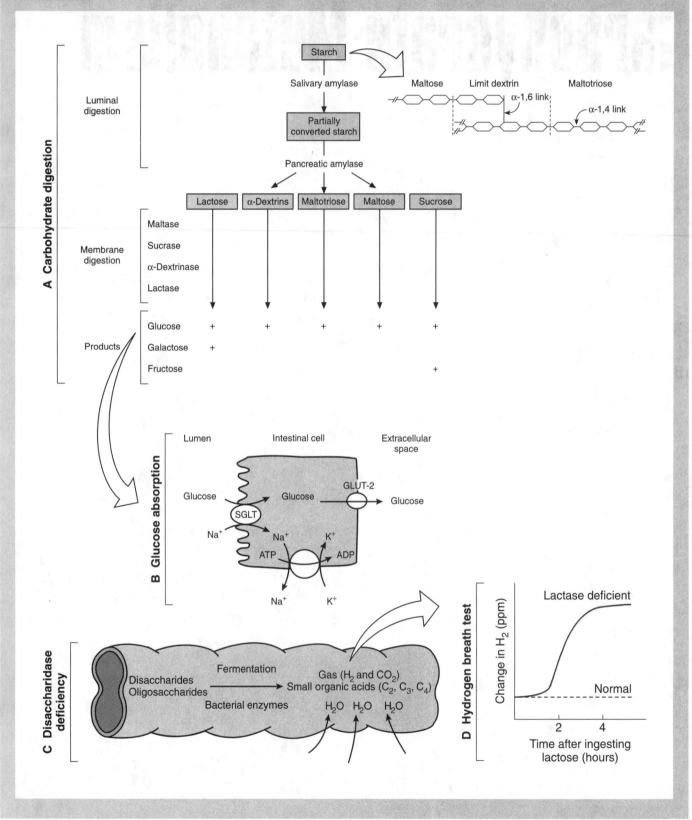

A Carbohydrate digestion

Luminal digestion

Starch

Salivary amylase

Partially converted starch

Pancreatic amylase

Maltose   Limit dextrin   Maltotriose
α-1,6 link   α-1,4 link

Lactose | α-Dextrins | Maltotriose | Maltose | Sucrose

Membrane digestion

Maltase
Sucrase
α-Dextrinase
Lactase

Products

	Lactose	α-Dextrins	Maltotriose	Maltose	Sucrose
Glucose	+	+	+	+	+
Galactose	+				
Fructose					+

B Glucose absorption

Lumen   Intestinal cell   Extracellular space

Glucose   Glucose   GLUT-2   Glucose

SGLT

Na⁺   Na⁺   K⁺

ATP   ADP

Na⁺   K⁺

C Disaccharidase deficiency

Disaccharides Oligosaccharides

Fermentation → Gas (H_2 and CO_2) Small organic acids (C_2, C_3, C_4)

Bacterial enzymes H_2O H_2O H_2O

D Hydrogen breath test

Lactase deficient

Normal

Change in H_2 (ppm)

Time after ingesting lactose (hours)

2   4

Currently accepted dietary guidelines recommend that 55% of calories come from carbohydrate. The source and approximate amount of carbohydrate in most diets are starch (60%), sucrose (30%), and lactose (5%). The sites of carbohydrate digestion are the mouth and small intestine, and the enzymes involved are located both in the lumen of the gastrointestinal tract and in the intestinal brush border membrane. The end products of carbohydrate digestion are glucose (80%), fructose (15%), and galactose (5%). Absorption of glucose requires a family of structurally related proteins, the GLUT transporters, which differ from one another in their tissue specificity and kinetic properties. Glucose and galactose are transported by the same proteins.

Carbohydrate Digestion

Starches are **complex carbohydrates**, consisting of hundreds of glucose residues linked together, forming branched polymers (**Part A**). The glucose residues are linked by **α-1,4 glycosidic bonds**, and branch points are created by **α-1,6 glycosidic bonds**. Digestion of carbohydrate occurs in two phases, the luminal and membrane phases. The luminal phase involves hydrolysis of α-1,4 glycosidic bonds. It starts in the mouth where **salivary α-amylase** randomly cleaves internal α-1,4 glycosidic bonds, producing oligosaccharides with an average chain length of 8 to 10 glucose residues. No significant digestion of carbohydrate occurs in the stomach. In the intestinal lumen, **pancreatic α-amylase** hydrolyzes α-1,4 glycosidic bonds in the oligosaccharides, producing a mixture of disaccharides (maltose), trisaccharides (maltotriose), and limit dextrins (small oligosaccharides, containing all of the original α-1,6 branch points). These products, together with sucrose and lactose (dietary disaccharides) are degraded to monosaccharides by enzymes in the **brush border membrane**. The α-1,6 bonds of dextrins are hydrolyzed by **α-dextrinase**. Maltose, sucrose, and lactose are hydrolyzed to monosaccharides by a family of disaccharidases, including **maltase, sucrase**, and **lactase**.

Absorption of Monosaccharides

Monosaccharides are absorbed from the small intestine into the portal blood (**Part B**). Absorption across intestinal epithelial cells involves **active transport** across the apical membrane into the cell and **facilitated diffusion** across the basolateral membrane into the extracellular space. Glucose moves from a lower to a higher concentration as it crosses the apical membrane. The transporter, **SGLUT**, cotransports Na^+ and glucose in the same direction. The energy for transporting glucose against a concentration gradient is provided by the movement of Na^+ down a concentration gradient. The Na^+ gradient is maintained by **Na^+/K^+ ATPase**, which pumps Na^+ out of the cell in exchange for K^+. Inhibitors of Na^+/K^+ ATPase, such as oubain, also inhibit the transport of glucose into intestinal cells. Glucose moves from a higher to a lower concentration as it is transported across the basolateral membrane, a process that is facilitated by the **GLUT-2** transporter. All cells contain GLUT transporters in their plasma membranes. Liver contains GLUT-2, which has a high K_m and is never saturated under physiologic conditions. Muscle and adipose tissue contain **GLUT-4**, an insulin-sensitive transporter. Excess GLUT-4 transporters are stored in the Golgi of these tissues. Binding of insulin to cell surface receptors results in translocation of GLUT-4 from the Golgi to the plasma membrane, thereby increasing the rate of glucose uptake by muscle and adipose tissue. Brain and red blood cells are rich in **GLUT-1**, which has a low K_m for glucose and is normally saturated, ensuring a constant supply of glucose to these tissues.

Disaccharidase Deficiency

Genetic deficiencies have been described for most of the disaccharidases, and the symptoms are similar in all cases (**Part C**). **Lactase deficiency** is the most common, with the frequency varying widely among different age and ethnic groups. It can also occur secondary to gastroenteritis or other diseases that damage the intestinal mucosa. Lactase is more sensitive to mucosal damage than maltase or sucrase. Normally, disaccharides are not absorbed, but when the mucosa is damaged some of the lactose may be absorbed and excreted in the urine. Undigested lactose is fermented by bacterial enzymes in the intestine, resulting in H_2, CO_2, and a mixture of acetic, propionic, and butyric acids. The accumulation of H_2 and CO_2 results in abdominal pain and flatulence. The small organic acids are osmotically active, and H_2O moves from the extracellular space into the lumen, resulting in diarrhea and dehydration. These symptoms disappear after eliminating milk and milk products from the diet.

The Hydrogen Breath Test

The least invasive and most reliable method for diagnosing lactase deficiency is the hydrogen breath test (**Part D**). This test measures H_2 gas in expired air following oral administration of a "lactose cocktail." The H_2 breath test can also be used to diagnose other disaccharidase deficiencies following ingestion of the appropriate "disaccharide cocktail."

Clinical Significance

Carbohydrates provide the most important source of energy for the body. Restriction of carbohydrate in the diet to less than about 0.5 g/kg body weight per day is likely to result in excessive breakdown of muscle protein, ketosis, cation depletion, and dehydration. Any condition that results in impaired digestion or absorption may result in bacterial fermentation in the large intestine, producing symptoms similar to those previously described for lactase deficiency.

For more information see Coffee C, *Metabolism*. Fence Creek, pp 141–150.

Effects of Insulin on Blood Glucose

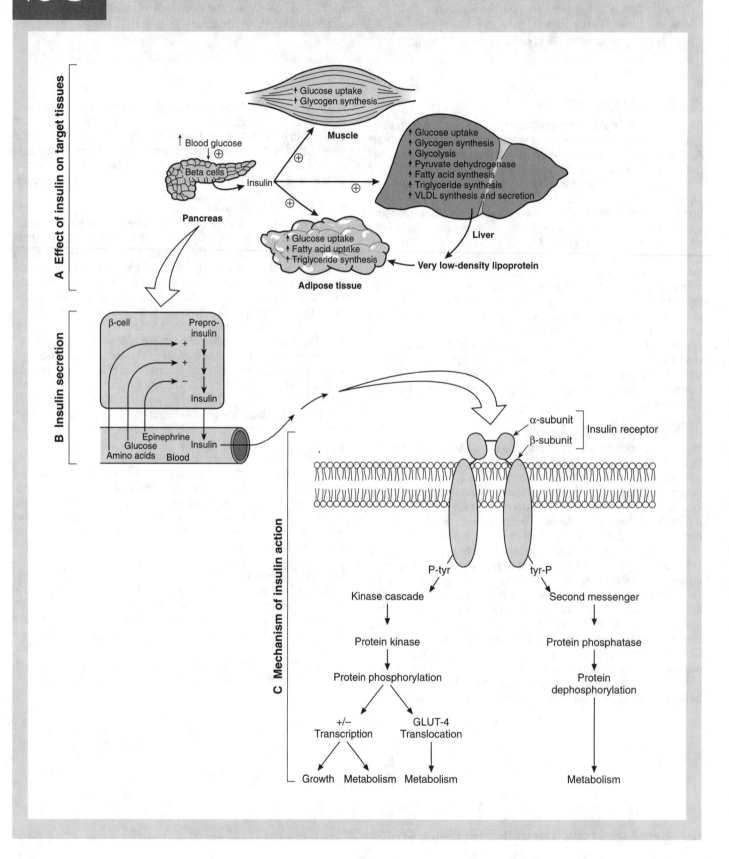

A Effect of insulin on target tissues

↑ Glucose uptake
↑ Glycogen synthesis

Muscle

↑ Blood glucose ⊕

Beta cells

Insulin

⊕

⊕

Pancreas

↑ Glucose uptake
↑ Glycogen synthesis
↑ Glycolysis
↑ Pyruvate dehydrogenase
↑ Fatty acid synthesis
↑ Triglyceride synthesis
↑ VLDL synthesis and secretion

Liver

↑ Glucose uptake
↑ Fatty acid uptake
↑ Triglyceride synthesis

Very low-density lipoprotein

Adipose tissue

B Insulin secretion

β-cell   Prepro-insulin

+

+

–

Insulin

Epinephrine
Glucose   Insulin
Amino acids   Blood

C Mechanism of insulin action

α-subunit] Insulin receptor
β-subunit

P-tyr   tyr-P

Kinase cascade   Second messenger

Protein kinase   Protein phosphatase

Protein phosphorylation   Protein dephosphorylation

+/–   GLUT-4
Transcription   Translocation

Growth   Metabolism   Metabolism   Metabolism

Glucose is an obligate fuel for the central nervous system and red blood cells. At rest, the body consumes between 160 and 200 g of glucose per day, with the brain consuming about 120 g per day. The blood is the major vehicle for transporting glucose, and since the body maintains blood glucose within a concentration range of 70 to 110 mg/dL, there must be mechanisms for lowering blood glucose following a meal and for releasing glucose into the blood between meals. The liver is the organ primarily responsible for controlling the concentration of blood glucose. It can rapidly take up and release glucose in response to the concentration of circulating glucose. The two major hormones that regulate blood glucose are insulin and glucagon. The function of insulin is to lower blood glucose.

Effect of Insulin on Target Tissues

Insulin is an **anabolic** hormone that lowers blood glucose and promotes its storage by stimulating the synthesis of glycogen and fatty acids (**Part A**). Following a meal, the digestion and absorption of carbohydrate result in a transient **hyperglycemia** that stimulates the pancreatic β-cells to release insulin. The three primary target tissues for insulin are liver, muscle, and adipose tissue.

Liver

Insulin lowers blood glucose by stimulating three pathways of glucose utilization in liver: **glycogen synthesis, glycolysis**, and **fatty acid synthesis**. After the glycogen stores have been filled, excess glucose is converted to acetyl CoA by glycolysis and the **pyruvate dehydrogenase** reaction. The acetyl CoA is used for fatty acid synthesis. The fatty acids are converted to triglycerides, packaged into very low density lipoproteins (VLDLs), and secreted into the blood.

Muscle

Insulin increases **glucose uptake** by muscle by stimulating **GLUT-4** translocation from the Golgi to the plasma membrane. The glucose is channeled into **glycogen synthesis**. Muscle glycogen is used exclusively by muscle as a source of energy.

Adipose Tissue

Insulin stimulates **glucose uptake** by adipose tissue by increasing the number of **GLUT-4 transporters** in the plasma membrane. Glucose is used primarily for synthesis of **α-glycerol phosphate**, which forms the glycerol backbone of triglyceride. Insulin also stimulates **fatty acids uptake** from both VLDL and chylomicron triglyceride by increasing the amount of **lipoprotein lipase** found in the capillary bed of adipose tissue. The synthesis of adipose lipoprotein lipase is induced by insulin. The coordinate increase in α-glycerol phosphate and fatty acids results in increased triglyceride synthesis.

Insulin Secretion

Proinsulin, the protein precursor of insulin, is synthesized in pancreatic β-cells and converted to insulin by **limited proteolysis (Part B)**. The products of proteolysis, **insulin** and **C-peptide**, are stored in vesicles in β-cells, and released into the blood upon stimulation. The most important stimulus of insulin secretion is **glucose**, although the amino acid **arginine** is also a powerful secretagogue. Insulin secretion is inhibited by **epinephrine**.

Mechanism of Insulin Action

The biologic effects of insulin are initiated by the binding of insulin to cell-surface receptors (**Part C**). The insulin receptor consists of two α-subunits and two β-subunits that are linked by disulfide bonds. The α-subunits form the insulin-binding domain, while the β-subunits span the membrane and have cytosolic domains with intrinsic **tyrosine kinase** activity. Binding of insulin to the receptor activates tyrosine kinase, leading to autophosphorylation and to the phosphorylation of several cellular proteins that transmit the insulin signal to the interior of the cell. Some of the effects of insulin are mediated by cellular protein kinases, while others are mediated by protein phosphatases. Responses mediated by **protein kinases** include the translocation of intracellular stores of GLUT-4 to the plasma membrane, an increase in the rate of transcription of some genes, and a decrease in the rate of transcription of others. The transcriptional effects can stimulate cell growth and alter the metabolism of cells. Insulin induces the synthesis of several enzymes involved in energy storage pathways, a mechanism that involves increased transcription of the genes that encode these enzymes (e.g., hepatic glucokinase, phosphofructokinase, pyruvate kinase, fatty acid synthase). Several metabolic responses to insulin are mediated by **protein phosphatases** and involve **dephosphorylation of key regulatory enzymes in carbohydrate and lipid metabolism**. Dephosphorylation results in **activation** of key enzymes in energy storage pathways (e.g., glycogen, fatty acid, triglyceride synthesis).

Clinical Significance

The importance of insulin in regulating blood glucose levels can be readily appreciated by considering the consequences of having either too little or too much insulin. Diabetes mellitus results from insulin insufficiency. The hallmark of this disease is sustained **hyperglycemia**, due to both overproduction and underutilization of glucose. Persistently elevated glucose results in glycosylation of proteins, which may be related to the pathologic changes in diabetics that develop in insulin-independent tissues such as the lens of the eye, peripheral nerve, and basement membrane of kidneys. Glucose is also reduced to sorbitol by aldol reductase in these tissues. Sorbitol accumulation in the lens causes osmotic damage, leading to cataract formation. Conversely, an elevation in insulin levels results in **hypoglycemia**, a condition arising when blood glucose drops below 40 to 45 mg/dL. The most common cause of hypoglycemia in insulin-dependent diabetics is induced by administration of insulin. It is estimated that patients with insulin-dependent diabetes taking one or two doses of insulin daily will experience approximately one mild episode of hypoglycemia each week.

For more information see Coffee C, *Metabolism*. Fence Creek, pp 129–131, 237–239.

Effects of Glucagon on Blood Glucose

24

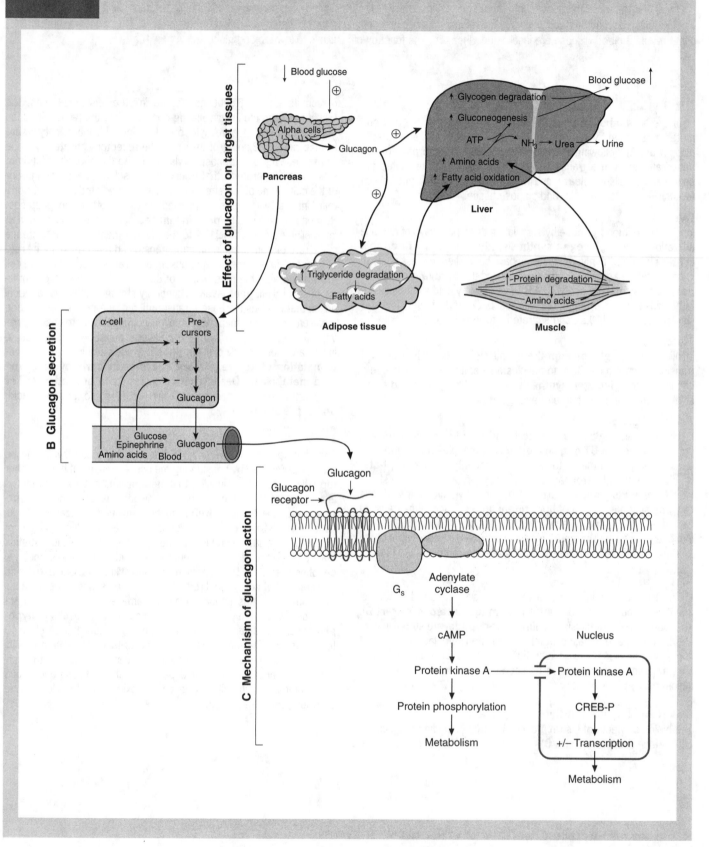

A Effect of glucagon on target tissues

↓ Blood glucose

⊕

Alpha cells

Glucagon

Pancreas

⊕

⊕

↑ Glycogen degradation

↑ Gluconeogenesis

ATP → NH₃ → Urea → Urine

↑ Amino acids

↑ Fatty acid oxidation

Blood glucose ↑

Liver

Triglyceride degradation

Fatty acids

Adipose tissue

↑ Protein degradation

↓ Amino acids

Muscle

B Glucagon secretion

α-cell   Pre-cursors

+

+

−

Glucose
Epinephrine
Amino acids

Glucagon

Glucagon
Blood

C Mechanism of glucagon action

Glucagon

Glucagon receptor →

Gs

Adenylate cyclase

cAMP

Protein kinase A → Protein kinase A

Protein phosphorylation

Metabolism

Nucleus

CREB-P

+/− Transcription

Metabolism

58   III. CARBOHYDRATE METABOLISM

OVERVIEW

The actions of glucagon oppose the actions of insulin. Glucagon is a catabolic hormone that results in mobilization, rather than storage, of fuels. Glucagon is synthesized by pancreatic α-cells and secreted into the blood in response to hypoglycemia. The major target tissues for glucagon are the liver and adipose tissue. Glucagon stimulates the release of glucose from liver by activating the pathways of glycogen degradation and gluconeogenesis. It stimulates the release of fatty acids from adipose tissue. The effects of glucagon are mediated by cAMP-dependent phosphorylation of key enzymes in carbohydrate and lipid metabolism. The opposing roles of insulin and glucagon in glucose homeostasis are often described by the insulin to glucagon ratio. A change in the ratio has two major effects on key regulatory enzymes in pathways of carbohydrate and lipid metabolism: 1) it alters the extent to which these enzymes are phosphorylated or dephosphorylated; and 2) it alters the absolute amount of specific enzymes present in target tissues by regulating the rate at which the corresponding genes are transcribed.

Effect of Glucagon on Target Tissues

The role of glucagon is to respond to hypoglycemia by stimulating the release of glucose into the blood (**Part A**). This response involves metabolic pathways in liver, adipose tissue, and skeletal muscle. Both liver and adipose tissue respond to glucagon, but skeletal muscle does not.

Liver

The most rapid way to increase blood glucose is to stimulate hepatic **glycogen degradation**. A slower, more sustained way is to activate **gluconeogenesis**, the de novo pathway of glucose synthesis. The activation of gluconeogenesis begins before hepatic glycogen stores are completely exhausted. The major precursors for gluconeogenesis are **amino acids** that are derived from muscle protein, and ATP that is derived from fatty acid oxidation. Amino groups are removed from amino acids and incorporated into urea, while the carbon skeletons that remain are incorporated into glucose.

Adipose Tissue

The role of adipose tissue in combating hypoglycemia is to supply the liver with fatty acids that can be oxidized to generate ATP for driving gluconeogenesis. The binding of glucagon to receptors on fat cells stimulates **triglyceride degradation**, resulting in release of fatty acids into the blood. Fatty acids are transported by albumin to the liver.

Skeletal Muscle

The major source of carbon for gluconeogenesis comes from amino acids that are derived from the breakdown of muscle protein. Muscle does *not* contain glucagon receptors, although there is an abundance of insulin receptors on the surface of muscle cells. When the insulin receptors are occupied, protein degradation is suppressed. However, when these receptors are unoccupied, protein degradation occurs. Thus, glucagon has no direct effect on the release of amino acids from muscle, although the use of amino acids by liver for glucose synthesis is stimulated by glucagon.

Glucagon Secretion

Glucagon is a small peptide hormone, containing 29 amino acids. It is synthesized by pancreatic α-cells as a larger precursor that is converted to the active hormone by **limited proteolysis (Part B)**. Glucagon is stored in vesicles and released into the blood upon stimulation of α-cells. The primary stimulus for glucagon secretion is a **decrease in blood glucose**. Glucagon secretion is also stimulated by **epinephrine** and a number of amino acids, particularly **alanine** and **arginine**. Secretion of glucagon is inhibited by an elevation in blood glucose and by insulin.

Mechanism of Glucagon Action

The effects of glucagon are initiated when it binds to its receptor (**Part C**). The glucagon receptor, like other receptors that interact with G proteins, spans the plasma membrane 7 times. The binding of glucagon to an extracellular domain induces a conformational change in the receptor, causing it to interact with a **G_s protein** and to activate **adenylate cyclase**. An increase in cellular cAMP activates protein kinase A, which catalyzes the phosphorylation of a specific serine residue in target proteins. All of the cellular effects of glucagon are mediated by **protein phosphorylation**. Key regulatory enzymes in pathways that lead to hepatic glucose release are activated by phosphorylation (e.g., hepatic glycogen phosphorylase, hepatic fructose-2,6-bisphosphatase, and hormone-sensitive lipase in adipose tissue). Glucagon also stimulates the synthesis of a number of enzymes that, either directly or indirectly, facilitate the release of glucose into the blood. This effect of glucagon on enzyme synthesis occurs in the nucleus and involves transcription of specific genes. Protein kinase A phosphorylates CREB, a protein that binds to a cAMP regulatory element (CRE) in DNA. When CREB-P binds to DNA, the rate of transcription of genes for PEPCK, fructose-1,6-bisphosphatase and glucose-6-phosphatase, is increased. Only the phosphorylated form of CREB will bind to CRE.

Clinical Significance

Hyperglucagonemia is a syndrome resulting from glucagon-secreting tumors of pancreatic α-cells. Circulating glucagon levels are usually between 10- and 100-fold higher than normal. This syndrome is usually diagnosed by the appearance of a characteristic rash in middle-aged patients that have mild diabetes mellitus. The elevated blood glucose levels in these patients results from increased glucose output by the liver due to high glucagon levels. Insulin levels are also increased secondary to elevated blood glucose. The diabetes is mild and is not accompanied by ketosis. There is sufficient insulin to suppress fatty acid release from adipose tissue. The rash in these patients progresses to lesions on the face, abdomen, and lower extremities. The lesions crust over and then resolve, leaving areas of marked hyperpigmentation.

For more information see Coffee C, *Metabolism*. Fence Creek, pp 130–132, 237–240.

25 Glycolysis

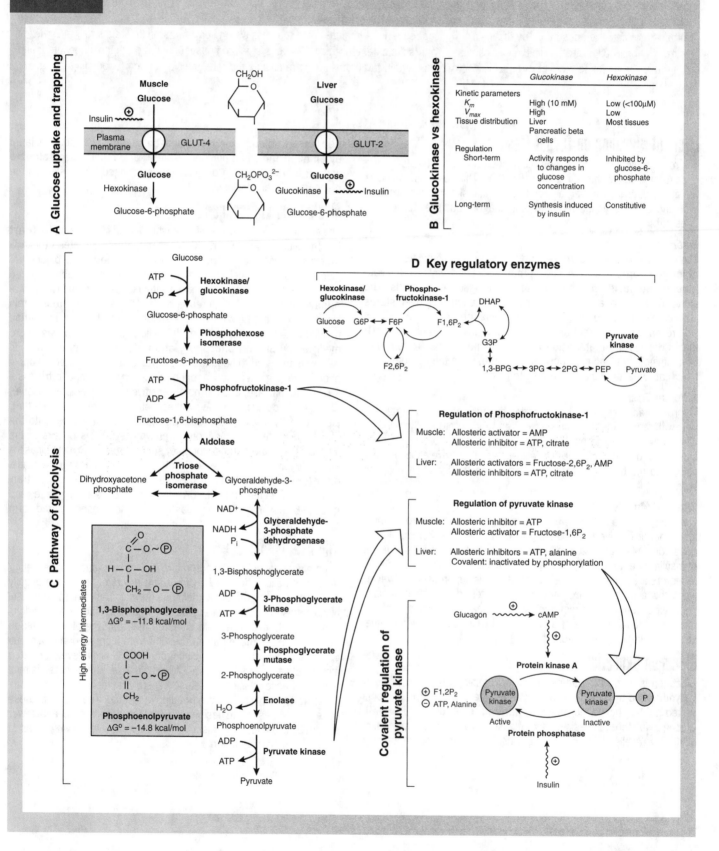

A Glucose uptake and trapping

Muscle
Glucose
Insulin ⊕
Plasma membrane | GLUT-4
Glucose
Hexokinase
Glucose-6-phosphate

Liver
Glucose
Plasma membrane | GLUT-2
Glucose
Glucokinase ⊕ Insulin
Glucose-6-phosphate

CH_2OH
O

$CH_2OPO_3^{2-}$
O

B Glucokinase vs hexokinase

	Glucokinase	Hexokinase
Kinetic parameters		
K_m	High (10 mM)	Low (<100µM)
V_{max}	High	Low
Tissue distribution	Liver Pancreatic beta cells	Most tissues
Regulation		
Short-term	Activity responds to changes in glucose concentration	Inhibited by glucose-6-phosphate
Long-term	Synthesis induced by insulin	Constitutive

C Pathway of glycolysis

Glucose
ATP
ADP
Hexokinase/ glucokinase
Glucose-6-phosphate
Phosphohexose isomerase
Fructose-6-phosphate
ATP
ADP
Phosphofructokinase-1
Fructose-1,6-bisphosphate
Aldolase
Dihydroxyacetone phosphate
Triose phosphate isomerase
Glyceraldehyde-3-phosphate
NAD^+
NADH
P_i
Glyceraldehyde-3-phosphate dehydrogenase
1,3-Bisphosphoglycerate
ADP
ATP
3-Phosphoglycerate kinase
3-Phosphoglycerate
Phosphoglycerate mutase
2-Phosphoglycerate
H_2O
Enolase
Phosphoenolpyruvate
ADP
ATP
Pyruvate kinase
Pyruvate

High energy intermediates

C=O~℗
H—C—OH
CH_2—O—℗
1,3-Bisphosphoglycerate
$\Delta G^0 = -11.8$ kcal/mol

COOH
C—O~℗
CH_2
Phosphoenolpyruvate
$\Delta G^0 = -14.8$ kcal/mol

D Key regulatory enzymes

Hexokinase/ glucokinase
Glucose ⇄ G6P ⇄ F6P
Phospho-fructokinase-1
F6P ⇄ F1,6P₂
$F2,6P_2$
DHAP
G3P
1,3-BPG ⇄ 3PG ⇄ 2PG ⇄ PEP
Pyruvate kinase
Pyruvate

Regulation of Phosphofructokinase-1

Muscle: Allosteric activator = AMP
Allosteric inhibitor = ATP, citrate

Liver: Allosteric activators = Fructose-2,6P₂, AMP
Allosteric inhibitors = ATP, citrate

Regulation of pyruvate kinase

Muscle: Allosteric inhibitor = ATP
Allosteric activator = Fructose-1,6P₂

Liver: Allosteric inhibitors = ATP, alanine
Covalent: inactivated by phosphorylation

Covalent regulation of pyruvate kinase

Glucagon ⇝ ⊕ ⇝ cAMP
⊕
Protein kinase A
⊕ F1,2P₂
⊖ ATP, Alanine
Pyruvate kinase (Active)
Pyruvate kinase (Inactive) — P
Protein phosphatase
⊕
Insulin

OVERVIEW

Glycolysis is the central pathway of carbohydrate metabolism, occurring in the cytosol of all cells. Under aerobic conditions, glycolysis converts 1 mol of glucose to 2 mols each of pyruvate, ATP, and NADH. Under anaerobic conditions, 2 mols each of lactate and ATP are formed. Three steps in glycolysis are irreversible: the rate-limiting step, catalyzed by phosphofructokinase-1 (PFK-1); the first step, catalyzed by glucokinase or hexokinase; and the last step, catalyzed by pyruvate kinase. These enzymes are also sites of regulation. The primary role of glycolysis varies in different tissues. RBCs have no mitochondria and depend entirely on glycolysis for ATP synthesis. Skeletal muscle generates ATP by oxidizing a variety of fuels, although glycolysis becomes the primary pathway of ATP synthesis when oxygen is limiting. Liver derives most of its ATP from oxidation of noncarbohydrate fuels. The role of hepatic glycolysis depends on the nutritional state. In the well-fed state, glycolysis is a part of the pathway for converting excess glucose to fatty acids for storage. In the fasting state, the reversible steps in glycolysis are used in the pathway of gluconeogenesis.

Glucose Uptake and Trapping

The entry of glucose into cells is mediated by tissue-specific **GLUT transporters (Part A)**. Inside the cell, glucose is converted to glucose-6-phosphate (G6P) by **glucokinase** or **hexokinase**, effectively trapping glucose in the cell. The conversion of glucose to G6P in both muscle and liver is enhanced by insulin, although the mechanism is different. In muscle, insulin increases the number of GLUT-4 transporters in the plasma membrane, whereas in liver the synthesis of glucokinase is induced by insulin.

Comparison of Glucokinase and Hexokinase

Glucokinase is found only in liver and pancreatic β-cells, while hexokinase is found in all cells **(Part B)**. The most significant differences in these isozymes are their kinetic properties. The high K_m and V_{max} of **glucokinase** allow the liver to function as an effective buffer of blood glucose. The K_m of glucokinase (10 mM) and GLUT-2 are approximately equal, thereby ensuring that glucose uptake is never saturated under physiologic conditions. Glucokinase and hexokinase are also regulated differently.

Pathway of Glycolysis

Glycolysis consists of ten sequential reactions that convert glucose to pyruvate **(Part C)**. All intermediates between glucose and pyruvate are phosphorylated, thereby ensuring they do not leave the cell. The **first stage** of glycolysis **requires ATP**. Glucose, a C_6 substrate, is converted to two C_3 intermediates, dihydroxyacetone phosphate (DHAP) and glyceraldehyde-3-phosphate (G3P). This sequence of reactions requires 2 mols of ATP per mol of glucose. G3P and DHAP are interconvertible, and both can be metabolized by a common pathway. The **second stage** of glycolysis results in **ATP synthesis**. The sequence of reactions that convert G3P to pyruvate produce 2 mols of ATP and 1 mol of NADH per mol of G3P. The only oxidation step in the pathway is catalyzed by G3P dehydrogenase, which converts G3P to 1,3-bisphosphoglycerate (1,3-BPG), producing NADH.

High-Energy Intermediates and ATP Synthesis

Two intermediates in glycolysis, **1,3-BPG** and **phosphoenolpyruvate (PEP)** have high-energy phosphate bonds that are used for ATP synthesis. **3-Phosphoglycerate kinase** and **pyruvate kinase** cat-alyze the transfer of P_i from 1,3-BPG and PEP, respectively, to ADP, forming ATP. The ΔG° for hydrolysis of the high-energy phosphate bond in 1,3-BPG and PEP are -11.8 kcal/mol and -14.8 kcal/mol, respectively, while the ΔG° for the synthesis of ATP from ADP and P_i is $+7.3$ kcal/mol. Although two ATPs per glucose are consumed in the first stage of glycolysis, four ATPs are produced in the second stage, giving a **net yield of two ATPs per glucose**.

Key Regulatory Enzymes

The primary target of regulation in glycolysis is **PFK-1**, which catalyzes the rate-limiting reaction in the pathway **(Part D)**. Allosteric inhibitors and activators increase and decrease the K_m for fructose-6-phosphate (F6P), respectively. Tissue-specific differences in the allosteric effectors reflect different functions of glycolysis in various tissues. In tissues where ATP synthesis is the major function, PFK-1 is **inhibited by ATP** and **activated by AMP**, compounds that are indicators of the energy state of the cell. In liver, the most important activator of PFK-1 is fructose-2,6-bisphosphate ($F2,6P_2$), a specialized compound that controls the flux between the opposing pathways of glycolysis and gluconeogenesis. **$F2,6P_2$ is an intracellular indicator of blood glucose levels**. When blood glucose is high, $F2,6P_2$ is high; when blood glucose is low, $F2,6P_2$ is low. The synthesis of $F2,6P_2$ is stimulated by insulin, and its degradation is stimulated by glucagon. The precursor for $F2,6P_2$ is F6P, an intermediate in glycolysis. **Pyruvate kinase**, another target of regulation, is controlled differently in muscle and liver. It is allosterically activated by $F1,6P_2$ and inhibited by ATP in muscle. In liver, it is regulated both covalently and allosterically. Covalent regulation involves phosphorylation and dephosphorylation, which is mediated by glucagon and insulin, respectively. The phosphorylated form of pyruvate kinase is inactive. ATP and alanine are allosteric inhibitors of the active form of the enzyme.

Clinical Significance

A deficiency in any enzyme in glycolysis can lead to **hemolytic anemia**, although the most common deficiency is in **pyruvate kinase**. The RBC depends on glycolysis for all its ATP, and most of it is used to maintain the integrity of the plasma membrane. Therefore, any condition that compromises ATP synthesis can lead to cell lysis.

For more information see Coffee C, *Metabolism*. Fence Creek, pp 155–163, 233–240.

26 Metabolic Fate of Pyruvate

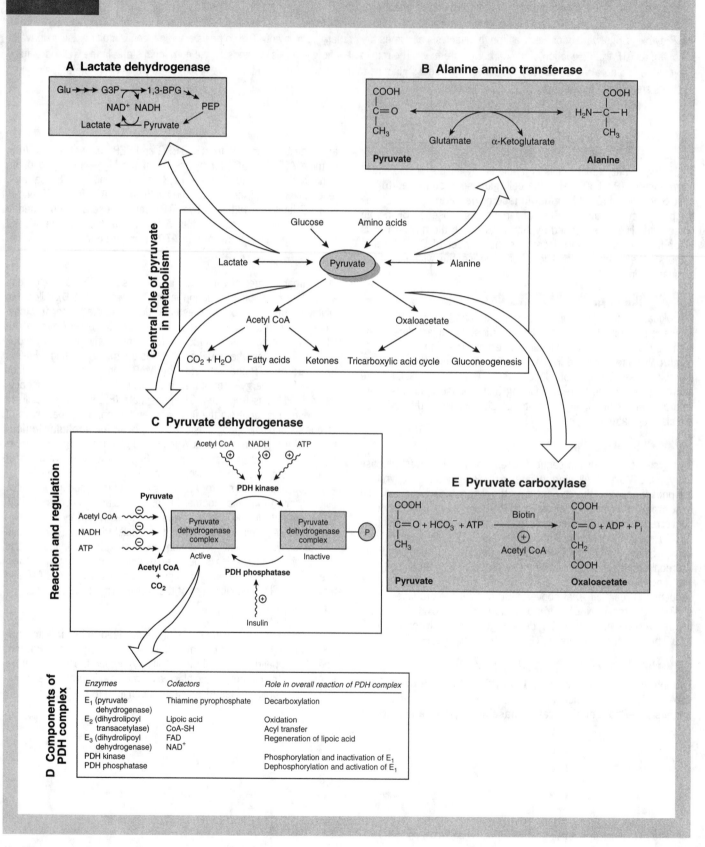

A Lactate dehydrogenase

Glu $\longrightarrow$ G3P $\rightleftharpoons$ 1,3-BPG $\longrightarrow$ PEP

NAD$^+$ NADH

Lactate $\longleftarrow$ Pyruvate

B Alanine amino transferase

Pyruvate $\longleftrightarrow$ Alanine

Glutamate α-Ketoglutarate

Central role of pyruvate in metabolism

Glucose   Amino acids

Lactate $\longleftrightarrow$ Pyruvate $\longleftrightarrow$ Alanine

Acetyl CoA   Oxaloacetate

$CO_2 + H_2O$ Fatty acids   Ketones   Tricarboxylic acid cycle   Gluconeogenesis

C Pyruvate dehydrogenase

Reaction and regulation

Acetyl CoA   NADH   ATP

PDH kinase

Pyruvate

Acetyl CoA ⊖
NADH ⊖
ATP ⊖

Pyruvate dehydrogenase complex → Pyruvate dehydrogenase complex — P

Active   Inactive

Acetyl CoA + CO_2

PDH phosphatase

Insulin

E Pyruvate carboxylase

$C=O + HCO_3^- + ATP \xrightarrow[\text{Acetyl CoA}]{\text{Biotin}} C=O + ADP + P_i$

Pyruvate   Oxaloacetate

D Components of PDH complex

Enzymes	Cofactors	Role in overall reaction of PDH complex
E$_1$ (pyruvate dehydrogenase)	Thiamine pyrophosphate	Decarboxylation
E$_2$ (dihydrolipoyl transacetylase)	Lipoic acid CoA-SH	Oxidation Acyl transfer
E$_3$ (dihydrolipoyl dehydrogenase)	FAD NAD$^+$	Regeneration of lipoic acid
PDH kinase		Phosphorylation and inactivation of E$_1$
PDH phosphatase		Dephosphorylation and activation of E$_1$

OVERVIEW

Pyruvate plays a central role in metabolism, occurring at a major crossroad of carbohydrate, lipid, and protein metabolism. Pyruvate can be converted to four products: lactate, alanine, acetyl CoA, and oxaloacetate. Lactate and alanine are produced in reactions that occur in the **cytosol** of most cells. Since both of these reactions are **reversible**, any condition that leads to elevated pyruvate will lead to an increase in blood lactate; and, in some cases, alanine will also be elevated. The conversion of pyruvate to acetyl CoA and oxaloacetate are **irreversible** reactions that occur in the **mitochondria**, and the enzymes catalyzing these reactions are highly regulated. Acetyl CoA is used either to generate energy (via oxidation by the tricarboxylic acid [TCA] cycle) or to store energy (via fatty acid or ketone synthesis). Oxaloacetate is used either as a substrate for gluconeogenesis or to replenish intermediates in the TCA cycle.

Lactate Dehydrogenase

The NADH-dependent reduction of pyruvate to lactate occurs only under **anaerobic** conditions (**Part A**). Most of the lactate found in blood is produced by rapidly contracting **skeletal muscle** and **red blood cells**, which are dependent on glycolysis for ATP synthesis. The reaction in glycolysis that converts glyceraldehyde-3-phosphate (G3P) to 1,3-bisphosphoglycerate (1,3-BPG) requires NAD^+ and produces NADH. Under anaerobic conditions, NADH cannot be converted back to NAD^+ by the electron transport chain. Therefore, NAD^+ regeneration is accomplished by the reduction of pyruvate to lactate, a reaction that allows glycolysis (and ATP synthesis) to continue. The reverse of the lactate dehydrogenase (LDH) reaction is the only metabolic option for lactate in human tissues. Most of the circulating lactate is taken up by liver and cardiac muscle. Liver uses the lactate as a **substrate for gluconeogenesis**, whereas cardiac muscle oxidizes it to CO_2 and H_2O. The properties of LDH isozymes differ significantly in skeletal muscle and cardiac muscle. The properties of the major skeletal muscle isozyme (M_4) favor the reduction of pyruvate to lactate, while the properties of the major cardiac muscle isozyme (H_4) favor the oxidation of lactate to pyruvate.

Alanine Aminotransferase

The reversible conversion of pyruvate to alanine is catalyzed by alanine aminotransferase (ALT) (**Part B**). The carbon skeletons of pyruvate and alanine differ only by the presence of an amino group at C-2 of alanine rather than the carbonyl group found at C-2 of pyruvate. Glutamate is the amino donor, producing alanine and α-ketoglutarate. This reaction operates in the direction of **alanine synthesis in skeletal muscle** and in the direction of **pyruvate synthesis in liver**. Alanine acts as a carrier of amino groups from skeletal muscle to liver, where they can be removed and incorporated into urea. The pyruvate resulting from transamination of alanine in liver can be used for gluconeogenesis. Different isozymes of ALT are found in skeletal muscle and liver. Differences in the isozyme properties allow the reaction to operate in opposite directions in the two tissues. A defect in any of the pathways of pyruvate utilization may lead to the accumulation of alanine in the blood. Similarly, conditions that lead to glutamate accumulation also shift the equilibrium from pyruvate toward alanine synthesis.

Pyruvate Dehydrogenase

The conversion of pyruvate to acetyl CoA and CO_2 is catalyzed by pyruvate dehydrogenase (PDH), a multienzyme complex found in mitochondria (**Part C**). This reaction links glycolysis with both the TCA cycle and fatty acid synthesis. PDH activity is **stringently regulated** because carbon that passes through this reaction can no longer be used for glucose synthesis. ATP, acetyl CoA, and NADH, compounds that indicate a high-energy state, are **allosteric inhibitors** of PDH. PDH is also subject to inactivation by **phosphorylation**. PDH kinase, which catalyzes the phosphorylation of PDH, is activated by ATP, NADH, and acetyl CoA. The dephosphorylation of PDH, catalyzed by PDH phosphatase, is stimulated by insulin. **Components of the PDH multienzyme complex** include three enzymes and five coenzymes (**Part D**): E_1 requires thiamine pyrophosphate; E_2 requires lipoic acid and CoA; and E_3 requires FAD and NAD^+. PDH kinase and phosphatase are also a part of the multienzyme complex. The mitochondrial enzymes, α-ketoglutarate dehydrogenase and branched-chain ketoacid dehydrogenase, are similar to PDH in both structure and function. They catalyze the oxidative decarboxylation of α-ketoacids, and are multienzyme complexes having E_1, E_2, and E_3 subunits that require the same five coenzymes as PDH. E_3 is identical in all three multienzyme complexes and is encoded by the same gene, whereas E_1 and E_2 are different in each complex.

Pyruvate Carboxylase

The carboxylation of pyruvate to oxaloacetate (**Part E**) has two major functions: 1) it is the primary reaction for **replenishing intermediates in the TCA cycle**; and 2) it is the **first step in gluconeogenesis**. Pyruvate carboxylase is located in the mitochondrial matrix and has an absolute requirement for acetyl CoA as an allosteric activator. Biotin is required as a transient carrier of carboxyl groups.

Clinical Significance

Lactic acidosis occurs when the metabolism of pyruvate is blocked. It is characterized by a decrease in the pH of arterial blood and an increase in circulating lactate levels to a concentration greater than 5 mM. The most common cause of lactic acidosis is tissue hypoxia, resulting from a decrease in tissue perfusion. Lactic acidosis is also associated with several enzyme deficiencies, including PDH, pyruvate carboxylase, and glucose-6-phosphatase.

For more information see Coffee C, *Metabolism*. Fence Creek, pp 163–167, 235–240.

27 Glycogen Metabolism

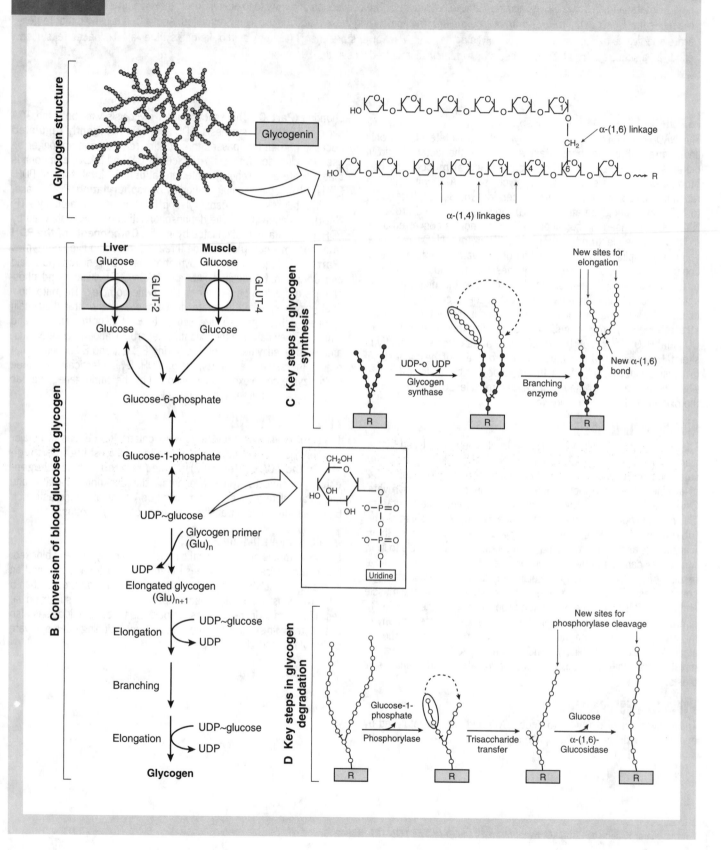

A Glycogen structure

Glycogenin

α-(1,6) linkage

α-(1,4) linkages

B Conversion of blood glucose to glycogen

Liver
Glucose
GLUT-2
Glucose

Muscle
Glucose
GLUT-4
Glucose

Glucose-6-phosphate

Glucose-1-phosphate

UDP~glucose

Glycogen primer (Glu)$_n$

UDP

Elongated glycogen (Glu)$_{n+1}$

Elongation — UDP~glucose → UDP

Branching

Elongation — UDP~glucose → UDP

Glycogen

CH_2OH

Uridine

C Key steps in glycogen synthesis

UDP-o UDP
Glycogen synthase

New sites for elongation

Branching enzyme

New α-(1,6) bond

R

D Key steps in glycogen degradation

Glucose-1-phosphate
Phosphorylase

Trisaccharide transfer

New sites for phosphorylase cleavage

Glucose
α-(1,6)-Glucosidase

R

OVERVIEW

Glycogen is the storage form of glucose in mammalian tissues. Although present in the cytoplasm of almost all tissues, it is most abundant in liver and muscle. The concentration of glycogen is greater in liver than in muscle. However, because muscle constitutes a larger mass, its total capacity for storage is 3 to 4 times that of liver. The functional role of glycogen is different in these two tissues. In muscle, glycogen acts as a store of glucose that can be rapidly mobilized to provide energy for muscle contraction. In liver, glycogen is important in buffering blood glucose levels. The synthesis and degradation of glycogen occur via different pathways, thereby allowing each pathway to be regulated independently of the other. All of the enzymes and regulatory proteins required for glycogen synthesis and degradation are associated with the glycogen particles.

Glycogen Structure

Glycogen is a **highly branched** polymer of glucose, with branching occurring at an average frequency of every ten glucose residues (**Part A**). Branching increases the solubility of glycogen, and it also increases the rate at which glucose can be stored and mobilized from glycogen. Each glycogen particle has a protein, **glycogenin**, that is covalently linked to the polysaccharide. Glucose residues are linked together by α-1,4 **glycosidic bonds**, forming linear chains, and at every branch point two glucose residues are linked together by α-1,6 **glycosidic bonds**. Glycogen is stored in muscle as granules, known as β-**particles**, that contain up to 60,000 glucose residues. Liver contains **large rosette-like granules** that are aggregates of β-particles.

Conversion of Blood Glucose to Glycogen

Following a meal, both liver and muscle convert blood glucose to glycogen (**Part B**). Glucose is transported into the cells by tissue-specific GLUT transporters, where glucose is converted to glucose-6-phosphate (G6P) by **glucokinase** in liver and **hexokinase** in muscle and other tissues. The conversion of G6P to glucose-1-phosphate (G1P) commits glucose to the pathway of glycogen synthesis. G6P and G1P are readily interconvertible by **phosphoglucomutase**. In order to add glucose onto the end of a glycogen chain, G1P has to be **activated**. Reaction of G1P with UTP produces **UDP-glucose**, which serves as a high-energy carrier of glucose in many types of transfer reactions. Cleavage of the bond between C-1 of glucose and UDP provides the energy required for linking one glucose residue to another in glycogen. Glycogen synthesis involves two types of reactions, **elongation** of the linear chains and **formation of branch points**.

The opposing pathway, glycogen degradation, occurs between meals when dietary glucose is unavailable. Glycogen degradation involves two types of reactions, the sequential removal of glucose (as G1P) from the ends of glycogen chains and the disassembly of branch points. Since the phosphoglucomutase reaction is reversible, G1P derived from glycogen degradation is converted to G6P. In muscle, G6P is channeled into glycolysis and oxidized for energy, whereas in liver it is hydrolyzed by **glucose-6-phosphatase (G6Pase)**, releasing free glucose into the blood. G6Pase is not found in muscle, thus explaining why muscle glycogen cannot contribute glucose to blood.

Key Steps in Glycogen Synthesis

The primary reaction in glycogen synthesis is the formation of α-1,4 glycosidic bonds, a reaction catalyzed by **glycogen synthase (Part C)**. In this reaction glucose is transferred from UDP $\sim$ glucose to an acceptor, which is usually a partially degraded glycogen chain. The chains are elongated by repeated addition of glucose. As the chains become longer, glycogen synthase binds less tightly and elongation eventually ceases. The **branching enzyme** transfers an oligosaccharide containing six to seven glucose residues from the end of a chain to a glucose residue in the interior of the chain, creating a new α-1,6 glycosidic bond and three shorter chains that can be elongated by glycogen synthase.

Key Steps in Glycogen Degradation

The primary reaction in glycogen degradation is the cleavage of α-1,4 glycosidic bonds, a reaction catalyzed by **glycogen phosphorylase (Part D)**. This reaction involves the **addition of P_i** rather than H_2O across the α-1,4 bond, resulting in the release of G1P from the end of the chains. This reaction is repeated until the distance from the branch point is four glucose residues, at which time the **debranching enzyme** begins to disassemble the branch points. Debranching occurs in two steps. In the first step, a trisaccharide is transferred from one shortened chain to another, creating a longer chain that can be further degraded by phosphorylase. Trisaccharide transfer also leaves a single glucose residue attached at the branch point in an α-1,6 linkage. In the second step, this glucose is hydrolyzed by α-1,6 **glucosidase**. The only glucose residues in glycogen that are released as free glucose are those at the branch points; all others are released as G1P.

Clinical Significance

Glycogen metabolism in the liver is an important mechanism for avoiding both **hyperglycemia** and **hypoglycemia**. Following a meal, the concentration of glucose in the portal blood can increase to almost twice the fasting level. Normally, this hyperglycemia is transient because the liver is very efficient at removing glucose from the blood and storing it as glycogen. Similarly, **hypoglycemia** can be avoided for several hours of fasting because glucose can be mobilized from liver glycogen and released into the blood.

For more information see Coffee C, *Metabolism*. Fence Creek, pp 173–179, 233–239.

Coordinate Regulation of Glycogen Metabolism

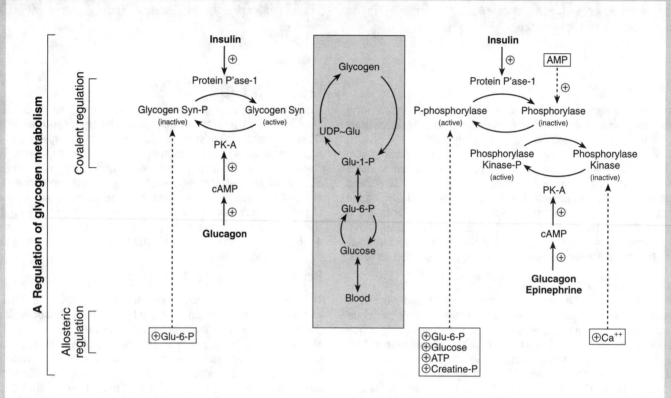

A Regulation of glycogen metabolism

B Avoiding a futile cycle

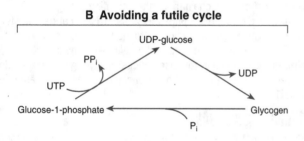

C Conditions affecting glycogen metabolism

	Glycogen synthesis	Glycogen degradation
Well-fed state	Increased	Decreased
Fasting	Decreased	Increased
Hyperglycemia	Increased	Decreased
Hypoglycemia	Decreased	Increased
Elevated		
Insulin	Increased	Decreased
Glucagon	Decreased	Increased
Epinephrine	Decreased	Increased
Cyclic adenosine monophosphate	Decreased	Increased
Enzyme phosphorylation		
Glycogen synthase	Decreased	...
Glycogen phosphorylase	...	Increased

OVERVIEW

The synthesis and degradation of glycogen occur via different pathways. The rate at which the pathways proceed is coordinately regulated by both covalent and allosteric mechanisms. The covalent regulation is under the hormonal control of insulin, glucagon, and epinephrine. In general, factors that promote glycogen synthesis inhibit glycogen degradation, and vice versa. Factors that contribute to the integrated control of these opposing pathways are hormonal signals, cellular cAMP levels, protein kinases, and protein phosphatase-1. Several enzyme deficiencies have been identified that lead to glycogen storage diseases.

Regulation of Glycogen Metabolism

The two key regulatory enzymes in glycogen metabolism are **glycogen synthase** and **phosphorylase**. Both enzymes are regulated by covalent and allosteric mechanisms (**Part A**).

Covalent Regulation

The primary mechanism for regulating glycogen synthase and phosphorylase is by phosphorylation and dephosphorylation, reactions that are mediated by **protein kinases** and **protein phosphatase-1**, respectively. The activities of protein kinases and protein phosphatase-1 are, in turn, under hormonal control. Following a meal, **insulin** is elevated, resulting in the activation of protein phosphatase-1, which removes phosphate groups from both glycogen synthase and phosphorylase. The dephosphorylated form of glycogen synthase is active, while that of phosphorylase is inactive. In the **fasting state**, glucagon is elevated, resulting in an increase in cAMP, initiating a series of reactions that result in the phosphorylation of both glycogen synthase and phosphorylase. The phosphorylated form of glycogen synthase is inactive, while that of glycogen phosphorylase is active. In **muscle**, cAMP synthesis is stimulated by **epinephrine**, whereas in **liver** both **glucagon** and **epinephrine** stimulate cAMP synthesis. The activation of phosphorylase involves two protein kinases, protein kinase A and phosphorylase kinase.

Allosteric Regulation

Under certain conditions, allosteric mechanisms can override covalent mechanisms. Allosteric inhibitors decrease the activity of the covalently active forms of the glycogen synthase and phosphorylase, whereas allosteric activators stimulate the covalently inactive forms. In glycogen metabolism, the primary target of allosteric regulation is **phosphorylase**, which is affected differently in muscle and liver. In muscle, the covalently active form of phosphorylase is inhibited by compounds that indicate a high-energy state (e.g., ATP, creatine phosphate, and G6P), while the covalently inactive form is allosterically activated by AMP, a compound indicating a low-energy state. In liver, the most important allosteric inhibitor of phosphorylase is glucose.

Avoiding a Futile Cycle

Futile cycles are created by opposing reactions or pathways that result in the net hydrolysis of high-energy phosphate bonds (**Part B**). Simultaneous operation of glycogen synthesis and degradation creates a futile cycle in which UTP is hydrolyzed to UDP, thereby wasting energy. This situation can be avoided by having **separate pathways** that are **coordinately controlled**, so that when glycogen synthesis occurs, glycogen degradation does not occur. The coordination is mediated both by hormones and allosteric effectors that exert opposite effects on glycogen synthase and phosphorylase.

Conditions Affecting Glycogen Metabolism

Glycogen synthesis is stimulated by feeding, hyperglycemia, and elevated insulin, conditions that decrease the concentration of intracellular cAMP and lead to dephosphorylation of cellular proteins (**Part C**). Conversely, glycogen degradation is stimulated by fasting, hypoglycemia, and elevated glucagon and/or epinephrine, conditions that increase the intracellular concentration of cAMP and lead to the phosphorylation of cellular proteins.

Clinical Significance

The glycogen storage diseases summarized in the following table are characterized by the accumulation of glycogen, resulting from a deficiency in an enzyme in glycogen metabolism. In some forms of glycogen storage disease, the structure of glycogen is abnormal. Most of the glycogen storage diseases are inherited as autosomal recessive traits. The clinical and biochemical findings are related to the nature of the defect involved and the site of glycogen storage. Glycogen storage disorders that affect the liver are associated with hepatomegaly and fasting hypoglycemia, whereas those that affect muscle are characterized by weakness, cramping, and muscle atrophy. Type I glycogen storage disease, also known as von Gierke disease, results from an inherited deficiency in glucose-6-phosphatase, an enzyme expressed only in liver, kidney, and intestine. The symptoms of von Gierke disease include hepatomegaly, hypoglycemia, lactic acidosis, hyperuricemia, and hyperlipidemia. Although this enzyme is not directly involved in glycogen degradation, its activity is required to complete both hepatic glycogenolysis and gluconeogenesis.

GLYCOGEN STORAGE DISEASES

Type	Name	Enzyme Deficiency	Characteristics
I	von Gierke disease[a]	Glucose-6-phosphatase (G6Pase)	Glycogen accumulation in liver and kidney; lactic acidemia, hypoglycemia, hyperuricemia, hyperlipidemia; ketosis; normal glycogen structure
II	Pompe disease	Lysosomal α-(1,4)-glucosidase	Glycogen accumulation in lysosomes; early death; normal blood glucose; normal glycogen structure; frequently heart is main organ involved
III	Cori disease, Forbes disease	Debranching enzyme	Abnormal glycogen, with short outer chains; hypoglycemia
IV	Andersen disease	Branching enzyme	Abnormal glycogen, with long outer chains; early death due to cardiac or liver failure
V	McArdle disease	Muscle glycogen phosphorylase	Abnormally high content of muscle glycogen; weakness, cramping, and decreased serum lactate after exercise; normal glycogen structure
VI	Hers disease	Liver glycogen phosphorylase	Abnormally high content of liver glycogen; mild hypoglycemia and acidosis; normal glycogen structure

[a] Different subtypes associated with deficiency in different subunits of G6Pase.

For more information see Coffee C, *Metabolism*. Fence Creek, pp 180–183, 233–239.

29 Gluconeogenesis

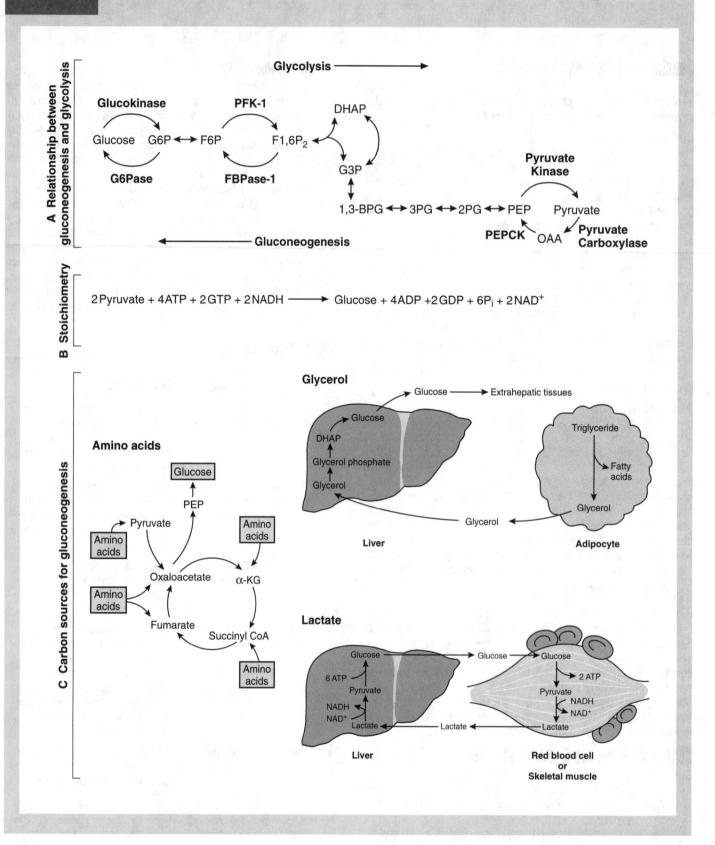

A Relationship between gluconeogenesis and glycolysis

Glycolysis ⟶

Glucokinase Glucose → G6P ⟷ F6P **PFK-1** → F1,6P$_2$ → DHAP

G6Pase **FBPase-1** G3P

1,3-BPG ⟷ 3PG ⟷ 2PG ⟷ PEP

Pyruvate Kinase → Pyruvate

PEPCK OAA **Pyruvate Carboxylase**

← Gluconeogenesis

B Stoichiometry

$$2\,\text{Pyruvate} + 4\,\text{ATP} + 2\,\text{GTP} + 2\,\text{NADH} \longrightarrow \text{Glucose} + 4\,\text{ADP} + 2\,\text{GDP} + 6\,P_i + 2\,\text{NAD}^+$$

C Carbon sources for gluconeogenesis

Amino acids

Glucose

PEP

Pyruvate

Amino acids → Oxaloacetate — α-KG ← Amino acids

Amino acids → Oxaloacetate

Fumarate ← Succinyl CoA ← Amino acids

Glycerol

Glucose ⟶ Extrahepatic tissues

DHAP ← Glucose

Glycerol phosphate

Glycerol

Liver

Triglyceride → Fatty acids → Glycerol

Adipocyte

Glycerol ⟶

Lactate

Glucose ⟶ Glucose ⟶ Glucose

6 ATP → Pyruvate   2 ATP → Pyruvate

NADH / NAD$^+$ → Lactate   NADH / NAD$^+$

Lactate ← Lactate ← Lactate

Liver

Red blood cell or Skeletal muscle

OVERVIEW

The major function of gluconeogenesis is to provide a source of glucose that can augment the role of liver glycogen in preventing hypoglycemia. Both liver and kidney contain all of the enzymes required for gluconeogenesis, although about 80% of the blood glucose derived from this pathway is made by the liver. Skeletal muscle can use small precursors to synthesize glucose-6-phosphate (G6P), but cannot release glucose into the blood due to the absence of glucose-6-phosphatase (G6Pase). Gluconeogenesis starts in the mitochondria, where pyruvate is converted to oxaloacetate, and the final step in the pathway occurs in the endoplasmic reticulum where G6P is hydrolyzed to glucose. All other steps occur in the cytosol. The carbon precursors for gluconeogenesis are lactate, glycerol, and amino acids. The energy for driving glucose synthesis comes from fatty acid oxidation.

Relationship Between Gluconeogenesis and Glycolysis

Gluconeogenesis and glycolysis are opposing pathways that share many of the same enzymes (**Part A**). There are four enzymes that are unique to gluconeogenesis: pyruvate carboxylase, phosphoenolpyruvate carboxykinase (PEPCK), fructose-1,6-bisphosphatase (FBPase-1), and G6Pase. These enzymes bypass the three irreversible steps in glycolysis.

The reaction catalyzed by **pyruvate carboxylase** is described by the equation shown below. Biotin functions as a transient carrier of the carboxyl group from HCO_3^- to pyruvate. The attachment of the carboxyl group to biotin requires energy that is supplied by ATP hydrolysis. Most of this energy is conserved in the newly formed C-C bond in oxaloacetate. Acetyl CoA, derived from fatty acid oxidation, is an allosteric activator of pyruvate carboxylase.

$$\text{Pyruvate} + HCO_3^- + ATP \xrightarrow[\oplus \text{acetyl CoA}]{\text{biotin}} \text{Oxaloacetate} + ADP + P_i$$

The conversion of oxaloacetate to phosphoenolpyruvate (PEP) is catalyzed by **PEPCK**, as shown in the following reaction:

$$\text{Oxaloacetate} + GTP \longrightarrow \text{Phosphoenolpyruvate} + CO_2 + GDP_2 + P_i$$

The formation of the high-energy phosphate bond in PEP requires more energy than is available from the hydrolysis of GTP. Additional energy comes from decarboxylation of oxaloacetate. This reaction cleaves the C-C bond that was formed in the previous reaction. The **sum of the first two reactions** can be described by the following equation:

$$\text{Pyruvate} + ATP + GTP \longrightarrow PEP + ADP + GDP + P_i$$

Two high-energy bonds are required to convert pyruvate to PEP. Under cellular conditions, where the concentration of PEP is extremely low, the ΔG for this reaction is -6 kcal/mol, rendering the conversion of pyruvate to PEP an irreversible reaction.

FBPase-1 catalyzes the hydrolysis of fructose-1,6-bisphosphate ($F1,6P_2$) to fructose-6-P (F6P). As shown below, this reaction is irreversible, and it bypasses the opposing reaction in glycolysis catalyzed by phosphofructokinase-1 (PFK-1):

$$F1,6P_2 + H_2O \longrightarrow F6P + P_i$$

The final step in gluconeogenesis is the hydrolysis of G6P to glucose and P_i, a reaction catalyzed by **G6Pase**. This enzyme is located in the lumen of the smooth endoplasmic reticulum. This reaction is irreversible, and it bypasses the opposing step in hepatic glycolysis catalyzed by glucokinase:

$$G6P + H_2O \longrightarrow \text{Glucose} + P_i$$

Stoichiometry of Gluconeogenesis

The synthesis of 1 mol of glucose requires 2 mols each of pyruvate, NADH, GTP, and 4 mols of ATP (**Part B**). The reactions requiring energy are catalyzed by pyruvate carboxylase, PEPCK, and 3-phosphoglycerate kinase, which also participates in glycolysis. NADH is required to reverse the reaction in glycolysis that is catalyzed by glyceraldehyde-3-phosphate dehydrogenase.

Carbon Skeletons for Gluconeogenesis

Any compound that can be converted to an **intermediate in glycolysis or the TCA cycle** can be used as a source of carbon for gluconeogenesis. The three sources of carbon for gluconeogenesis are amino acids, glycerol, and lactate (**Part C**). The turnover of **skeletal muscle** supplies the liver with **glucogenic amino acids** that are degraded to either pyruvate or an intermediate in the TCA cycle. All of the amino acids found in proteins can supply carbon for glucose synthesis except leucine and lysine. Triglyceride hydrolysis in **adipose tissue** releases **glycerol** into the blood. The presence of **glycerol kinase** in liver converts glycerol to glycerol-3-phosphate, which is oxidized to dihydroxyacetone phosphate (**DHAP**), an intermediate in glycolysis. Glycerol kinase is absent in adipose tissue. **Anaerobic muscle and red blood cells** release lactate into the blood. It is removed by liver, where it is oxidized to pyruvate and used for glucose synthesis. The cycle between anaerobic glycolysis in red blood cells and muscle and gluconeogenesis in liver is known as the **Cori cycle**. This cycle does not result in net glucose synthesis, but it recycles C_3 precursors.

Clinical Significance

The major function of gluconeogenesis is to prevent fasting hypoglycemia. The daily glucose requirement for an adult is 160 to 200 g, most of which is consumed by the brain. The liver contains a limited reserve of glycogen (about 75 g), which can supply glucose to other tissues for a few hours. Synthesis of glucose from amino acids and other small precursors begins before the supply of glycogen is exhausted.

For more information see Coffee C, *Metabolism*. Fence Creek, pp 187–194, 233–239.

30 Coordinate Regulation of Glycolysis and Gluconeogenesis

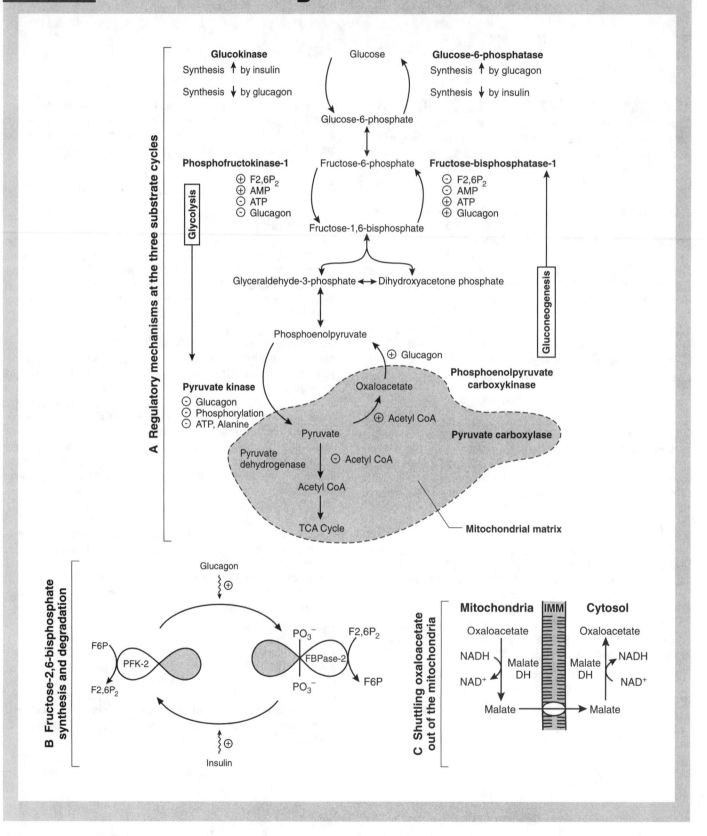

A Regulatory mechanisms at the three substrate cycles

Glucokinase
Synthesis ↑ by insulin
Synthesis ↓ by glucagon

Glucose

Glucose-6-phosphatase
Synthesis ↑ by glucagon
Synthesis ↓ by insulin

Glucose-6-phosphate

Phosphofructokinase-1
⊕ F2,6P$_2$
⊕ AMP
⊖ ATP
⊖ Glucagon

Fructose-6-phosphate

Fructose-bisphosphatase-1
⊖ F2,6P$_2$
⊖ AMP
⊕ ATP
⊕ Glucagon

Glycolysis

Fructose-1,6-bisphosphate

Gluconeogenesis

Glyceraldehyde-3-phosphate ⟷ Dihydroxyacetone phosphate

Phosphoenolpyruvate

⊕ Glucagon

Pyruvate kinase
⊖ Glucagon
⊖ Phosphorylation
⊖ ATP, Alanine

Oxaloacetate

Phosphoenolpyruvate carboxykinase

⊕ Acetyl CoA

Pyruvate carboxylase

Pyruvate

Pyruvate dehydrogenase   ⊖ Acetyl CoA

Acetyl CoA

TCA Cycle

Mitochondrial matrix

B Fructose-2,6-bisphosphate synthesis and degradation

Glucagon
⊕

F6P
PFK-2
F2,6P$_2$

PO$_3^-$ F2,6P$_2$
FBPase-2
PO$_3^-$ F6P

Insulin
⊕

C Shuttling oxaloacetate out of the mitochondria

Mitochondria   IMM   **Cytosol**

Oxaloacetate   Oxaloacetate

NADH   Malate   Malate   NADH
DH   DH
NAD$^+$ NAD$^+$

Malate ⟶   ⟶ Malate

Gluconeogenesis and glycolysis are regulated in close coordination. Most of the conditions that activate gluconeogenesis inhibit glycolysis and vice versa. The targets of regulation are the pairs of enzymes that catalyze opposing reactions at the irreversible steps in these pathways. The direction in which substrate flows through each of these substrate cycles is dependent on the activity of the opposing enzymes. Regulatory mechanisms that coordinate gluconeogenesis and glycolysis include allosteric effects, short-term hormonal effects mediated by phosphorylation and dephosphorylation, and adaptive effects mediated by induction and repression of enzyme synthesis.

Regulatory Mechanisms at the Three Substrate Cycles

The enzymes unique to gluconeogenesis and glycolysis catalyze **irreversible reactions**. To avoid futile cycling of substrate at the expense of ATP, the enzymes at these points are reciprocally regulated (**Part A**).

Glucose/Glucose-6-Phosphate Cycle

Both glucose-6-phosphatase (G6Pase) and glucokinase (GK) have a high K_m for their respective substrates, and neither enzyme is saturated at physiologic concentrations of substrate. Therefore, the short-term regulation of these enzymes is due primarily to substrate concentration. Long-term regulation is mediated by insulin and glucagon, which alter the rate of transcription of the genes encoding these enzymes in a reciprocal fashion. An elevation in glucagon induces the synthesis of G6Pase and represses the synthesis of GK, whereas insulin has the opposite effect.

Fructose-6-Phosphate/Fructose-1,6-Bisphosphate Cycle

The most important factor in determining the net direction at which substrates move through this substrate cycle is the concentration of fructose-2,6-bisphosphate ($F2,6P_2$). The only known function of $F2,6P_2$ is the reciprocal regulation of glycolysis and gluconeogenesis. $F2,6P_2$ simultaneously stimulates glycolysis by activating phosphofructokinase-1 (PFK-1) and decreases gluconeogenesis by inhibiting fructose-bisphosphatase-1 (FBPase-1). The cellular concentration of $F2,6P_2$ is a reflection of the blood glucose level, increasing and decreasing as blood glucose levels increase and decrease. PFK-1 and FBPase-1 are also allosterically regulated reciprocally by ATP and AMP, compounds that are indicators of the energy state of the cell.

Phosphoenolpyruvate/Pyruvate Cycle

Phosphoenolpyruvate carboxykinase (PEPCK) and pyruvate kinase are reciprocally regulated by glucagon. Glucagon stimulates gluconeogenesis by increasing the rate of transcription of the gene encoding PEPCK. Simultaneously, glucagon leads to phosphorylation and inactivation of pyruvate kinase, thereby inhibiting glycolysis. Pyruvate kinase is also allosterically inhibited by ATP and alanine, which are substrates for gluconeogenesis. The activity of pyruvate carboxylase is coordinated with that of pyruvate dehydrogenase (PDH) by acetyl CoA, which activates pyruvate carboxylase and inhibits PDH. Inhibition of PDH conserves pyruvate for gluconeogenesis rather than removing it from the pool of glucogenic substrates.

Fructose-2,6-Bisphosphate Synthesis and Degradation

The primary factor in determining whether glycolysis or gluconeogenesis is operating in liver is the cellular concentration of $F2,6P_2$, which activates glycolysis and inhibits gluconeogenesis. The synthesis and degradation of $F2,6P_2$ are catalyzed by different domains on a single **bifunctional enzyme (Part B)**. The PFK-2 domain catalyzes the ATP-dependent conversion of F6P to $F2,6P_2$, whereas the FBPase-2 domain hydrolyzes $F2,6P_2$ to F6P. The catalytic activity of PFK-2 is coordinated with that of FBPase-2 so that both are not active at the same time. Glucagon stimulates the phosphorylation of the bifunctional enzyme, resulting in activation of FBPase-2, whereas insulin promotes dephosphorylation, resulting in activation of PFK-2. Thus, elevated insulin leads to increased $F2,6P_2$ and increased glycolysis, whereas elevated glucagon leads to decreased $F2,6P_2$ and increased gluconeogenesis.

Shuttling Oxaloacetate Out of the Mitochondria

The first step in gluconeogenesis occurs in the mitochondria where pyruvate is converted to oxaloacetate. The inner mitochondrial membrane is impermeable to oxaloacetate, and transport to the cytosol requires the malate shuttle, which consists of a transport protein and two malate dehydrogenase isozymes that are located on opposite sides of the membrane (**Part C**). Oxaloacetate is first reduced to malate by NADH in the mitochondria, and after being transported into the cytosol, malate is oxidized back to oxaloacetate, producing NADH. Therefore, malate acts as a carrier of both oxaloacetate and reducing equivalents to the cytosol, where both NADH and oxaloacetate are available for gluconeogenesis.

Clinical Significance

A plasma glucose level below 40 mg/dL represents severe hypoglycemia. There are two general types of hypoglycemia: postprandial and fasting hypoglycemia. **Postprandial hypoglycemia** is caused by an exaggerated release of insulin following a meal. Although plasma glucose returns to normal without intervention, small meals eaten frequently are recommended. **Fasting hypoglycemia**, resulting from decreased gluconeogenesis, is often seen in patients with liver damage or adrenal insufficiency. Alternatively, fasting hypoglycemia, due to increased glucose uptake and utilization, is seen in patients with pancreatic β-cell tumors who experience uncontrolled insulin secretion. In contrast, **hyperglycemia** can result from increased gluconeogenesis, secondary to secretion of glucagon, catecholamines, or cortisol.

For more information see Coffee C, *Metabolism*. Fence Creek, pp 195–197, 233–239.

Pentose Phosphate Pathway

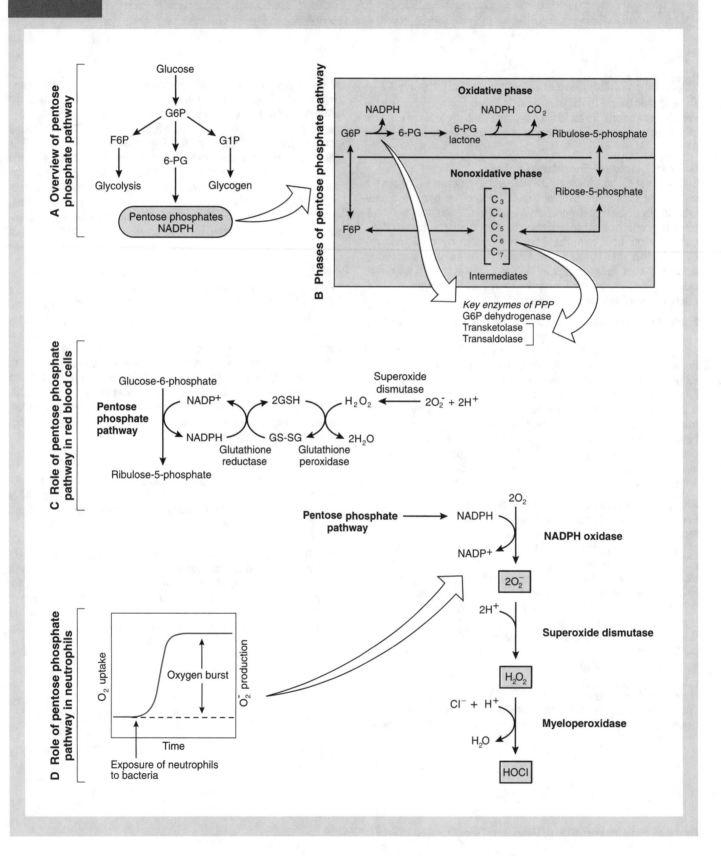

A Overview of pentose phosphate pathway

B Phases of pentose phosphate pathway

Oxidative phase

Nonoxidative phase

Intermediates

Key enzymes of PPP
G6P dehydrogenase
Transketolase
Transaldolase

C Role of pentose phosphate pathway in red blood cells

Pentose phosphate pathway

Glutathione reductase

Glutathione peroxidase

Superoxide dismutase

D Role of pentose phosphate pathway in neutrophils

Oxygen burst

Exposure of neutrophils to bacteria

Pentose phosphate pathway

NADPH oxidase

Superoxide dismutase

Myeloperoxidase

OVERVIEW

The pentose phosphate pathway, also known as the hexose monophosphate shunt, provides an alternative pathway for the oxidation of glucose (**Part A**). In most tissues, 80% to 90% of glucose oxidation is by glycolysis, and the remaining 10% to 20% is oxidized by the pentose phosphate pathway. Glucose-6-phosphate (G6P) is an important branch point in glucose metabolism. The oxidation of G6P to 6-phosphogluconate (6-PG) commits glucose to the pentose phosphate pathway. The pathway does not require oxygen, and it neither requires nor generates ATP. It is found in the cytosol of all cells and has two major functions: 1) synthesis of ribose phosphate, which is required for nucleotide and nucleic acid synthesis; and 2) synthesis of NADPH, which is used as a reducing agent in many biosynthetic pathways. NADPH is also important in preventing oxygen insult to the RBC, and it participates in the bactericidal function of neutrophils.

Phases of the Pentose Phosphate Pathway

The steps in the pathway can be divided into two sequences of reactions (**Part B**). The **oxidative phase** consists of the first three reactions, which result in NADPH and pentose phosphate production. This phase of the pathway is **irreversible**. The **nonoxidative phase** of the pathway converts excess pentose phosphates back to G6P so that they can be recycled. This phase consists of a series of **reversible** reactions that are in equilibrium with intermediates in glycolysis. The intermediates in the nonoxidative phase range from C_3 to C_7 in length. Two of the intermediates, **fructose-6-phosphate** and **glyceraldehyde-3-phosphate**, are also intermediates in glycolysis.

Key Enzymes in the Pentose Phosphate Pathway

The reactions catalyzed by **G6P dehydrogenase** (G6PD) and **6-PG dehydrogenase** generate almost all of the NADPH in cells (**Part B**). **G6PD** also catalyzes the **rate-limiting step** in the pathway. It is allosterically inhibited by NADPH. The two enzymes responsible for most of the reactions in the nonoxidative phase are **transketolase** and **transaldolase**. Transketolase requires **thiamine pyrophosphate** as a coenzyme. Measurement of transketolase activity in RBC lysates is used for the clinical assessment of thiamine deficiency. The validity of this test resides in the fact that transketolase is the only enzyme in the RBC that requires thiamine pyrophosphate.

Role of Pentose Phosphate Pathway in the RBC

NADPH is essential for protection of the RBC against oxidative damage by superoxide (O_2^-) and hydrogen peroxide (H_2O_2), strong oxidizing agents that can cause irreversible damage to the cell and result in lysis. Superoxide is produced by the reduction of hemoglobin-bound oxygen, which occurs spontaneously in the RBC. Oxidative damage is minimized by the sequential action of three enzyme-catalyzed reactions that maintain the concentration of superoxide and hydrogen peroxide at low levels (**Part C**). Superoxide is converted to hydrogen peroxide by the action of **superoxide dismutase**, an enzyme found in all cells. Hydrogen peroxide is reduced to water in a reaction catalyzed by **glutathione peroxidase**. This reaction requires two molecules of reduced glutathione (GSH), which is oxidized to the dimer GS-SG. GSH is regenerated by the NADPH-dependent reduction of GS-SG, a reaction catalyzed by **glutathione reductase**. Thus, the role of NADPH in the RBC is to maintain the concentration of reduced glutathione at about 5 mM.

Role of Pentose Phosphate Pathway in Neutrophils

Neutrophils and other phagocytic cells use superoxide, hydrogen peroxide, and hypochlorous acid (HOCl) to kill bacteria that have been engulfed by the cell. If a suspension of resting neutrophils is presented with bacteria, phagocytosis is accompanied by a rapid uptake of oxygen, known as the **oxygen burst** (**Part D**). The oxygen taken up by neutrophils is reduced to superoxide by NADPH in a reaction catalyzed by **NADPH oxidase**. Hydrogen peroxide and HOCl are produced in sequential reactions catalyzed by **superoxide dismutase** and **myeloperoxidase**, respectively.

Role of Pentose Phosphate Pathway in Other Cells and Tissues

All nucleated cells require pentose phosphates for **nucleotide, DNA**, and **RNA synthesis**. However, the tissues most enriched in enzymes of this pathway are those that have the greatest demand for NADPH. Biosynthetic pathways requiring NADPH and the major tissues in which they occur are **fatty acid synthesis** (liver and lactating mammary gland); **cholesterol** and **bile acid synthesis** (liver); **steroid hormone synthesis** (adrenal cortex, ovaries, testes); and **cytochrome P_{450}-dependent detoxification reactions** (liver).

Clinical Significance

The NADPH required for reduction of hydrogen peroxide in the RBC is generated entirely by the pentose phosphate pathway. Therefore, a deficiency in G6PD, the enzyme catalyzing the first step in the pathway, drastically impairs NADPH production. The clinical features of **G6PD deficiency** are **hemolytic anemia** and **chronic bacterial infection**. Many individuals with partial G6PD activity are asymptomatic under most conditions. However, several commonly used drugs, including **antibiotics, antimalarials**, and **antipyretics**, stimulate superoxide production. The increased use of NADPH for superoxide production diminishes the ability to maintain reduced glutathione levels and can precipitate an oxidative crisis, resulting in hemolytic anemia. G6PD deficiency is inherited as an X-linked recessive trait. A deficiency in **NADPH oxidase** in neutrophils results in **chronic granulocytic disease (CGD)**. In individuals with CGD, neutrophils can take up bacteria but their bactericidal capacity is impaired. NADPH oxidase is a complex enzyme consisting of several subunits encoded by different genes that are located on different chromosomes, accounting for the observation that CGD disorders show both autosomal recessive and X-linked inheritance.

For more information see Coffee C, *Metabolism*. Fence Creek, pp 201–208, 234–235.

32 Galactose, Fructose, and Glucuronic Acid Metabolism

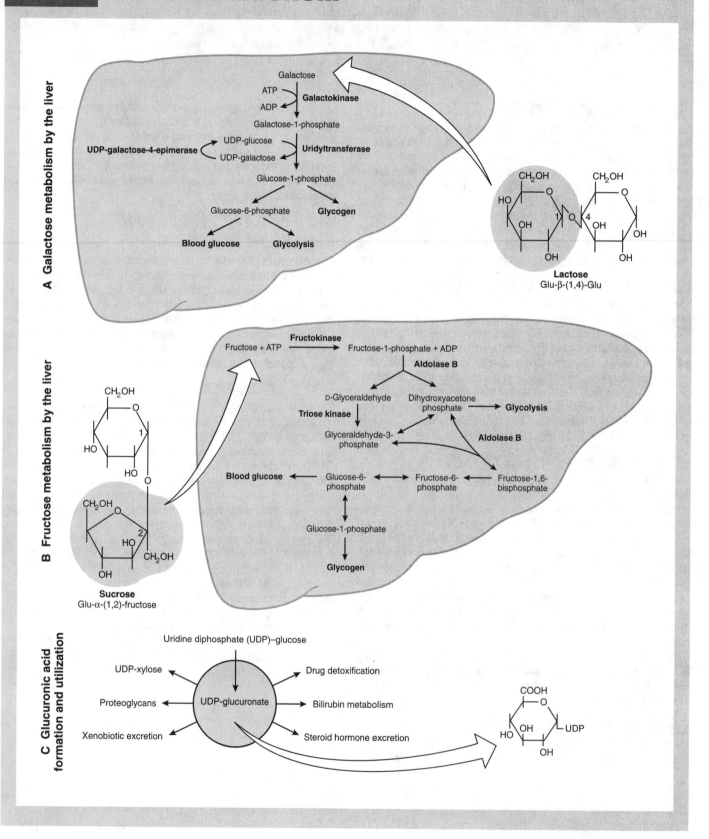

A Galactose metabolism by the liver

Galactose
ATP → **Galactokinase** → ADP
Galactose-1-phosphate
UDP-galactose-4-epimerase ⇄ UDP-glucose / UDP-galactose — **Uridyltransferase**
Glucose-1-phosphate
Glucose-6-phosphate → Blood glucose / Glycolysis
Glycogen

Lactose
Glu-β-(1,4)-Glu

B Fructose metabolism by the liver

Fructokinase
Fructose + ATP → Fructose-1-phosphate + ADP
Aldolase B
D-Glyceraldehyde   Dihydroxyacetone phosphate → **Glycolysis**
Triose kinase
Glyceraldehyde-3-phosphate
Aldolase B
Blood glucose ← Glucose-6-phosphate ⇄ Fructose-6-phosphate ← Fructose-1,6-bisphosphate
Glucose-1-phosphate
Glycogen

Sucrose
Glu-α-(1,2)-fructose

C Glucuronic acid formation and utilization

Uridine diphosphate (UDP)–glucose
UDP-xylose
Proteoglycans
Xenobiotic excretion
UDP-glucuronate
Drug detoxification
Bilirubin metabolism
Steroid hormone excretion

COOH—O—UDP

OVERVIEW

Interconversion of hexoses is important in several metabolic pathways. Dietary galactose and fructose can be efficiently converted to intermediates in the pathways of glucose metabolism. Under normal conditions, dietary galactose and fructose are cleared almost entirely by the liver. The conversion of UDP-glucose to UDP-galactose allows the lactating mammary gland to synthesize lactose from glucose. UDP-glucose is oxidized to UDP-glucuronic acid, providing an activated form of glucuronic acid that can be used by connective tissue for proteoglycan synthesis and by the liver for conjugating insoluble compounds with glucuronic acid, a process that allows these compounds to be excreted.

Galactose Metabolism by the Liver

Most dietary galactose is derived from lactose, the major disaccharide in milk (**Part A**). Hydrolysis by **lactase** in the intestinal brush border membrane results in a mixture of galactose and glucose. Following absorption, galactose is delivered to the liver by the portal blood, where it is assimilated into the pathways of **glycolysis, gluconeogenesis**, and **glycogen synthesis**. Three unique enzymes allow galactose to be metabolized by the liver. **Galactokinase** converts galactose to galactose-1-phosphate; **galactose-1-phosphate uridyltransferase** converts galactose-1-phosphate to glucose-1-phosphate in an exchange reaction that requires UDP-glucose and generates UDP-galactose. UDP-galactose is converted to UDP-glucose by **UDP-galactose-4-epimerase**. This series of reactions effectively converts galactose-1-phosphate to glucose-1-phosphate, which can be either used for glycogen synthesis or converted to glucose-6-phosphate that can be channeled into glycolysis, or used to replenish blood glucose.

The lactating mammary gland synthesizes lactose, the major milk sugar from glucose by the sequence of reactions shown below:

$$\text{UDP-Glucose} \xrightarrow{\text{epimerase}} \text{UDP-galactose} \xrightarrow[\text{Glucose}]{\text{Lactose synthase}} \text{Galactose-}\beta\text{-(lactose) (1,4)-glucose}$$

Lactose synthase consists of two subunits, **galactosyl transferase** and **α-lactalbumin**. During pregnancy, the synthesis of α-lactalbumin is inhibited by progesterone. Shortly after birth, synthesis of lactalbumin is stimulated by prolactin, thereby initiating synthesis of lactose.

Fructose Metabolism by the Liver

Most dietary fructose is consumed as sucrose, a disaccharide containing fructose and glucose (**Part B**). Three liver enzymes allow fructose to be assimilated into pathways of glycolysis, gluconeogenesis, and glycogen synthesis. **Fructokinase** converts fructose to fructose-1-phosphate, which is cleaved by **aldolase B**, generating glyceraldehyde and dihydroxyacetone phosphate (DHAP), an intermediate in glycolysis. **Triose kinase** catalyzes the conversion of glyceraldehyde to glyceraldehyde-3-phosphate (G3P), also an intermediate in glycolysis. Condensation of DHAP and G3P produces fructose-1,6-bisphosphate, which can be used either for glycogen synthesis or for blood glucose replenishment.

Seminal fluid sperm use fructose as the major source of energy. Glucose is converted to fructose by seminal vesicles and released into seminal fluid. The reactions that convert glucose to fructose are shown below:

$$\text{Glucose} \xrightarrow[\text{NADPH} \;\to\; \text{NADP}^+]{\text{Aldol reductase}} \text{Sorbitol} \xrightarrow[\text{NAD}^+ \;\to\; \text{NADH}]{\text{Sorbitol dehydrogenase}} \text{Fructose}$$

Formation and Utilization of Glucuronic Acid

Glucuronic acid metabolism in human tissues involves UDP-glucuronic acid (**Part C**). UDP-glucose is converted to UDP-glucuronic acid by two sequential oxidation reactions catalyzed by UDP-glucose dehydrogenase. These two reactions oxidize C-6 of glucose to a carboxyl group. Most of the UDP-glucuronic acid is used either by connective tissue for **proteoglycan synthesis** or by the liver in **detoxification reactions**. Many highly insoluble compounds such as bilirubin, steroid hormones, various drugs, and xenobiotics are toxic if allowed to accumulate. These compounds are made soluble enough to be excreted by conjugation with glucuronic acid. A family of liver enzymes known as UDP-glucuronyltransferases catalyze the conjugation reactions, as shown below:

$$\underset{\text{(insoluble)}}{\text{R-OH + UDP-glucuronate}} \xrightarrow{\text{UDP-glucuronyltransferase}} \underset{\text{(soluble)}}{\text{R-O-glucuronide + UDP}}$$

Clinical Significance

Several inherited disorders occur in galactose and fructose metabolism. **Galactosemia** results from a deficiency in either galactokinase or galactose-1-phosphate uridyltransferase. Symptoms include cataracts that can lead to blindness. Galactose accumulation in the blood is accompanied by increased uptake by the lens, where aldol reductase reduces galactose to galactitol. **Galactitol** is a dead end product that is trapped in the cell and cannot be further metabolized. Its formation alters the osmotic conditions of the lens and depletes NADPH and glutathione, factors that contribute to cataract formation. Other symptoms include diarrhea and vomiting when milk or milk products are consumed. **Hereditary fructose intolerance** results from a genetic deficiency in aldolase B. The accumulation of fructose-1-phosphate leads a depletion of intracellular phosphate, disruption of oxidative phosphorylation, and inhibition of energy-dependent processes. Fructose-1-phosphate inhibits glycogen phosphorylase and phosphoglucomutase, resulting in impaired glycogen degradation and hypoglycemia. **Essential fructosuria**, a relatively benign condition, results from a genetic deficiency in fructokinase and is characterized by elevated fructose in the blood and urine. Fructose can be taken up by extrahepatic tissues and converted to fructose-6-phosphate by hexokinase.

For more information see Coffee C, *Metabolism*. Fence Creek, pp 211–215, 233–239.

33 Glycosylation of Proteins

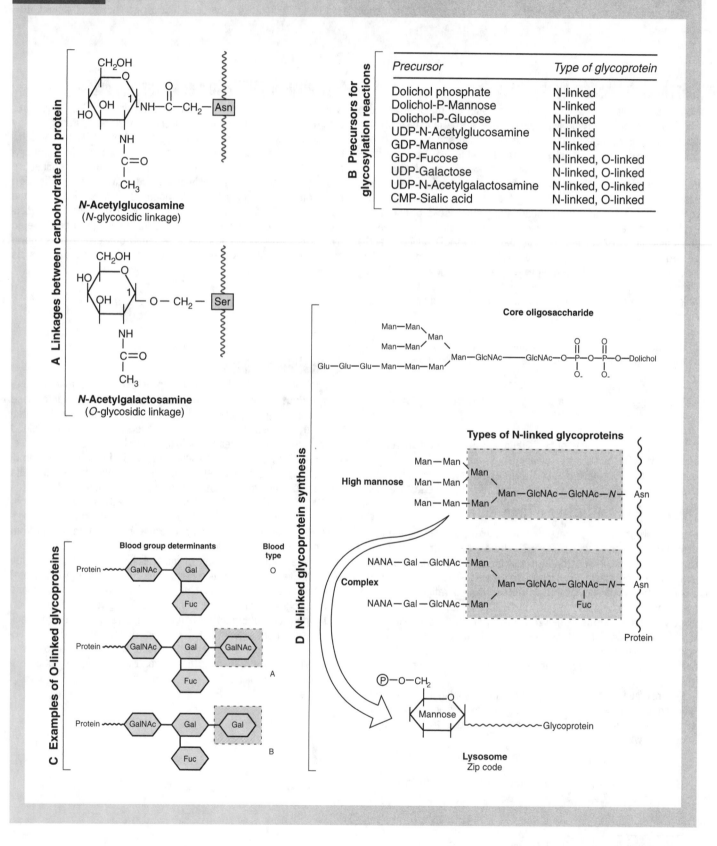

A Linkages between carbohydrate and protein

N-Acetylglucosamine
(*N*-glycosidic linkage)

N-Acetylgalactosamine
(*O*-glycosidic linkage)

B Precursors for glycosylation reactions

Precursor	Type of glycoprotein
Dolichol phosphate	N-linked
Dolichol-P-Mannose	N-linked
Dolichol-P-Glucose	N-linked
UDP-N-Acetylglucosamine	N-linked
GDP-Mannose	N-linked
GDP-Fucose	N-linked, O-linked
UDP-Galactose	N-linked, O-linked
UDP-N-Acetylgalactosamine	N-linked, O-linked
CMP-Sialic acid	N-linked, O-linked

C Examples of O-linked glycoproteins

Blood group determinants

Blood type

D N-linked glycoprotein synthesis

Core oligosaccharide

Types of N-linked glycoproteins

High mannose

Complex

Lysosome
Zip code

Glycoproteins are widely distributed in nature. They are found embedded in membranes and in lysosomes, extracellular matrix, and mucus. Serum proteins, with the notable exception of albumin, are glycoproteins. Many enzymes, structural proteins, hormones, antigens, immunoglobulins, receptors, and transport proteins contain covalently linked oligosaccharide chains. Although the precise role of the carbohydrate is not clear in many cases, some functions that have been attributed to the carbohydrate moiety of proteins include cell–cell interactions, embryonic development and differentiation, cell migration, blood group determinants, and targeting proteins to specific destinations.

Linkages Between Carbohydrate and Protein

Oligosaccharide chains are attached to protein by N-glycosidic and O-glycosidic bonds (**Part A**). **N-glycosidic bonds** are formed between the amide group of an asparagine (Asn) side chain and C-1 of N-acetylglucosamine (GlcNAc). The enzyme that catalyzes the formation of the N-glycosidic bond recognizes Asn residues having the sequence Asn-X-Thr or Asn-X-Ser, where X can be any amino acid. This sequence is necessary but insufficient for defining glycosylation sites. Some Asn residues with this sequence do not become glycosylated. **O-glycosidic bonds** are formed between the side-chain hydroxyl group of serine or threonine and C-1 of either N-acetylgalactosamine (GalNAc) or xylose. In collagen, a special type of O-glycosidic linkage is found where galactose is attached to hydroxylysine residues. A Gal-Glu disaccharide is attached to collagen, whereas the oligosaccharide in most glycoproteins is branched and contains 12 to 15 monosaccharides.

Precursors for Glycosylation Reactions

The sugars found in glycoproteins are mannose, glucose, galactose, fucose, GlcNAc, GalNAc, and sialic acid (**Part B**). Synthesis of the oligosaccharide chains requires two types of high-energy donors, **nucleotide-linked sugars** (e.g., UDP-GlcNAc, GDP-mannose, CMP-sialic acid) and **dolichol phosphate-linked sugars** (e.g., dolichol-P-mannose, dolichol-P-glucose). Dolichol phosphate is a **lipid carrier** that is used only in the synthesis of N-linked oligosaccharides.

O-Linked Glycoproteins

O-linked oligosaccharide synthesis occurs in the Golgi. It begins with the addition of GalNAc or xylose to a serine or threonine side chain of the protein. Additional sugars are added one at a time to produce a mature oligosaccharide, which is usually branched. The enzymes involved are a family of membrane-bound proteins known as **glycosyltransferases**. Clinically important O-linked oligosaccharides include the **blood group determinants (Part C)**. The external surface of the red blood cell contains hundreds of antigens that have been classified into several genetically distinct blood group systems. The A, B, and O antigens constitute the ABO blood group system. The specificity of the ABO blood group is determined by a few key monosaccharides located near the end of the oligosaccharide chain. The O antigen is a precursor for both the A and B antigens, which differ by a single monosaccharide at the end of the oligosaccharide chain. The A antigen has GalNAc at the end of the chain, the B antigen has galactose in the corresponding position, while the O antigen has neither galactose nor GalNAc.

N-Linked Glycoproteins

The synthesis of N-linked oligosaccharides is considerably more complex and strikingly different from the synthesis of O-linked oligosaccharides (**Part D**). A **core oligosaccharide** consisting of two molecules of GlcNAc, nine molecules of mannose, and three molecules

of glucose is assembled on dolichol phosphate and subsequently transferred to an asparagine residue in the acceptor protein. Diverse classes of N-linked glycoproteins are created by modification of the oligosaccharide after it is attached to the protein. Modification reactions start in the endoplasmic reticulum and proceed as the protein moves through the Golgi. The ends of the oligosaccharide chains are trimmed and extended in different ways to generate two major classes of N-linked glycoproteins, **high mannose** and **complex glycoproteins**. All mature N-linked glycoproteins retain five of the original monosaccharides. The last step in N-linked oligosaccharide modification is sorting or targeting, which occurs in the Golgi. This step puts specific **zip codes** onto different glycoproteins that specify their final destination. The zip code that directs lysosomal hydrolases to lysosomes is the presence of **mannose-6-phosphate** in the oligosaccharide chain. Mannose-6-phosphate binds to receptors in the Golgi, and vesicles containing these proteins pinch off and fuse with lysosomes. A deficiency in **N-acetylglucosaminylphosphotransferase** results in the inability to phosphorylate mannose and leads to **I-cell disease**, in which lysosomal enzymes are synthesized but are secreted into the plasma rather than being incorporated into lysosomes. Lysosomes are filled **inclusion bodies** containing material that cannot be degraded.

Clinical Significance

The correlation between antigens, enzymes, and antibodies for the ABO blood group is summarized in the table below. The type of antigen on the surface of RBCs can be correlated with the presence or absence of specific enzymes. For example, **N-acetylgalactosaminyltransferase** is required to form type A antigen, whereas **galactosyltransferase** is required to form type B antigen. If neither enzyme is present, the O antigen accumulates, and if both enzymes are present, both A and B antigens are found on RBCs. Blood types can also be correlated with antibodies in the serum. Individuals with type A antigen have antibodies against antigen B and vice versa. Individuals with type O have neither antigen A nor B on their RBCs, and they have antibodies to both A and B antigens in their serum. In blood transfusions, in which packed red blood cells are transfused, type O individuals are considered to be universal donors.

Blood Type	Antigen on Red Blood Cell	Glycosyltransferase Present	Antibodies in Serum
Type A	A	N-acetylgalactosaminyl-transferase	Anti-B
Type B	B	Galactosyltransferase	Anti-A
Type AB	A and B	Both	Neither
Type O	O[a]	Neither	Anti-A and anti-B

[a] Also known as the H antigen.

For more information see Coffee C, *Metabolism*. Fence Creek, pp 221–226.

34 Proteoglycans

A Proteoglycan structure

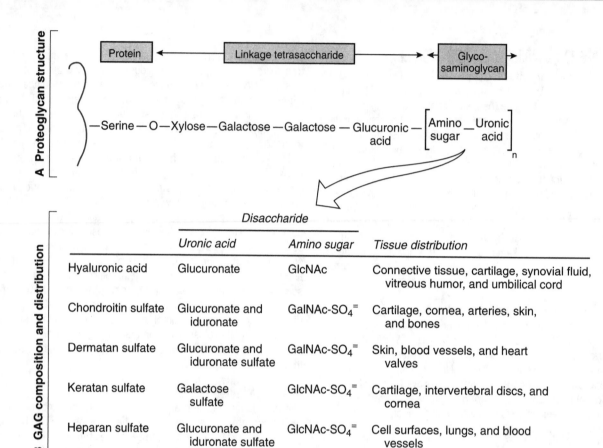

| Protein | ↔ | Linkage tetrasaccharide | ↔ | Glyco-saminoglycan |

—Serine—O—Xylose—Galactose—Galactose—Glucuronic acid—[Amino sugar — Uronic acid]$_n$

B GAG composition and distribution

| | Disaccharide | | Tissue distribution |
	Uronic acid	Amino sugar	
Hyaluronic acid	Glucuronate	GlcNAc	Connective tissue, cartilage, synovial fluid, vitreous humor, and umbilical cord
Chondroitin sulfate	Glucuronate and iduronate	GalNAc-SO$_4^=$	Cartilage, cornea, arteries, skin, and bones
Dermatan sulfate	Glucuronate and iduronate sulfate	GalNAc-SO$_4^=$	Skin, blood vessels, and heart valves
Keratan sulfate	Galactose sulfate	GlcNAc-SO$_4^=$	Cartilage, intervertebral discs, and cornea
Heparan sulfate	Glucuronate and iduronate sulfate	GlcNAc-SO$_4^=$	Cell surfaces, lungs, and blood vessels
Heparin	Glucuronate and iduronate sulfate	GlcNAc-SO$_4^=$	Mast cells (lung, liver, skin)

C Cartilage aggregan

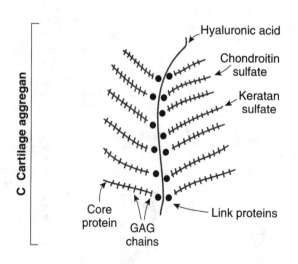

Hyaluronic acid

Chondroitin sulfate

Keratan sulfate

Core protein

GAG chains

Link proteins

OVERVIEW

The major components of the extracellular space in mammalian tissues are the proteoglycans, also known as mucopolysaccharides, and the fibrous proteins, collagen and elastin. Proteoglycans are found in high concentrations in cartilage, bone, blood vessels, heart valves, synovial fluid, vitreous humor, and skin. They are composed of heterogeneous carbohydrate polymers known as glycosaminoglycans (GAGs) that are covalently linked to protein. The GAGs have a high density of negative charge and are highly hydrated, with associated water constituting more than 50% of the weight. GAGs and proteoglycans can associate to form highly organized complexes in the extracellular matrix, providing a gel-like matrix in which cells are embedded to form tissues.

Proteoglycan Structure

GAGs are long linear carbohydrate polymers that are covalently linked to protein by an O-glycosidic bond (**Part A**). The GAGs are tethered to the protein by a **linkage tetrasaccharide** containing xylose, galactose, and glucuronic acid. Extending from the linkage tetrasaccharide is a **repeating disaccharide**, which is usually composed of an amino sugar, either N-acetylglucosamine (GlcNAc) or N-acetylgalactosamine (GalNAc), and a uronic acid, either glucuronic acid or its 5-epimer, iduronic acid. The polymer may be as long as 1000 residues or more. The amino sugars are usually sulfated, and in some cases the uronic acid may also be sulfated. The sulfate groups and the carboxylate groups on the uronic acids give the polymer a high density of **negative charge**. A protein may have many GAGs extending from it, in the way that bristles extend from a test-tube brush. Synthesis of the repeating disaccharide requires UDP-GlcNAc, UDP-GalNAc, and UDP-glucuronic acid. Iduronic acid is formed by the epimerization of glucuronic acid after it has been incorporated into the chain. Sulfation requires 3'-phosphoadenosine-5'-phosphosulfate (PAPS) as an activated sulfate donor, and it occurs only after the monosaccharides are polymerized.

Glycosaminoglycan Composition and Distribution

The five classes of proteoglycans found in the extracellular matrix are hyaluronic acid, chondroitin sulfate, dermatan sulfate, keratan sulfate, and heparan sulfate (**Part B**). Hyaluronic acid differs from the other classes in three ways: it is found in both prokaryotic and eukaryotic systems, it contains no sulfate, and it is not covalently linked to protein. Heparin, a polymer structurally similar to heparan sulfate, is an intracellular compound rather than a component of the extracellular matrix. Heparin is found in mast cells that line the arteries of lungs, liver, and skin, and when secreted into the blood, it acts as an anticoagulant. Antithrombin III binds heparin, making it a better inhibitor of thrombin.

Cartilage Aggregan

Large aggregates of proteoglycans, known as aggregan, are found in cartilage (**Part C**). Aggregan is a highly organized macromolecular complex having a mass of 10^8 daltons or more. It consists of a central **hyaluronic acid** polymer that is associated with numerous **chondroitin sulfate and keratan sulfate polymers**. The chondroitin and keratan sulfates are noncovalently anchored to hyaluronic acid by proteins known as **link proteins**. Because of the structure and negative charge of aggregan, the associated water greatly increases its volume. The large volume of aggregan provides cartilage with the ability to cushion against mechanical stress.

Clinical Significance

Deficiencies in the enzymes that degrade proteoglycans result in a family of diseases known as the **mucopolysaccharidoses**. In adult tissues, the turnover of proteoglycans is relatively slow, having half-lives ranging from days to weeks. Proteoglycans are taken up from the extracellular matrix by invagination of the cell membrane. The vacuoles, which contain components of the extracellular matrix, fuse with lysosomes and the proteoglycans are degraded by lysosomal hydrolases. Degradation of GAGs requires the concerted action of several specific **endoglycosidases, exoglycosidases, and sulfatases**. Diseases resulting from deficiencies in these enzymes are listed in the following table, together with the clinical findings and the characteristic degradation product that accumulates with each disease. Most of the mucopolysaccharidoses are characterized by skeletal deformities and varying degrees of mental illness. Methods are available for the prenatal diagnosis of each of these diseases. All of the mucopolysaccharidoses except Hunter syndrome have an autosomal recessive inheritance pattern. Hunter syndrome shows X-linked inheritance.

Type	Enzyme Defect	Urinary Metabolites	Clinical Findings
MPS I: Hurler syndrome	α-L-Iduronidase	Dermatan sulfate, heparan sulfate	Skeletal deformities, mental retardation, and corneal clouding
MPS II: Hunter syndrome	Iduronidate sulfatase	Dermatan sulfate and heparan sulfate	Skeletal deformities, mental retardation, and deafness
MPS III: Sanfilippo syndrome, type A	Heparan sulfatase	Heparan sulfate	Mental retardation and mild skeletal changes
Sanfilippo syndrome, type B	α-N-Acetylglucosaminidase	Heparan sulfate	Mental retardation and mild skeletal changes
MPS IV: Morquio syndrome, type A	N-Acetylgalactosamine-6-sulfatase	Keratan sulfate	Severe skeletal deformities and corneal clouding
Morquio syndrome, type B	β-Galactosidase	Keratan sulfate	Severe skeletal deformities
MPS VII: Sly syndrome	β-D-Glucuronidase	Dermatan sulfate and heparan sulfate	Mental retardation

For more information see Coffee C, *Metabolism*. Fence Creek, pp 226–229, 234–236.

Directions: For each of the following questions, choose the **one best** answer.

1. All of the following compounds are reducing sugars **except:**

(A) Glucose

(B) Sucrose

(C) Lactose

(D) Fructose

(E) Galactose

2. An 8-year-old patient whose intestinal mucosa was deficient in iso-maltase activity was given a hydrogen breath test. Which of the following dietary carbohydrates would give a positive test?

(A) Milk

(B) Amylose

(C) Amylopectin

(D) Sucrose

(E) Maltose

3. Which of the following glucose transporters is located in the plasma membrane of muscle?

(A) GLUT-1

(B) GLUT-2

(C) GLUT-4

(D) GLUT-5

(E) SGLUT

4. Which of the following pathways in the liver is inhibited by insulin?

(A) Glycolysis

(B) Fatty acid synthesis

(C) Pentose phosphate pathway

(D) Fatty acid oxidation

(E) Glycogen synthesis

5. The secretion of glucagon by pancreatic α-cells is inhibited by an increase in the serum concentration of:

(A) Glucose

(B) Epinephrine

(C) Alanine

(D) Lysine

(E) All of the above

6. Which of the following enzymes is most directly activated by insulin?

(A) Glycogen synthase

(B) Acetyl CoA carboxylase

(C) Protein phosphatase

(D) Pyruvate dehydrogenase

(E) Glycogen phosphorylase

7. Which of the following pairs of enzymes is allosterically regulated in skeletal muscle?

(A) Phosphofructokinase-1 and glucokinase

(B) Hexokinase and pyruvate kinase

(C) 3-Phosphoglycerate kinase and phosphofructokinase-1

(D) Lactate dehydrogenase and pyruvate kinase

(E) Pyruvate kinase and aldolase

8. Glycolysis would be compromised by a deficiency in which of the following vitamins?

(A) Pantothenic acid

(B) Thiamine

(C) Biotin

(D) Niacin

(E) Riboflavin

9. Which of the following enzymes catalyzes a reaction that is irreversible under the conditions that exist within the cell?

(A) Lactate dehydrogenase

(B) Pyruvate carboxylase

(C) Alanine aminotransferase

(D) 3-Phosphoglycerate kinase

(E) Aldolase

10. Pyruvate dehydrogenase is:

(A) Phosphorylated by a protein kinase that is activated by acetyl CoA

(B) Active in its phosphorylated form

(C) Activated by NADH

(D) Most active when the insulin/glucagon ratio is low

(E) Located in the inner mitochondrial membrane

11. Which of the following statements about glycogenolysis is true?

(A) Glycogenolysis is enhanced by the activity of protein phosphatase.

(B) Glycogenolysis is allosterically activated by ATP.

(C) Glycogenolysis involves cleavage of both α-1,4 and β-1,6 glycosidic bonds.

(D) Glycogenolysis is stimulated by the binding of epinephrine to either α- or β-adrenergic receptors.

(E) Glycogenolysis in muscle supplies glucose that can be oxidized by the brain.

12. The most important allosteric effectors of glycolysis in muscle are:

(A) Isocitrate and glucose-6-phosphate

(B) Fructose-2,6-bisphosphate and ATP

(C) ATP and AMP

(D) Fructose-1,6-bisphosphate and alanine

(E) AMP and NADH

13. Which of the following enzymes is required to form branch points in glycogen?

(A) α-1,4 $\rightarrow$ α-1,6 Glucan transferase

(B) UDP-glucose pyrophosphorylase

(C) Glycogen phosphorylase

(D) α-1,4 $\rightarrow$ α-1,4 Glucan transferase

(E) Phosphoglucomutase

Questions 14–15 are based on the following clinical case:

A 6-month-old child was brought to the emergency room in a coma. His abdomen was swollen and his blood glucose was 28 mg/dL. Serum analysis showed a pH of 7.2 and elevated levels of lactate, fatty acids, and uric acid. His serum bicarbonate level was lower than normal.

14. The most likely diagnosis for this patient is:

(A) McArdle disease

(B) von Gierke disease

(C) Pompe disease

(D) Her disease

(E) Cori disease

15. Measurement of serum hormone levels in this patient would show:

(A) Elevated insulin

(B) Decreased glucagon

(C) Decreased epinephrine

(D) Elevated glucagon

(E) Decreased cortisol

16. A deficiency in which of the following vitamins would markedly compromise the ability to convert lactate to glucose?

(A) Pyridoxine

(B) Thiamine

(C) Biotin

(D) Riboflavin

(E) Folic acid

17. Which of the following pairs of enzymes are required for gluconeogenesis?

(A) Glucose-6-phosphatase and phosphofructokinase-1

(B) Pyruvate kinase and pyruvate carboxylase

(C) Fructose-1,6-bisphosphatase and pyruvate kinase

(D) Phosphoenolpyruvate carboxykinase and glucose-6-phosphatase

(E) Glucokinase and pyruvate carboxylase

18. Which of the following sets of amino acids are used as carbon sources for the de novo synthesis of glucose?

(A) Serine, alanine, leucine

(B) Aspartate, histidine, glutamate

(C) Glutamine, leucine, valine

(D) Tryptophan, glycine, lysine

(E) All of the above

19. Which of the following enzymes is active in its phosphorylated state?

(A) Glycogen synthase

(B) Fructose-2,6-bisphosphatase

(C) Pyruvate kinase

(D) Pyruvate dehydrogenase

(E) Phosphofructokinase-2

20. The most important allosteric activator of hepatic gluconeogenesis is:

(A) Acetyl CoA

(B) Glucose-6-phosphate

(C) Fructose-2,6-bisphosphate

(D) AMP

(E) Fructose-6-phosphate

21. A deficiency in which of the following enzymes is most likely to result in hemolytic anemia?

(A) Transketolase

(B) Glucose-6-phosphate dehydrogenase

(C) Myeloperoxidase

(D) NADPH oxidase

(E) Glucose-6-phosphatase

22. A deficiency in thiamine would impair the activity of which of the following enzymes?

(A) Glucose-6-phosphate dehydrogenase

(B) Glutathione peroxidase

(C) Transaldolase

(D) Glutathione reductase

(E) Transketolase

23. A deficiency in glucose-6-phosphate dehydrogenase would affect all of the following processes **except:**

(A) Cytochrome P_{450}-dependent detoxification reactions

(B) Gluconeogenesis from lactate

(C) Steroid hormone synthesis

(D) Fatty acid synthesis

(E) Superoxide production in phagocytes

24. Hereditary fructose intolerance results from a genetic deficiency in which of the following enzymes?

(A) Sorbitol dehydrogenase

(B) Phosphofructokinase

(C) Fructokinase

(D) Aldolase B

(E) Aldol reductase

25. Which of the following processes requires UDP-glucuronic acid as a substrate?

(A) Glycogen synthesis

(B) Glycoprotein synthesis

(C) Detoxification of bilirubin

(D) Synthesis of keratin sulfate

(E) Metabolism of galactose

26. The formation of cataracts is most commonly associated with a deficiency in which of the following enzymes?

(A) Fructokinase

(B) Galactokinase

(C) Aldol reductase

(D) Sorbitol dehydrogenase

(E) Aldolase B

27. The monosaccharide that links the asparagine side chain to oligosaccharide chains in N-linked glycoproteins is:

(A) Fucose

(B) Mannose

(C) N-Acetylglucosamine

(D) Glucose

(E) N-Acetylneuraminic acid

28. Which of the following descriptions applies to individuals with I-cell disease?

(A) Transfer of an oligosaccharide from dolichol phosphate to protein is impaired.

(B) Lysosomal enzymes are incorrectly targeted to mitochondria.

(C) Large inclusion bodies are found in the extracellular space.

(D) The formation of mannose-6-phosphate is impaired.

(E) Lysosomal enzymes cleave carbohydrate from serum glycoproteins.

29. All of the following characteristics describe glycosaminoglycans **except:**

(A) They are found in the extracellular matrix

(B) They have a high density of negative charge

(C) They contain N-acetylneuraminic acid

(D) They contain a repeating disaccharide

(E) They frequently contain iduronic acid

30. Hurler's syndrome results from a deficiency in which of the following enzymes?

(A) Heparin N-sulfatase

(B) α-L-iduronidase

(C) β-Glucuronidase

(D) Iduronidate sulfatase

(E) Arylsulfatase

PART III: ANSWERS AND EXPLANATIONS

1. The answer is B.

Reducing sugars must have an unsubstituted anomeric carbon atom. The C-1 of glucose and galactose and C-2 of fructose are unsubstituted anomeric carbon atoms that can reduce copper. In the disaccharide lactose, the C-1 of glucose is an unsubstituted anomeric carbon atom. In sucrose, the C-1 anomeric carbon of glucose is linked to the C-2 anomeric carbon of fructose, making sucrose unable to reduce copper.

2. The answer is C.

Isomaltase cleaves α-1,6 glycosidic bonds. Amylopectin is a form of plant starch that contains both α-1, 4 and α-1,6 glycosidic bonds. The deficiency of isomaltase in this patient will result in partially degraded amylopectin which will be further degraded by intestinal bacteria, releasing H_2 gas. Amylose and maltose contain only α-1,4 glycosidic

bonds, while milk sugar (lactose) contains β-1,4 glycosidic bonds and sucrose contains α-1,2 glycosidic bonds.

3. The answer is C.

GLUT-4 is the insulin-sensitive transporter that is found in muscle and adipose tissue. GLUT-2 is found in the basolateral membrane of intestinal cells and in the plasma membrane of liver. GLUT-5 is a fructose transporter, and SGLUT is the sodium-dependent glucose transporter that is found in the brush border membrane of intestinal and kidney cells.

4. The answer is D.

Insulin inhibits fatty acid oxidation by decreasing the rate of fatty acid entry into the mitochondria. Insulin activates pathways that allow energy in glucose to be stored as glycogen and fatty acids. For glucose to be converted to fatty acids, it must first be converted to pyruvate by glycolysis, followed by the oxidative decarboxylation of pyruvate to produce acetyl CoA. The substrates for fatty acid synthesis are acetyl CoA, ATP, and NADPH. Most of the NADPH is provided by the pentose phosphate pathway.

5. The answer is A.

The secretion of glucagon is inhibited by an increase in the concentration of blood glucose. Epinephrine and amino acids, particularly alanine and lysine, stimulate glucagon secretion.

6. The answer is C.

The binding of insulin to its receptor generates a second messenger that activates protein phosphatase, which in turn catalyzes the dephosphorylation and concomitant activation of a group of enzymes involved in energy storage pathways, including glycogen synthase, acetyl CoA carboxylase, and pyruvate dehydrogenase. In contrast, glycogen phosphorylase is inhibited by insulin and is active in the phosphorylated form.

7. The answer is B.

Hexokinase is allosterically inhibited by glucose-6-phosphate. Pyruvate kinase is allosterically activated by fructose-1,6-bisphosphate and allosterically inhibited by ATP. Phosphofructokinase-1 is activated by AMP and inhibited by ATP. Glucokinase is not present in skeletal muscle. 3-Phosphoglycerate kinase, lactate dehydrogenase, and aldolase are not subject to allosteric regulation.

8. The answer is D.

Niacin is the vitamin precursor of NAD^+. The only enzyme in the pathway of glycolysis that requires a coenzyme is glyceraldehyde-3-phosphate dehydrogenase. This enzyme catalyzes the oxidation of glyceraldehyde-3-phosphate to 1,3-bisphosphoglycerate and produces NADH.

9. The answer is B.

The reaction catalyzed by pyruvate carboxylase is irreversible under cellular conditions. Pyruvate carboxylase, the enzyme that converts pyruvate to oxaloacetate, is located in mitochondria where it catalyzes the first step in gluconeogenesis and is the major enzyme for replenishing intermediates in the tricarboxylic acid cycle.

10. The answer is A.

The pyruvate dehydrogenase complex is a multienzyme complex that is located in the mitochondrial matrix. It consists of three types of subunits that require five types of coenzymes to catalyze the oxidative decarboxylation of pyruvate to acetyl CoA. The complex also contains a specific protein kinase and protein phosphatase that regulate its activity. Pyruvate dehydrogenase is most active in the dephosphorylated state, a condition that exists when the insulin/glucagon ratio is high. Pyruvate dehydrogenase phosphatase is activated by insulin and pyruvate dehydrogenase kinase is activated by NADH and acetyl CoA.

11. The answer is D.

Hormones can activate glycogenolysis by either stimulating cAMP synthesis or increasing the intracellular Ca^{2+} concentration. Ca^{2+} allosterically activates phosphorylase kinase, whereas cAMP-dependent protein kinase A initiates a cascade of phosphorylation reactions that lead to the activation of glycogen phosphorylase, the enzyme that cleaves α-1,4 glycosidic bonds, releasing glucose-i-phosphate. Glycogenolysis can also be activated by the accumulation of AMP,

which allosterically activates the nonphosphorylated form of phosphorylase. Muscle glycogen cannot serve as a source of glucose for other tissues because glucose-6-phosphatase is absent in muscle. The two types of bonds found in glycogen are α-1,4 and α-1,6 glycosidic bonds.

12. The answer is C.

The rate-limiting step in glycolysis is catalyzed by phosphofructokinase-1. In muscle, the most important allosteric activator of this enzyme is AMP, whereas in liver the most important activator is fructose-2,6-bisphosphate. In both tissues, ATP and citrate are allosteric inhibitors. Isocitrate, glucose-6-phosphate, alanine, NADH, and fructose-1,6-phosphate are not significant allosteric effectors of phosphofructokinase-1 in either muscle or liver.

13. The answer is A.

Branch points in glycogen are created by α-1,4 → α-1,6 glucan transferase, which transfers an oligosaccharide containing 6-7 glucose residues from the nonreducing end of a chain to a glucose residue in the interior of the chain, where a new α-1,6 glycosidic bond is formed. In contrast, α-1,4 → α-1,4 glucan transferase is involved in the debranching of glycogen.

14. The answer is B.

These symptoms are consistent with von Gierke's disease, which results from a deficiency in glucose-6-phosphatase. The swollen abdomen, together with hypoglycemia, suggest that the patient is unable to degrade glycogen. A deficiency in this enzyme also prevents gluconeogenesis from being completed. Lactate, an important substrate for gluconeogenesis, accumulates. The accumulation of glucose-6-phosphate results in an increase in the pentose phosphate pathway and the synthesis of ribose-5-phosphate, which is used for purine nucleotide synthesis. When more purine nucleotides are made than are needed, the excess is degraded, resulting in the production of uric acid.

15. The answer is D.

The hypoglycemia would result in secretion of glucagon, epinephrine, and cortisol. Normally, glucagon stimulates hepatic glycogenolysis and gluconeogenesis, while epinephrine stimulates glycogenolysis and lipolysis and inhibits insulin secretion. Cortisol is less important in the short-term regulation of blood glucose, but it plays a key role in long-term regulation of blood glucose.

16. The answer is C.

The conversion of lactate to glucose involves oxidation to pyruvate and the subsequent carboxylation of pyruvate to oxaloacetate, the first step in gluconeogenesis. Pyruvate carboxylase requires biotin as a coenzyme. The only other coenzyme that is required to convert oxaloacetate to glucose is NADH, which is synthesized from niacin.

17. The answer is D.

There are four enzymes that are unique for gluconeogenesis: pyruvate carboxylase, phosphoenolpyruvate carboxykinase, fructose-1,6-bisphosphatase, and glucose-6-phosphatase. These four enzymes are required to bypass the three irreversible steps in glycolysis. The other enzymes listed are required for gluconeogenesis, but also participate in glycolysis.

18. The answer is B.

The only two amino acids found in proteins that cannot provide carbon for the net synthesis of glucose are leucine and lysine. These two amino acids are strictly ketogenic. The aromatic amino acids and isoleucine are both glucogenic and ketogenic. All of the other amino acids are strictly glucogenic.

19. The answer is B.

The synthesis and degradation of fructose-2,6-bisphosphate are catalyzed by phosphofructokinase-2 and fructose-2,6-bisphosphatase, respectively. The activity of these two enzymes is coordinately regulated by phosphorylation. cAMP-dependent phosphorylation inhibits the synthesis of fructose-2,6-bisphosphate and stimulates its degradation. The level of fructose-2,6-bisphosphate in liver is controlled by the insulin/glucagon ratio. When insulin is elevated, the intracellular concentration of fructose-2,6-bisphosphate is elevated, and vice versa.

20. The answer is A.

Acetyl CoA is required for the activation of pyruvate carboxylase. Fructose-2,6-bisphosphate and AMP are allosteric inhibitors of fructose-1,6-bisphosphatase.

21. The answer is B.

NADPH plays an important role in preventing lysis of red blood cells by helping maintain a high level of reduced glutathione. The first enzyme in the pathway for generating NADPH is glucose-6-phosphate dehydrogenase, which is very active in red blood cells. Glucose-6-phosphatase is found only in liver and kidney where it participates in gluconeogenesis, and NADPH oxidase and myeloperoxidase are found in neutrophils where they participate in bactericidal mechanisms. Transketolase is found in red blood cells where it is a component of the pentose phosphate pathway, but it is not involved in NADPH production.

22. The answer is E.

Transketolase, a key enzyme in the pentose phosphate cycle, requires thiamine pyrophosphate for activity. It is the only enzyme in the nonoxidative phase of the pentose phosphate pathway that requires a coenzyme.

23. The answer is B.

All of the pathways listed except gluconeogenesis require NADPH, which is provided primarily from the pentose phosphate pathway. The first reaction in the pentose phosphate pathway is catalyzed by glucose-6-phosphate dehydrogenase. Gluconeogenesis requires NADH but not NADPH.

24. The answer is D.

Aldolase B cleaves fructose-1-phosphate to dihydroxyacetone phosphate and glyceraldehyde. A deficiency in this enzyme results in the accumulation of fructose-1-phosphate.

25. The answer is C.

The liver conjugates bilirubin with glucuronic acid, rendering it sufficiently soluble to be excreted in the bile. This conjugation reaction uses UDP-glucuronic acid as the activated donor of glucuronic acid. Glycogen synthesis, glycoprotein synthesis, and the metabolism of galactose require UDP-glucose, but not UDP-glucuronic acid. Keratin sulfate is the only glycosaminoglycan whose synthesis does not require UDP-glucuronic acid as a substrate.

26. The answer is B.

A deficiency in galactokinase results in the accumulation of blood galactose, which is taken up by the lens where aldol reductase reduces it to galactitol. Galactitol is a dead end product that can neither be metabolized nor transported out of the cell. Its formation depletes NADPH, resulting in the inability to maintain reduced glutathione levels, conditions that eventually lead to cataract formation.

27. The answer is C.

The linkage between carbohydrate and protein in all N-linked glycoproteins is between C-1 of N-acetylglucosamine and the amide N of an asparagine side chain.

28. The answer is D.

The step in glycoprotein synthesis that targets certain enzymes to the lysosomes is the phosphorylation of selected mannose residues in the oligosaccharide chain of glycoproteins. In I cell disease, the formation of mannose-6-phosphate does not occur due to a deficiency in N-acetylglucosaminylphosphotransferase. Instead of ending up in the lysosomes, these proteins are secreted into the plasma, where they are inactive because of their low pH optimum. However, if a sample of plasma is acidified, these enzymes are fully active. The lysosomes of patients with I-cell disease contain inclusion bodies that are filled with glycosaminoglycans that have been taken up from the extracellular space but cannot be degraded.

29. The answer is C.

N-acetylneuraminic acid is not found in glycosaminoglycans, although it is present in both glycoproteins and glycolipids. Glycosaminoglycans are made up of repeating disaccharide units that usually consist of an amino sugar and a uronic acid. They have a high degree of negative charge due to the presence of sulfate and carboxyl groups, and approximately 50% of the weight of glycosaminoglycans can be attributed to associated water. The glycosaminoglycans are found in the extracellular space where they act as shock absorbers and lubricants.

30. The answer is B.

Hurler's syndrome, also known as type I mucopolysaccharidosis, results from an inherited deficiency in α-L-iduronidase. It is characterized by skeletal deformities, mental retardation, and corneal clouding.

PART IV
Lipid Metabolism

Lipid Digestion and Absorption

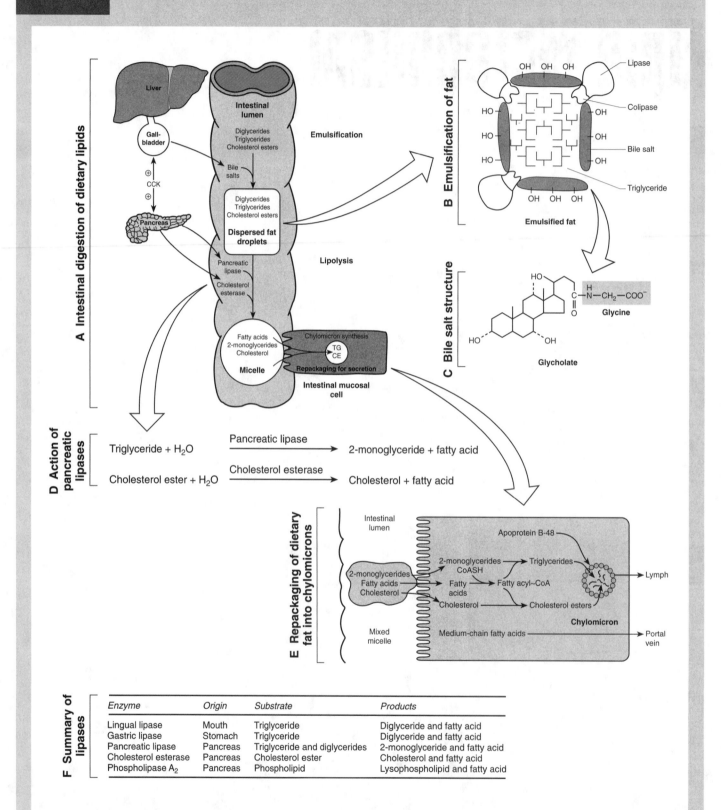

A Intestinal digestion of dietary lipids

Liver

Gall-bladder

CCK

Pancreas

Intestinal lumen

Diglycerides
Triglycerides
Cholesterol esters

Bile salts

Emulsification

Diglycerides
Triglycerides
Cholesterol esters

Dispersed fat droplets

Pancreatic lipase

Cholesterol esterase

Lipolysis

Fatty acids
2-monoglycerides
Cholesterol

Micelle

Chylomicron synthesis

TG
CE

Repackaging for secretion

Intestinal mucosal cell

B Emulsification of fat

OH OH OH

Lipase

Colipase

HO — OH

HO — OH

HO — OH

Bile salt

Triglyceride

OH OH OH

Emulsified fat

C Bile salt structure

HO

H—N—CH₂—COO⁻

Glycine

HO — OH

Glycholate

D Action of pancreatic lipases

$$\text{Triglyceride} + H_2O \xrightarrow{\text{Pancreatic lipase}} \text{2-monoglyceride} + \text{fatty acid}$$

$$\text{Cholesterol ester} + H_2O \xrightarrow{\text{Cholesterol esterase}} \text{Cholesterol} + \text{fatty acid}$$

E Repackaging of dietary fat into chylomicrons

Intestinal lumen

Apoprotein B-48

2-monoglycerides
Fatty acids
Cholesterol

2-monoglycerides
CoASH → Triglycerides

Fatty acids → Fatty acyl~CoA

Cholesterol → Cholesterol esters

Lymph

Chylomicron

Mixed micelle

Medium-chain fatty acids → Portal vein

F Summary of lipases

Enzyme	Origin	Substrate	Products
Lingual lipase	Mouth	Triglyceride	Diglyceride and fatty acid
Gastric lipase	Stomach	Triglyceride	Diglyceride and fatty acid
Pancreatic lipase	Pancreas	Triglyceride and diglycerides	2-monoglyceride and fatty acid
Cholesterol esterase	Pancreas	Cholesterol ester	Cholesterol and fatty acid
Phospholipase A₂	Pancreas	Phospholipid	Lysophospholipid and fatty acid

OVERVIEW

Dietary fat consists mainly of triglyceride, with smaller amounts of cholesterol, cholesterol esters, and phospholipids. Digestion of triglyceride begins in the mouth with lingual lipase and continues in the stomach with gastric lipase, which together hydrolyze small amounts of triglyceride to fatty acids and diglycerides. The hydrolysis of fat in the mouth and stomach is slow because the fat has not been emulsified. Most of the digestion of dietary fat occurs in the small intestine, where emulsification is followed by hydrolysis, which is catalyzed by pancreatic enzymes. The products of fat digestion diffuse into intestinal mucosal cells, where they are reesterified and then assembled into chylomicrons, which are secreted into the lymphatics. Failure to digest and absorb lipids leads to the excretion of excessive amounts of fat in the feces.

Intestinal Digestion of Dietary Lipids

Cholecystokinin (CCK), a hormone secreted by the intestinal mucosa, initiates two events leading to lipolysis (**Part A**): 1) it binds to receptors on the gall bladder, resulting in contraction and release of bile salts into the lumen; and 2) it stimulates the release of pancreatic enzymes from the exocrine pancreatic cells into the intestinal lumen. The bile salts disperse the large lipid droplets, providing smaller particles that are more easily hydrolyzed by the pancreatic enzymes.

Emulsification of Fat

The fat globules entering the small intestine are too large to be hydrolyzed efficiently by lipases. The **bile salts** act as emulsifying agents, dispersing large fat globules into smaller particles that have a larger surface area for the lipolytic enzymes to bind. The dispersed particles (**Part B**) consist of bile salts that surround a core of neutral lipid consisting primarily of triglyceride. The bile salts are **amphipathic molecules** having two or three hydroxyl groups that project from the same side of the hydrophobic steroid ring system. They also have a side chain attached to the five-membered ring that is completely ionized at the pH in the small intestine (**Part C**). These structural properties make the bile salts good detergents and effective emulsification agents. The bile salts are synthesized from cholesterol in the liver and are stored in the gall bladder. One of the primary bile salts is **glycocholate**, which has three hydroxyl groups attached to the ring system and a side chain carboxyl group that is conjugated with glycine.

Action of Pancreatic Enzymes

The pancreatic enzymes that are most important in digestion of dietary lipids are **pancreatic lipase** and **cholesterol esterase (Part D)**. Pancreatic lipase requires **colipase**, a small protein secreted by the pancreas, which anchors pancreatic lipase to the surface of dispersed lipid particles (**Part B**). The products derived from the action of pancreatic lipase and cholesterol esterase are **fatty acids, 2-monoglyceride**, and **unesterified cholesterol**. The products form mixed micelles with bile salts. At the surface of the brush border membrane, the products diffuse into the intestinal mucosal cell.

Repacking of Dietary Fat into Chylomicrons

Fatty acids, unesterified cholesterol, and 2-monoglyceride diffuse into the intestinal cell, leaving the bile salts in the lumen (**Part E**). Once inside the cell, triglycerides and cholesterol esters are reformed, packaged into chylomicrons and secreted. Esterification of fatty acids requires that they first be converted to fatty acyl CoA, a reaction catalyzed by **fatty acyl CoA synthetase**. This reaction, shown below, requires ATP as a source of energy.

$$R\text{-COOH} + CoASH + ATP \xrightarrow{\substack{\text{Fatty acyl CoA} \\ \text{synthetase}}} R\text{-}\overset{\displaystyle O}{\overset{\displaystyle \|}{C}}\text{-SCoA} + AMP + 2P_i$$

Triglycerides are reformed by the action of **fatty acyl CoA transferase**, which transfers fatty acids from CoA to the glycerol backbone of 2-monoglyceride. Similarly, cholesterol esters are reformed in a reaction catalyzed by **acyl CoA:cholesterol acyltransferase (ACAT)**. Fatty acids having ten carbons or less are not reesterified, but are released into the portal blood where they are transferred by albumin to the liver. Triglycerides and cholesterol esters, together with **apoprotein B-48** and **phospholipids**, are packaged into chylomicrons, which are secreted into the lymphatic capillaries and carried to the thoracic duct, where they enter the general circulation.

Summary of Lipases Involved in Digestion of Dietary Fat

The lipases involved in digestion of dietary fat originate in the mouth, stomach, and pancreas (**Part F**). Triglyceride hydrolysis in the mouth and stomach by lingual and gastric lipases accounts for about 10% of triglyceride hydrolysis in adults and as much as 40% to 50% in infants and small children whose major source of fat is milk. Milk is rich in medium chain triglycerides, which are highly emulsified in homogenized milk.

Clinical Significance

Failure to digest and absorb fat leads to the excretion of an excessive amount of fat in the feces, a condition known as **steatorrhea**. Quantitative determination of fecal fat is commonly used to establish the presence of steatorrhea. Normally, fecal fat excretion is less than 10% of the ingested fat. Malabsorption can occur either from 1) **pancreatic insufficiency**, which is usually secondary to cystic fibrosis; 2) **bile salt deficiency** due to either liver disease or obstruction in the bile duct; or 3) **defective chylomicron synthesis** due to the inability to synthesize apoprotein B-48, a condition known as **abetalipoproteinemia**. Since fat-soluble vitamins are absorbed and transported along with dietary fat, malabsorption syndromes frequently result in a deficiency of one or more of the fat-soluble vitamins.

For more information see Coffee C, *Metabolism*. Fence Creek, pp 243–253.

36 Structure and Function of Lipoproteins

A Lipoprotein structure

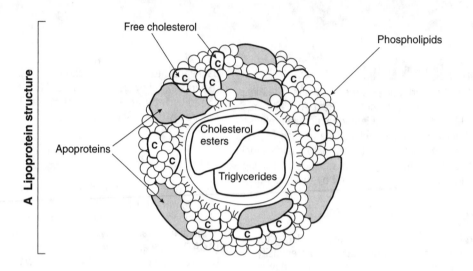

Free cholesterol

Phospholipids

Cholesterol esters

Triglycerides

Apoproteins

B Separation of lipoproteins

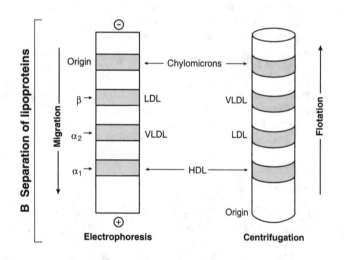

⊖

Origin

Migration

β → LDL

α₂ → VLDL

α₁

⊕

Electrophoresis

← Chylomicrons →

VLDL

LDL

← HDL →

Flotation

Origin

Centrifugation

C Physical properties

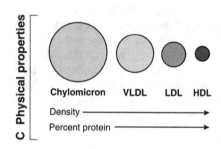

Chylomicron   **VLDL**   **LDL**   **HDL**

Density ——————→

Percent protein ——————→

E Apoprotein function

Apo A	Reverse cholesterol transport
Apo B	LDL receptor binding and clearance
Apo C	Regulation of lipoprotein lipase
Apo E	Remnant receptor binding and clearance

D Source, function, and apoprotein content

Lipoprotein	Source	Function	Apoproteins
Chylomicron	Intestine	Transport dietary triglyceride to peripheral tissues	Apo B-48, apo C-II, and apo E
Very-low-density lipoprotein (VLDL)	Liver	Transport endogenous triglyceride to peripheral tissues	Apo B-100, apo C-II, and apo E
Intermediate-density lipoprotein (IDL)	Plasma VLDLs	Triglyceride transport and precursor of LDL	Apo B-100, apo C-II, and apo E
Low-density lipoprotein (LDL)	Plasma IDLs	Transport cholesterol to peripheral tissues	Apo B-100
High-density lipoprotein	Liver and intestine	Reservoir of apoproteins and reverse cholesterol transport	Apo A, apo C, and apo E

The plasma lipoproteins are large water-soluble macromolecular complexes that transport insoluble lipids in the blood. The protein components of lipoproteins are known as apoproteins or apolipoproteins. Although each lipoprotein is characterized as belonging to one of four or five major classes, the classes do not have a static composition, and heterogeneity exists within each class. The metabolic fate of a lipoprotein is usually determined by its complement of apoproteins.

Lipoprotein Structure

In general, the structures of the lipoproteins are very similar, being roughly spherical in shape (**Part A**). The hydrophobic components, triglycerides and cholesterol esters, are located in the core, which is surrounded by a monolayer of amphipathic components consisting of apoproteins, phospholipids, and unesterified cholesterol. The polar head groups of the amphipathic components interact with the aqueous surroundings, thereby rendering the particle soluble. The lipoprotein classes differ primarily in size and density, properties that are related to the relative content of lipid and protein.

Separation of Major Lipoproteins

Four classes of lipoproteins can be separated from one another by either centrifugation or electrophoresis (**Part B**). Separation by **centrifugation** is based on **density**. When placed in a centrifugal field, the rate at which each lipoprotein floats upward through a salt solution depends on the relative amount of triglyceride. Chylomicrons have the lowest density and have the greatest flotation rate, followed by very-low-density lipoproteins (VLDLs), low-density lipoproteins (LDLs), and high-density lipoproteins (HDLs). Separation by **electrophoresis** is based on the **charge/size ratio** of the lipoprotein. Chylomicrons remain at the origin. LDLs migrate with the plasma β-globulins, VLDLs migrate with the α_2-globulins, and LDLs migrate with the α_1-globulins.

Physical Properties

Chylomicrons have the largest diameter, the lowest proportion of protein, and the lowest density (0.92 to 0.96 g/mL), while HDLs have the smallest diameter, the highest proportion of protein, and the highest density (1.063 and 1.125) (**Part C**). The diameter, proportion of protein, and density of VLDLs and LDLs are intermediate, respectively, between chylomicrons and HDLs.

Source, Function, and Apoprotein Content

Chylomicrons are synthesized only in the intestinal mucosal cells, where they are assembled as vehicles for transporting dietary fat (**Part D**). Lipids make up about 98% of chylomicrons, with 88% of the lipid being triglyceride. Nascent chylomicrons contain apo B-48. The other apoproteins found in chylomicrons (apo C-II and apo E) are acquired from HDLs after the chylomicrons enter the circulation. **VLDLs** are synthesized only in the liver, and their function is to transport endogenous triglycerides to extrahepatic tissues. Lipids make up about 90% of VLDLs, with about 55% of the lipid being triglyceride and 15% cholesterol esters. Nascent VLDLs contain only apo B-100. Other apoproteins (apo C-II and apo E) are acquired from HDL after entering

the blood. The progressive release of fatty acids from VLDL triglyceride results in a heterogeneous population of intermediate-density lipoproteins (**IDLs**), which can be further degraded to **LDLs**. The transformation of VLDLs to IDLs and LDLs is accompanied by a change in the neutral lipid core, which is progressively depleted of triglyceride and enriched in cholesterol esters. The apoprotein composition also changes as VLDLs are hydrolyzed to IDLs and LDLs. As the lipoproteins become smaller, apo C and apo E return to HDLs. LDL, the end product of VLDL, contains only apo B-100, and cholesterol esters make up about 50% of the total lipid. The major function of **LDLs** is to deliver cholesterol to extrahepatic tissues. **HDLs** are synthesized by both liver and intestinal cells. HDLs play a major role in transporting cholesterol from extrahepatic tissues to the liver, where it can be metabolized and excreted. HDLs also act as a circulating reservoir of apo C and apo E, which are readily exchanged with other lipoproteins. HDLs also contain apo A, which is not exchanged.

Apoprotein Function

The four major classes of apoproteins are apo A, apo B, apo C, and apo E (**Part E**). All four classes are synthesized by the liver, while only apo A and apo B-48 are synthesized by intestinal cells. Although several subtypes of apoproteins have been identified, the functions of all the subtypes are not completely understood. It is clear, however, that the complement of apoproteins in a particular lipoprotein is primarily responsible for the fate of the lipoprotein. **Apo A** is required for HDL to participate in reverse cholesterol transport from extrahepatic tissues back to the liver. **Apo B** binds to LDL receptors on the surface of cells, allowing LDLs to be taken up and cleared from the blood. **Apo C** regulates the activity of lipoprotein lipase, the extracellular enzyme that hydrolyzes chylomicron and VLDL triglyceride. **Apo E** binds to remnant receptors on the liver, allowing chylomicron remnants and IDLs to be cleared from the blood.

Clinical Significance

Both electrophoresis and centrifugation are used in clinical laboratories for diagnosis of hyperlipidemia and hypolipidemia. The measurement of serum cholesterol and triglyceride levels in plasma is not sufficient for making a diagnosis because these lipids are present in several different interactive lipoproteins. **Qualitative data** on the relative proportion of each lipoprotein can be obtained by electrophoretic separation. However, **quantitative analysis of the lipid composition** of each lipoprotein requires prior separation of the lipoprotein by centrifugation.

For more information see Coffee C, *Metabolism*. Fence Creek, pp 257–260.

37 Chylomicron Metabolism

A Lipid composition of chylomicrons

Triglyceride	88%
Phospholipid	8%
Cholesterol ester	3%
Cholesterol	1%

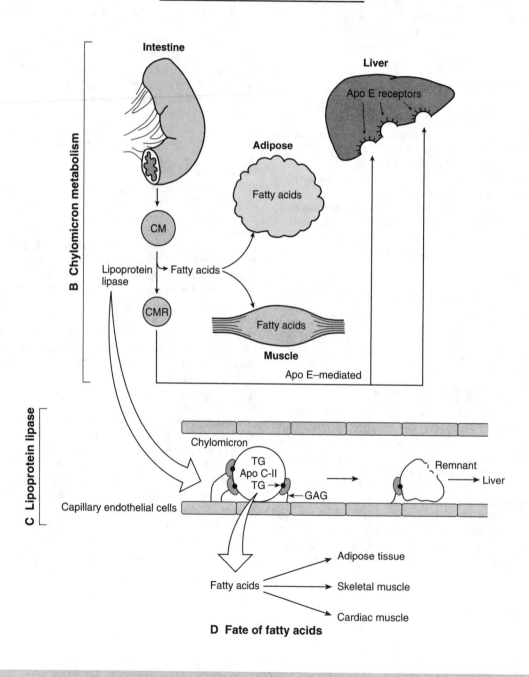

B Chylomicron metabolism

Intestine

Liver

Apo E receptors

Adipose

Fatty acids

CM

Lipoprotein lipase → Fatty acids

CMR

Fatty acids

Muscle

Apo E–mediated

C Lipoprotein lipase

Chylomicron

TG
Apo C-II
TG → ← GAG

Capillary endothelial cells

Remnant → Liver

Fatty acids → Adipose tissue
→ Skeletal muscle
→ Cardiac muscle

D Fate of fatty acids

OVERVIEW

Chylomicrons transport dietary triglyceride from the gastrointestinal tract to various tissues. Chylomicrons are rapidly cleared from the blood, having a half-life of less than an hour, and after an overnight fast they have normally disappeared from the plasma. Chylomicrons are synthesized in the Golgi of intestinal mucosal cells and delivered to the blood via the lymphatic system. Hydrolysis of chylomicron triglyceride by lipoprotein lipase releases fatty acids that are taken up by tissues. Since the chylomicrons are delivered to the blood by the lymphatic system and do not enter the portal blood, they are hydrolyzed by peripheral tissues before being presented to the liver. Following triglyceride hydrolysis, the chylomicron remnants bind to remnant receptors on the liver and are taken up by endocytosis.

Composition of Chylomicrons

Chylomicrons are composed of more than 98% lipid and less than 2% protein. Triglyceride constitutes about 88% of the total lipid (**Part A**). The nascent chylomicrons secreted by the intestinal mucosal cells contain **apo B-48**, an essential structural component that is required for secretion. After entering the circulation, the chylomicrons acquire apo C-II and apo E from high-density lipoprotein (HDL).

Metabolism of Chylomicrons

Nascent chylomicrons can neither be metabolized nor cleared from the blood because they do not contain apo C-II and apo E. However, after acquiring apo C-II from HDL, chylomicron triglyceride can be hydrolyzed to fatty acids and glycerol by **lipoprotein lipase (Part B)**. Triglyceride hydrolysis occurs in the capillary bed of tissues, with most of the hydrolysis occurring in adipose tissue, heart, and skeletal muscle. The fatty acids released from triglyceride diffuse into the tissues, where they are either converted to triglycerides for storage (adipose tissue) or oxidized for energy (heart and skeletal muscle). The liver does not metabolize circulating chylomicrons. The **chylomicron remnants** produced by triglyceride hydrolysis are about half the size of the nascent chylomicrons. They contain about 20% of the original dietary triglycerides and all of the dietary cholesterol esters. Apo E, present on the surface of the chylomicron remnants, binds to receptors on the liver, allowing the remnants to be taken up by receptor-mediated endocytosis. Liver is the only tissue having remnant receptors.

Lipoprotein Lipase

Lipoprotein lipase (**Part C**) is specific for lipoprotein triglyceride, and hydrolyzes triglyceride in chylomicrons, very-low-density lipoproteins and intermediate-density lipoproteins. All of these circulating lipoproteins contain **apo C-II**, which is essential for catalytic activity. Lipoprotein lipase is an extracellular enzyme that is attached to the luminal walls of the capillaries. It is anchored to the surface of endothelial cells by **glycosaminoglycan (GAG)** chains of heparan sulfate. Lipoprotein lipase is found in highest concentrations in the capillary bed of adipose tissue, heart, and skeletal muscle where triglycerides in chylomicrons are hydrolyzed, releasing fatty acids that are taken up by these tissues (**Part D**). Smaller amounts of lipoprotein lipase have been found in most other tissues except liver. Lipoprotein lipase is synthesized by parenchymal cells of most tissues and subsequently transferred to the luminal surface of vascular endothelial cells. Different tissues synthesize **different isozymes** of lipoprotein lipase. The isozyme synthesized in adipose tissue has a K_m for triglycerides that is about 10 times higher than that of the heart and skeletal muscle isozyme. Therefore, as the triglyceride concentration decreases during the transition between the fed and fasting state, the heart and skeletal muscle isozyme remains saturated, while the level of activity in adipose tissue diminishes. Additionally, the expression of lipoprotein lipase activity is **hormonally controlled**. The synthesis of the adipose tissue isozyme is increased by insulin in the well-fed state and declines in the fasting state. In contrast, the isozyme in other tissues is increased in the fasting state and declines in the well-fed state. These regulatory patterns are effective in **redirecting the uptake of fatty acids from adipose tissue to other tissues during the fasting state**.

Clinical Significance

Several types of **primary hyperlipidemia** result from inherited defects in the synthesis, metabolism, or clearance of lipoproteins. These diseases are characterized by elevated plasma lipids. There are three broad categories of primary hyperlipidemia, based on the type of lipid that accumulates in the plasma. In **type I** hyperlipidemia, triglyceride accumulates; in **type II**, cholesterol accumulates; and in **type III**, both triglyceride and cholesterol accumulate. Each of these classes can be subdivided, based on the nature of the lipoproteins that accumulate. Type I hyperlipidemia, also known as hyperchylomicronemia, is usually caused by a genetic deficiency in either lipoprotein lipase (type Ia) or in apo C-II (type Ib). The accumulation of chylomicrons gives the plasma a **milky appearance**, and, if stored at 4° C overnight, a characteristic **creamy layer** is found at the top of clear plasma. The most common clinical findings associated with hyperchylomicronemia are **recent memory loss, abdominal pain**, and **eruptive xanthomas**. It is also noteworthy that hyperlipidemia results secondary to many other diseases and is not necessarily limited to defects in the synthesis, metabolism, or uptake of lipoproteins.

For more information see Coffee C, *Metabolism*. Fence Creek, pp 261–268.

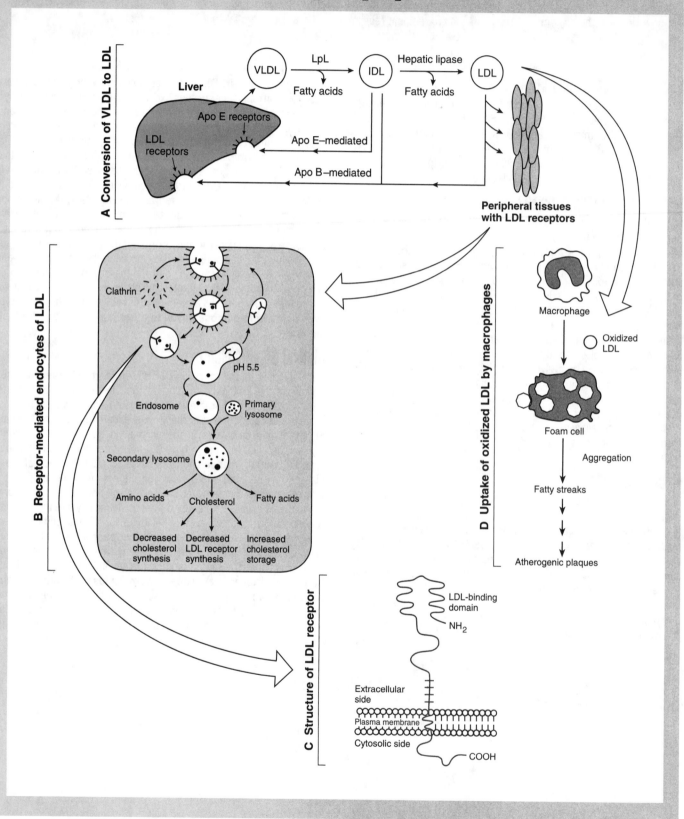

A Conversion of VLDL to LDL

Liver

VLDL → (LpL) → IDL → (Hepatic lipase) → LDL

Fatty acids

Fatty acids

Apo E receptors

LDL receptors

Apo E–mediated

Apo B–mediated

Peripheral tissues with LDL receptors

B Receptor-mediated endocytes of LDL

Clathrin

pH 5.5

Endosome

Primary lysosome

Secondary lysosome

Amino acids

Cholesterol

Fatty acids

Decreased cholesterol synthesis

Decreased LDL receptor synthesis

Increased cholesterol storage

C Structure of LDL receptor

LDL-binding domain

NH₂

Extracellular side

Plasma membrane

Cytosolic side

COOH

D Uptake of oxidized LDL by macrophages

Macrophage

Oxidized LDL

Foam cell

Aggregation

Fatty streaks

Atherogenic plaques

OVERVIEW

Very-low-density lipoproteins (VLDLs) are synthesized by the liver, whereas intermediate-density lipoproteins (IDLs) and low-density lipoproteins (LDLs) are derived from circulating VLDLs by the progressive hydrolysis of triglyceride. The function of VLDLs and LDLs is to transport triglyceride and cholesterol, respectively, from the liver to extrahepatic tissues. The metabolism of VLDLs is similar to that of chylomicrons, with the major difference being that VLDL triglyceride hydrolysis occurs primarily in the capillary bed of cardiac and skeletal muscle rather than adipose tissue. Approximately 25% of the IDLs are converted to LDLs, and the remainder are taken up by the liver. LDLs deliver cholesterol to cells by binding to LDL receptors and being internalized by receptor-mediated endocytosis. Oxidized LDLs bind to scavenger receptors on macrophages. The uncontrolled uptake of LDLs by macrophages is an early step in the development of atherogenic plaques.

Conversion of VLDL to LDL

Triglyceride and cholesterol esters constitute about 55% and 15%, respectively, of the lipid in the nascent VLDLs secreted by the liver. The only apoprotein present in nascent VLDLs is apo B-100. Circulating VLDLs acquire apo C-II and apo E from HDL after secretion into the plasma. VLDLs that contain apo C-II can be hydrolyzed by **lipoprotein lipase (Part A)**, releasing free fatty acids and producing IDLs. The fatty acids are taken up by cardiac and skeletal muscle where they are oxidized. IDLs have two possible fates: 1) they can bind to either remnant receptors or LDL receptors on liver and be cleared from the circulation; or 2) they can be further metabolized to LDLs. As IDLs get progressively smaller, the apoprotein content changes, with apo C-II and apo E being donated back to HDL. IDLs that have been depleted of apo C-II have a low affinity for lipoprotein lipase and are hydrolyzed to LDL by **hepatic lipase**, an extracellular enzyme located on the sinusoidal surfaces of the liver. About 70% of the total plasma cholesterol is found in the LDL particle. LDL has an oily core that contains about 1500 molecules of cholesterol ester. The core is surrounded by a surface monolayer containing phospholipid, unesterified cholesterol, and apo B-100. Apo B-100 interacts with the LDL receptor, allowing LDLs to be cleared from the plasma.

Receptor-Mediated Endocytosis of LDL

The primary function of LDL is to deliver cholesterol to extrahepatic tissues. Cells require cholesterol for the synthesis of plasma membranes, and some cells require additional cholesterol for the synthesis of specialized products. Cellular cholesterol can be obtained either from de novo synthesis or from receptor-mediated endocytosis of LDL (**Part B**). All nucleated cells contain **LDL receptors** that bind **apo B-100** of the LDL particle. LDL receptors are located in discrete regions of the plasma membrane known as "**coated pits.**" The cytosolic surface of the pit is coated with **clathrin**, a protein that polymerizes to form a scaffold that stabilizes the "coated pit" structure. Internalization of the receptor–LDL complex begins within 2 to 5 minutes after binding and occurs in several steps: 1) endocytosis of the receptor–LDL complex releases a clathrin-coated vesicle into the cytosol; 2) the clathrin coat is shed, forming an endosome; 3) the endosome is acidified to a pH between 5.0 and 5.5, resulting in dissociation of LDL from its receptor; 4) the regions of the endosome containing receptor bud off and are recycled to the plasma membrane; and 5) the regions of the endosome containing LDL fuse with lysosomes, where the LDL particle is degraded to amino acids, fatty acids, and unesterified cholesterol. The unesterified cholesterol affects three intracellular processes that reduce further accumulation of cholesterol: 1) **3-hydroxy-3-methylglutaryl coenzyme A (HMG CoA) reductase**, the rate-limiting enzyme in cholesterol synthesis, is inhibited; 2) **Acyl CoA:cholesterol acyltransferase (ACAT)**, the enzyme that converts intracellular cholesterol to cholesterol esters, is stimulated; and 3) **LDL receptor synthesis** is inhibited, thereby decreasing additional cholesterol uptake.

LDL Receptor Structure

All nucleated cells have cell-surface receptors that bind LDL and allow the particle to be internalized (**Part C**). The LDL receptor has several domains, including an extracellular domain that binds LDL, a membrane-spanning domain that anchors the receptor in the membrane, and a cytosolic domain that interacts with clathrin. The gene for the LDL receptor is located on chromosome 19.

Uptake of Oxidized LDL by Macrophages

Macrophages have **scavenger receptors** that have a high affinity for chemically modified forms of LDL, particularly **oxidized LDL (Part D)**. The synthesis of scavenger receptors, unlike that of LDL receptors, is not regulated by the accumulation of intracellular cholesterol. Therefore, uncontrolled uptake of oxidized LDL occurs, resulting in the transformation of macrophages into **foam cells**. The accumulation of foam cells in the walls of blood vessels results in **fatty streaks**. If foam cells continue to form over a long period of time, they become a part of **atherogenic plaques**.

Clinical Significance

Familial hypercholesterolemia (FH), the most common type II hyperlipidemia, results from an inherited defect in the LDL receptor. This disease occurs in about 1 in 500 people and is inherited as an autosomal dominant disorder. Individuals heterozygous for the FH gene have serum cholesterol levels that are approximately twice the normal value. In individuals homozygous for FH, plasma levels may reach 5 to 8 times the normal level. Affected individuals frequently have xanthomas and premature coronary artery disease. **Abetalipoproteinemia** results from the inability to synthesize apo B-100 and apo B-48, a truncated form of apo B-100. Serum levels of chylomicrons and VLDLs are low. Clinical symptoms include retinitis pigmentosa and the accumulation of acantocytes in the blood.

For more information see Coffee C, *Metabolism*. Fence Creek, pp 261–268.

39 High-Density Lipoprotein Metabolism

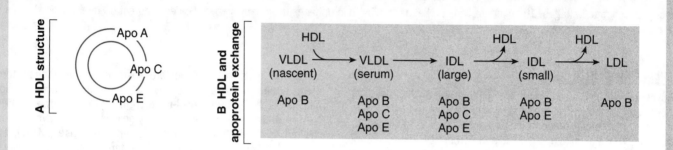

A HDL structure

Apo A
Apo C
Apo E

B HDL and apoprotein exchange

HDL → HDL → HDL

VLDL (nascent) → VLDL (serum) → IDL (large) → IDL (small) → LDL

Apo B	Apo B	Apo B	Apo B	Apo B
	Apo C	Apo C	Apo E	
	Apo E	Apo E		

C HDL and reverse cholesterol transport

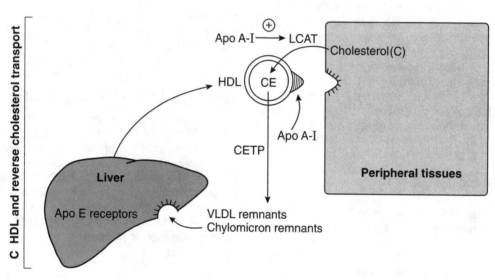

Apo A-I → LCAT ⊕

Cholesterol(C)

HDL CE

Apo A-I

CETP

Liver

Apo E receptors

VLDL remnants
Chylomicron remnants

Peripheral tissues

D HDL heterogeneity

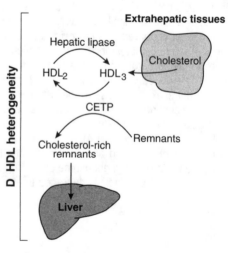

Extrahepatic tissues

Hepatic lipase

HDL₂ ← HDL₃ ← Cholesterol

CETP

Cholesterol-rich remnants ← Remnants

Liver

OVERVIEW

The primary source of high-density lipoproteins (HDLs) is the liver, although a small amount is derived from intestinal mucosal cells. HDLs contain apo A, apo C, and apo E. Two enzymes, lecithin-cholesterol acyltransferase (LCAT) and cholesterol ester transfer protein (CETP), are also associated with circulating HDL particles. Two major functions are attributed to HDLs: 1) they exchange apo E and apo C with other lipoproteins; and 2) they are essential for reverse cholesterol transport from extrahepatic tissues to the liver, where cholesterol can be degraded to bile acids and excreted. High levels of HDL offer protection from coronary heart disease.

HDL Structure

Approximately 50% of the mass of HDLs is protein. The nascent HDLs synthesized by the liver are **disc-like particles** that resemble membrane bilayers. They contain phospholipids and unesterified cholesterol, but very few cholesterol esters. The nascent HDLs are transformed into **spherical particles** as they accumulate cholesterol esters. HDLs contain apo A, C, and E (**Part A**). The most abundant apoprotein is apo A, which acts both as an essential structural component of the HDL particle and as a mediator of reverse cholesterol transport.

HDL and Apoprotein Exchange

HDLs serve as a circulating reservoir of apoproteins, with apo C and apo E being readily exchanged with other lipoproteins (**Part B**). Chylomicrons and VLDLs cannot be metabolized or cleared from the blood until apoproteins C and E have been acquired from HDL. **Apo C-II**, present in the surface monolayer of mature chylomicrons and VLDLs, is required for triglyceride hydrolysis by **lipoprotein lipase**. Similarly, **apo E** must be present in intermediate-density lipoproteins (IDLs) and chylomicron remnants for these particles to bind to **remnant receptors** and be cleared by the liver. As large IDLs are transformed to smaller particles, apo C and apo E are returned to HDLs.

HDL and Reverse Cholesterol Transport

The pathway of reverse cholesterol transport results in the net transfer of free cholesterol from peripheral tissues to the liver, where it can be processed for excretion (**Part C**). HDL acquires free cholesterol from peripheral tissues and transfers it to lipoprotein remnants, which can be readily taken up by the liver. Three proteins associated with HDL are essential for reverse cholesterol transport: apo A-I, LCAT, and CETP, also known as apo D.

Reverse cholesterol transport is initiated by **HDL binding** to the surface of a cell, a process that requires **apo A-I**. Unesterified cholesterol is transferred from intracellular sites to the surface of HDL, where it is converted to cholesterol ester by LCAT in the reaction shown below:

$$\text{Cholesterol} + \text{Lecithin} \xrightarrow[\oplus \text{Apo A-I}]{\text{LCAT}} \text{Cholesterol ester} + \text{Lysolecithin}$$

LCAT transfers a fatty acid from the 2-position of lecithin (phosphatidylcholine) to cholesterol, producing cholesterol ester and lysolecithin. **Apo A-I is required for LCAT activity.** Most of the cholesterol esters formed in this reaction are transferred from HDLs to the interior of remnants lipoproteins. The remnants have empty space that was created by the hydrolysis of triglyceride. This space can be filled with cholesterol esters. The transfer of cholesterol esters from HDL to remnants is catalyzed by **CETP**. The remnants are taken up by the liver, where cholesterol is converted to bile acids and excreted.

HDL Heterogeneity

HDLs are a heterogeneous group of lipoproteins, consisting of several forms (**Part D**). The two major forms are HDL_2 and HDL_3, which differ in size, density, and cholesterol content. HDL_2 particles are larger and have a higher cholesterol content than HDL_3. Hepatic lipase can convert the larger HDL_2 to the smaller HDL_3, which can then acquire more cholesterol from peripheral tissues. Both HDL_3 and HDL_2 can transfer cholesterol esters to remnant lipoproteins. A minor form, HDL_1, contains apo E and can bind to remnant receptors and be taken up by the liver.

Clinical Significance

HDL cholesterol is sometimes referred to as "good cholesterol" because high levels of HDL reduce the risk of atherosclerosis. A level of HDL cholesterol greater than 60 mg/dL is considered protective, while a level less than 35 mg/dL is considered a risk for atherosclerosis. The protective effect is related to the ability of HDL to transport cholesterol from extrahepatic tissues to the liver, where it can be converted to bile acids and excreted. In **Tangier disease** there is almost a complete absence of apo A-I and HDL in the serum. Serum lipid analysis shows abnormally high triglyceride and very low cholesterol levels. The serum lipoprotein profiles shows high levels of chylomicrons and VLDLs that cannot be degraded by lipoprotein lipase because of the absence of apo C-II, which is normally acquired from HDL. The tonsils of patients with Tangier disease are large and orange in color, due to the accumulation of foam cells that are filled with cholesterol esters. Cholesterol esters also accumulate in the spleen and in the rectal mucosa. There is no known treatment for this disease. The chief cause of morbidity is progressive neuropathy associated with cholesterol accumulation in nerve tissue.

For more information see Coffee C, *Metabolism*. Fence Creek, pp 261–268.

40 Cholesterol and Bile Acid Metabolism

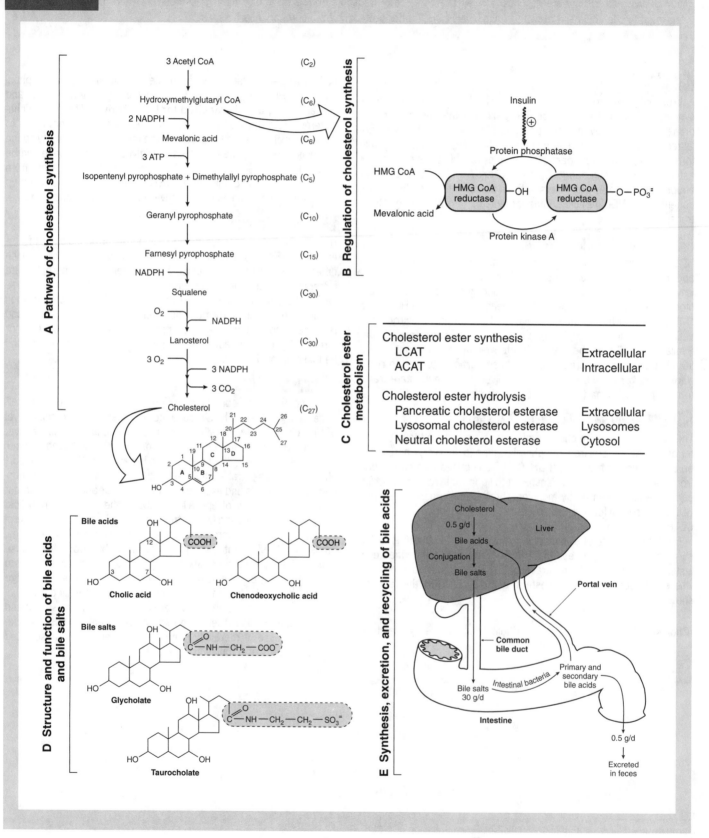

A Pathway of cholesterol synthesis

3 Acetyl CoA   (C_2)

Hydroxymethylglutaryl CoA   (C_6)

2 NADPH

Mevalonic acid   (C_6)

3 ATP

Isopentenyl pyrophosphate + Dimethylallyl pyrophosphate (C_5)

Geranyl pyrophosphate   (C_{10})

Farnesyl pyrophosphate   (C_{15})

NADPH

Squalene   (C_{30})

O_2 NADPH

Lanosterol   (C_{30})

3 O_2 3 NADPH   3 CO_2

Cholesterol   (C_{27})

B Regulation of cholesterol synthesis

Insulin

Protein phosphatase

HMG CoA

HMG CoA reductase — OH

HMG CoA reductase — O — $PO_3^=$

Mevalonic acid

Protein kinase A

C Cholesterol ester metabolism

Cholesterol ester synthesis	
LCAT	Extracellular
ACAT	Intracellular
Cholesterol ester hydrolysis	
Pancreatic cholesterol esterase	Extracellular
Lysosomal cholesterol esterase	Lysosomes
Neutral cholesterol esterase	Cytosol

D Structure and function of bile acids and bile salts

Bile acids

COOH

COOH

Cholic acid

Chenodeoxycholic acid

Bile salts

C=O — NH — CH_2 — COO

Glycholate

C=O — NH — CH_2 — CH_2 — $SO_3^=$

Taurocholate

E Synthesis, excretion, and recycling of bile acids

Cholesterol
0.5 g/d
Bile acids
Conjugation
Bile salts

Liver

Portal vein

Common bile duct

Bile salts
30 g/d

Intestinal bacteria

Primary and secondary bile acids

Intestine

0.5 g/d

Excreted in feces

OVERVIEW

Cholesterol is essential to the survival of animals, where it is a structural component of membranes and the precursor for bile acids, vitamin D, and steroid hormones. It is not found in plants or prokaryotes. Most normal adults synthesize about 1 g of cholesterol each day. The primary site of synthesis is the liver, although other tissues have a limited capacity for cholesterol synthesis. The rate-limiting step in cholesterol synthesis is catalyzed by 3-hydroxy-3-methylglutaryl coenzyme A (HMG CoA) reductase, an enzyme that is the target of many drugs designed to reduce serum cholesterol levels. Several enzymes interconvert cholesterol ester, the major storage and transport form, with unesterified cholesterol. The major excretory forms of cholesterol are bile acids, which are synthesized from cholesterol in the liver and converted to bile salts by conjugation with glycine or taurine. The bile salts are secreted by the liver as a component of bile.

Cholesterol Synthesis

Cholesterol synthesis requires acetyl CoA, ATP, NADPH, and O_2. The overall reaction is described by the following equation:

$$18 \text{ Acetyl CoA} + 18 \text{ ATP} + 16 \text{ NADPH} + 4 \text{ } O_2 \longrightarrow$$
$$\text{Cholesterol} + 9 \text{ } CO_2 + 16 \text{ } NADP^+ + 18 \text{ ADP} + 18 P_i$$

The pathway (**Part A**) can be described in four stages. The first stage is the formation of **HMG CoA** by the sequential condensation of three molecules of acetyl CoA. The second stage is the conversion of HMG CoA to two types of activated isoprenoids, **isopentenyl pyrophosphate** and **dimethylallyl pyrophosphate**. The synthesis of each isoprenoid requires three molecules of ATP. These C_5 compounds readily polymerize and are used as building blocks in several synthetic pathways. The third stage is the condensation of six isoprenoids to form **squalene**, a process that involves C_{10} and C_{15} intermediates. The fourth stage is the conversion of squalene, a linear C_{30} compound, to cholesterol, a cyclic C_{27} compound. **Lanosterol** is the first intermediate with a steroid nucleus.

Regulation of Cholesterol Synthesis

The rate-limiting step in cholesterol synthesis is catalyzed by **HMG CoA reductase**. Cholesterol synthesis is **increased by insulin and T_3 and inhibited by glucagon, cortisol, and cholesterol**. The effects of insulin and glucagon are mediated by phosphorylation and dephosphorylation (**Part B**). The dephosphorylated form that predominates when insulin is elevated is the active form. T_3, cortisol, and cholesterol regulate the rate of transcription of the gene for HMG CoA reductase.

Cholesterol Ester Metabolism

About 70% of the total cholesterol in the body exists as cholesterol esters. Several enzymes are involved in the interconversion of cholesterol and cholesterol ester (**Part C**). The two major enzymes involved in the formation of cholesterol esters are lecithin-cholesterol acyltransferase (LCAT) and acyl CoA:cholesterol acyltransferase (ACAT). Extracellular cholesterol is converted to cholesterol esters by **LCAT**, an enzyme associated with HDL. This reaction is essential for reverse cholesterol transport. LCAT transfers a fatty acid from lecithin to the 3-OH group of cholesterol. **ACAT**, an intracellular enzyme, transfers a fatty acid from fatty acyl CoA to cholesterol. ACAT is enriched in the liver, adrenal cortex, ovaries, and testes, where cholesterol esters are stored as oil droplets. The hydrolysis of cholesterol esters is catalyzed by three esterases. **Neutral cholesterol esterase**, found in the cytosol of liver, adrenal cortex, ovaries, and testes, hydrolyzes cholesterol esters, providing cholesterol for synthesis of bile acids or steroid hormones. **Pancreatic cholesterol esterase** is found in the intestinal lumen, where it hydrolyzes dietary cholesterol esters. **Lysosomal cholesterol esterase** hydrolyzes cholesterol esters that are taken up by receptor-mediated endocytosis of lipoproteins, especially LDL.

Structure and Function of Bile Acids and Salts

The primary bile acids, **cholic acid** and **chenodeoxycholic acid**, are synthesized by the liver (**Part D**). These compounds are C_{24} derivatives of cholesterol that have a side-chain carboxyl group and either two or three hydroxyl groups attached to the steroid nucleus. The side-chain carboxyl group is conjugated with either glycine or taurine, resulting in **bile salts**, which are completely ionized at physiologic pH. **Glycholate** and **taurocholate**, the bile salts of cholic acid, are the major emulsifying agents of dietary fat. The ionized side chain and all the hydroxyl groups project from the same side of the ring, resulting in an amphipathic structure that has excellent detergent properties.

Excretion and Recycling of Bile Acids

The bile salts are secreted by the liver as a component of bile (**Part E**). They are converted to **secondary bile acids** by intestinal bacteria, which remove the C-7 hydroxyl group and deconjugate the side chain. Reabsorption of bile acids from the small intestine into the portal blood is very efficient. Although the total pool of bile acids is only about 3 g, the pool is recycled about 10 times each day. Approximately 0.5 g of bile acids are excreted in the feces each day. These are replaced by the liver which converts about 0.5 g of cholesterol to bile acids each day.

Clinical Significance

Lovastatin and **mevinolin**, inhibitors of HMG CoA reductase, are commonly used to lower serum cholesterol. **Cholestyramine**, a resin that binds bile acids in the intestine and prevents them from being reabsorbed by the portal circulation, is also used to treat hypercholesterolemia. The decreased return of bile acids to the liver results in increased bile acid synthesis, thereby lowering cellular cholesterol. The decrease in cellular cholesterol results in increased synthesis of LDL receptors and increased clearance of plasma LDL.

For more information see Coffee C, *Metabolism*. Fence Creek, pp 291–299.

Steroid Hormone Metabolism

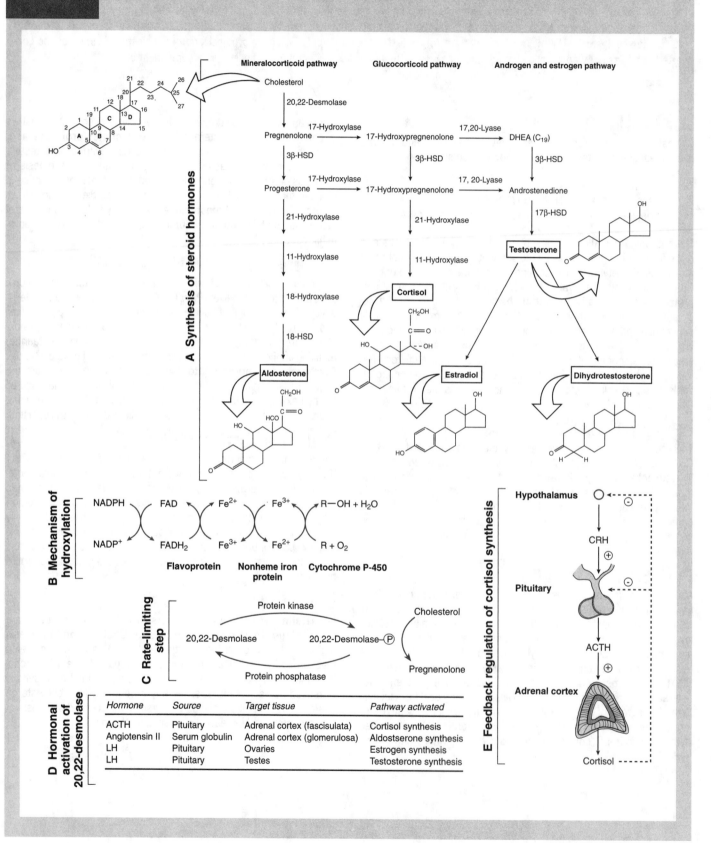

A Synthesis of steroid hormones

Mineralocorticoid pathway   Glucocorticoid pathway   Androgen and estrogen pathway

Cholesterol

20,22-Desmolase

Pregnenolone → 17-Hydroxypregnenolone → DHEA (C_{19})

17-Hydroxylase   17,20-Lyase

3β-HSD   3β-HSD   3β-HSD

Progesterone → 17-Hydroxypregnenolone → Androstenedione

17-Hydroxylase   17, 20-Lyase

21-Hydroxylase   21-Hydroxylase   17β-HSD

11-Hydroxylase   11-Hydroxylase   Testosterone

18-Hydroxylase   Cortisol

18-HSD

Aldosterone   Estradiol   Dihydrotestosterone

B Mechanism of hydroxylation

$$NADPH \rightarrow FAD \rightarrow Fe^{2+} \rightarrow Fe^{3+} \rightarrow R-OH + H_2O$$
$$NADP^+ \rightarrow FADH_2 \rightarrow Fe^{3+} \rightarrow Fe^{2+} \rightarrow R + O_2$$

Flavoprotein   Nonheme iron protein   Cytochrome P-450

C Rate-limiting step

Protein kinase

20,22-Desmolase → 20,22-Desmolase–Ⓟ   Cholesterol

Protein phosphatase   Pregnenolone

D Hormonal activation of 20,22-desmolase

Hormone	Source	Target tissue	Pathway activated
ACTH	Pituitary	Adrenal cortex (fasciculata)	Cortisol synthesis
Angiotensin II	Serum globulin	Adrenal cortex (glomerulosa)	Aldosterone synthesis
LH	Pituitary	Ovaries	Estrogen synthesis
LH	Pituitary	Testes	Testosterone synthesis

E Feedback regulation of cortisol synthesis

Hypothalamus

CRH

Pituitary

ACTH

Adrenal cortex

Cortisol

OVERVIEW

Steroid hormones are synthesized from cholesterol in the adrenal cortex, ovaries, and testes. The major adrenal cortical hormones are C_{21} derivatives of cholesterol, whereas androgens and estrogens are C_{19} and C_{18} derivatives, respectively. The conversion of cholesterol to adrenal steroids involves shortening the side chain to two carbons, whereas the synthesis of androgens and estrogens requires the complete removal of the side chain. In converting androgens to estrogens, an additional carbon is removed from the ring system. Most of the reactions in steroid hormone synthesis involve hydroxylation of carbon atoms. The synthesis of each class of steroid hormones is activated by a specific hormone that stimulates the activity of 20,22-desmolase, the rate-limiting enzyme in steroid synthesis.

Synthesis of Steroid Hormones

The adrenal cortex is organized into layers of cells that have different enzymes leading to the synthesis of different steroid hormones (see columns in **Part A**). All cells that synthesize steroid hormones contain 20,22-desmolase and 3β-hydroxysteroid dehydrogenase (HSD), the enzymes required to convert cholesterol to progesterone. **Mineralocorticoids** are made in the **zona glomerulosa**, the outermost cells of the adrenal cortex. Hydroxylation of progesterone by 21-hydroxylase and 11-hydroxylase results in 11-deoxycorticosterone and corticosterone, respectively. The sequential action of 18-hydroxylase and 18-HSD oxidizes the C-18 methyl group to an aldehyde, producing **aldosterone**, the major mineralocorticoid. 11-Deoxycorticosterone also has weak mineralocorticoid activity. The mineralocorticoids promote Na^+ retention and K^+ excretion by the kidney.

Glucocorticoid synthesis occurs in the **zona fasciculata** and **zona reticularis**. The hydroxylation of progesterone by 17-hydroxylase, 21-hydroxylase, and 11-hydroxylase produces **cortisol**, the major glucocorticoid. Glucocorticoids stimulate **gluconeogenesis** in the liver, **protein degradation** in skeletal muscle, and **mobilization of fatty acids** from adipose tissue.

Adrenal androgen synthesis occurs in the **zona reticularis**, the innermost layer of cells, where pregnenolone and progesterone are converted to **dehydroepiandrosterone (DHEA)** and **androstenedione** by 17-hydroxylase and 17,20-lyase. DHEA is converted to a sulfate ester, which has no androgen activity. Testes convert cholesterol to androstenedione by reactions identical to those in the adrenal cortex. Additionally, testes contain 17β-HSD, which reduces androstenedione to testosterone. Androstenedione, which is secreted by the adrenal cortex, is reduced to testosterone in the testes. Tissues that use **dihydrotestosterone** as the preferred androgen contain **5α-reductase**, which reduces testosterone to dihydrotestosterone. The immediate precursor for **estradiol** is testosterone. The ovaries contain all of the enzymes for testosterone synthesis plus **aromatase**, an enzyme that converts testosterone to estradiol.

Mechanism of Hydroxylation Reactions

Most reactions in steroid hormone synthesis involve hydroxylation of carbon atoms, including those catalyzed by specific hydroxylases, 20,22-desmolase and 17,20-lyase (**Part B**). These enzymes require O_2 and NADPH and are called **mixed function oxidases**. They consist of three types of subunits: a flavoprotein containing FAD, a non-

heme iron protein, and cytochrome P_{450}. They form an electron transport chain that uses NADPH to reduce O_2 to hydroxyl groups. One hydroxyl group is added to a carbon atom in the steroid and the other forms water. Most hydroxylation occurs in the smooth endoplasmic reticulum, although 20,22-desmolase, 17,20-lyase, 11-hydroxylase, and 18-hydroxylase are in mitochondria.

Rate-Limiting Step

The rate-limiting enzyme in each of the pathways is **20,22-desmolase (Part C)**. It is activated by **phosphorylation** of the cytochrome P_{450} subunit. The hormones, second messengers, and protein kinases involved are unique to each pathway, as described below.

Hormonal Activation of 20,22-Desmolase

Cells that synthesize different steroids have unique cell-surface receptors that bind specific peptide hormones (**Part D**). Cells that synthesize **cortisol** bind **adrenocorticotropic hormone (ACTH)**, a pituitary hormone, that stimulates cAMP synthesis, leading to phosphorylation and activation of 20,22-desmolase. Cells that synthesize **aldosterone** bind **angiotensin II**, which increases **diacylglycerol** and **calcium** levels, leading to phosphorylation and activation of 20,22-desmolase and 18-hydroxylase. Angiotensin II is formed by proteolysis of **angiotensinogen**, a plasma protein. The proteases, **renin** and **angiotensin-converting enzyme (ACE)** sequentially release angiotensin I and angiotensin II. Cells that synthesize **androgens and estrogens** are stimulated by **luteinizing hormone (LH)**, a pituitary hormone that increases intracellular cAMP.

Feedback Regulation of Cortisol Synthesis

Cortisol synthesis and secretion are controlled by both pituitary and hypothalamic hormones (**Part E**). Stress stimulates the hypothalamus to release **corticotropin-releasing hormone (CRH)**, which, in turn, stimulates the release of ACTH from the pituitary. As plasma cortisol levels rise in response to ACTH, receptors in the hypothalamus and pituitary bind cortisol, resulting in decreased release of CRH and ACTH. Similar feedback mechanisms exist for estrogen synthesis.

Clinical Significance

Several diseases involving abnormalities in steroid hormone metabolism are described in the following table:

Disease	Cause	Symptoms
Congenital adrenal hyperplasia	21-Hydroxylase deficiency	Elevated ACTH, virilization, salt wasting
Congenital adrenal hyperplasia	17-Hydroxylase deficiency	Elevated ACTH, hypertension, abnormal sexual maturation
Congenital adrenal hyperplasia	11-Hydroxylase	Elevated ACTH, hypertension, virilization
Testicular feminization	Androgen receptor deficiency	Male genotype, female-appearing genitalia
Male pseudohermaphroditism	5α-Reductase deficiency	Female appearance prior to puberty; virilization at puberty
Cushing disease	ACTH hypersecretion	Excess adrenal androgens, truncal obesity, glucose intolerance
Cushing syndrome	Adrenal carcinoma, adenoma	Excess adrenal androgens, truncal obesity, glucose intolerance

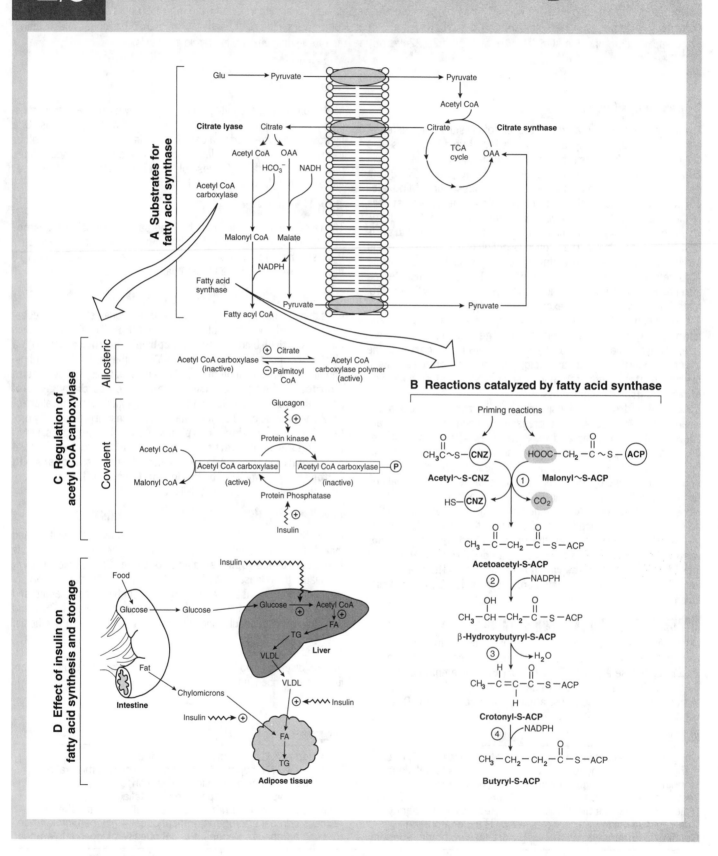

A Substrates for fatty acid synthesis

Glu → Pyruvate | Pyruvate

Acetyl CoA

Citrate lyase | Citrate ← Citrate | **Citrate synthase**

Acetyl CoA | OAA

HCO₃⁻ | NADH

Acetyl CoA carboxylase

TCA cycle | OAA

Malonyl CoA | Malate

NADPH

Fatty acid synthase

Fatty acyl CoA | Pyruvate | Pyruvate

C Regulation of acetyl CoA carboxylase

Allosteric

⊕ Citrate

Acetyl CoA carboxylase (inactive) ⇌ Acetyl CoA carboxylase polymer (active)

⊖ Palmitoyl CoA

Covalent

Glucagon ⊕

Protein kinase A

Acetyl CoA → Acetyl CoA carboxylase (active) → Acetyl CoA carboxylase (inactive) —Ⓟ

Malonyl CoA

Protein Phosphatase ⊕

Insulin

B Reactions catalyzed by fatty acid synthase

Priming reactions

$CH_3C\sim S-$ CNZ | HOOC$-CH_2-C\sim S-$ ACP

Acetyl~S-CNZ | ① | **Malonyl~S-ACP**

HS— CNZ ← | → CO_2

$CH_3-C-CH_2-C-S-ACP$

Acetoacetyl-S-ACP

② → NADPH

OH

$CH_3-CH-CH_2-C-S-ACP$

β-Hydroxybutyryl-S-ACP

③ → H_2O

H   O

$CH_3-C=C-C-S-ACP$

H

Crotonyl-S-ACP

④ → NADPH

$CH_3-CH_2-CH_2-C-S-ACP$

Butyryl-S-ACP

D Effect of insulin on fatty acid synthesis and storage

Insulin

Food

Glucose → Glucose → Glucose ⊕ → Acetyl CoA ⊕

FA

TG

VLDL | **Liver**

Fat

VLDL

Chylomicrons

Insulin ⊕

Intestine

Insulin ⊕

FA

TG

Adipose tissue

OVERVIEW

The pathways of fatty acid synthesis and storage are active in the well-fed state. Following a meal, the transient rise in blood glucose stimulates the release of insulin which, in turn, stimulates fatty acid synthesis in the liver and fatty acid storage in adipose tissue. The primary source of carbon for fatty acid synthesis is dietary glucose. The substrates for fatty acid synthesis are acetyl CoA, malonyl CoA, NADPH, and ATP. Translocation of acetyl CoA from mitochondria, where it is formed, to the cytosol, where fatty acid synthesis occurs, requires the citrate shuttle. The product of fatty acid synthesis in the liver is palmitic acid. Other fatty acids are generated by elongation and desaturation of palmitic acid. The rate-limiting enzyme in fatty acid synthesis is acetyl CoA carboxylase, which is regulated by both allosteric and covalent mechanisms. Most fatty acids that are derived from dietary lipid are stored as triglycerides in adipose tissue.

Generating Substrates for Fatty Acid Synthesis

The synthesis of palmitic acid, a C_{16} saturated fatty acid, can be described by the following equation:

$$8 \text{ Acetyl CoA} + 7 \text{ ATP} + 14 \text{ NADPH} \longrightarrow$$
$$\text{Palmitic acid} + 7 \text{ ADP} + 7 \text{ P}_i + 14 \text{ NADP}^+ + 8 \text{ CoA}$$

The major carbon source for fatty acid synthesis is dietary glucose that is converted to pyruvate by glycolysis (**Part A**). Following transport into mitochondria, pyruvate is decarboxylated to **acetyl CoA** in mitochondria, where it condenses with oxaloacetate, forming citrate in a reaction catalyzed by **citrate synthase** (**Part A**). Citrate acts as a carrier of acetyl CoA across the inner mitochondrial membrane into the cytosol, where it is cleaved by **citrate lyase**, regenerating acetyl CoA and oxaloacetate. These reactions constitute the citrate shuttle. Seven of the eight molecules of acetyl CoA required for palmitic acid synthesis are first carboxylated to **malonyl CoA**, an activated form of acetyl CoA. The formation of malonyl CoA is described by the following reaction, which is catalyzed by **acetyl CoA carboxylase**, a biotin-requiring enzyme.

$$\text{Acetyl CoA} + \text{HCO}_3^- + \text{ATP} \xrightarrow{\text{biotin}} \text{Malonyl CoA} + \text{ADP} + \text{P}_i$$

The **NADPH**, required for fatty acid synthesis, is derived from two sources, the citrate shuttle and the pentose phosphate pathway. Oxaloacetate (OAA) produced in the citrate lyase reaction is returned to the mitochondria as pyruvate. The conversion of oxaloacetate to pyruvate involves two sequential reactions catalyzed by cytosolic malate dehydrogenase and malic enzyme. **Malate dehydrogenase** catalyzes the NADH-dependent reduction of oxaloacetate to malate, and **malic enzyme** converts malate to pyruvate in a reaction that generates NADPH. The **glucose-6-phosphate dehydrogenase (G6PD)** and **6-phosphogluconate dehydrogenase (6-PGD)** reactions of the pentose phosphate pathway also supply NADPH.

Reactions Catalyzed by Fatty Acid Synthase

Fatty acid synthesis is an elongation process in which C_2 fragments are added sequentially to the carboxyl end of a fatty acid. The C_2 fragment at the ω-end of a fatty acid comes directly from acetyl CoA, whereas all other carbons are donated by malonyl CoA. Fatty acid synthase (FAS) is a multienzyme complex consisting of seven enzymes and acyl carrier protein (ACP), to which intermediates are attached during elongation (**Part B**). Each elongation step involves four sequential reactions: 1) **condensation,** 2) **reduction**, 3) **dehydration**, and 4) **reduction**. Both reduction reactions require NADPH. The initial condensation reaction involves an acetyl group attached to the condens-

ing enzyme (CNZ) and a malonyl group attached to ACP. Each group is linked to the respective protein by a **high-energy thioester bond**. Condensation of acetyl CoA with malonyl CoA releases CO_2 and produces a C_4 intermediate, which undergoes reduction, dehydration, and reduction, producing a fully reduced C_4 fatty acid that is linked by a thioester bond to ACP (butyryl-S-ACP). In preparation for the next elongation cycle, butyric acid is transferred from ACP to the condensing enzyme, and ACP is primed with another malonyl group. The cycle is repeated until the fatty acid is C_{16} in length, when it is released as palmitic acid or transferred to CoA, producing palmitoyl CoA.

Regulation of Acetyl CoA Carboxylase

Acetyl CoA carboxylase catalyzes the rate-limiting step in fatty acid synthesis (**Part C**). The enzyme is allosterically activated by **citrate** and inhibited by **palmitoyl CoA**. Citrate induces polymerization of the enzyme to highly active filaments, whereas palmitoyl CoA prevents the polymerization. Acetyl CoA carboxylase is also covalently regulated by phosphorylation and dephosphorylation, which is mediated by glucagon and insulin. **Insulin** activates protein phosphatase, resulting in **dephosphorylation** and **activation** of acetyl CoA carboxylase.

Effect of Insulin on Fatty Acid Synthesis and Storage

Insulin exerts its effects on fatty acid synthesis and storage by affecting several pathways in liver and adipose tissue (**Part D**). 1) **Hepatic glycolysis** and **pyruvate dehydrogenase** are activated by insulin, resulting in the conversion of glucose to acetyl CoA. 2) The synthesis of several enzymes involved in fatty acid synthesis is induced by insulin. These enzymes include **acetyl CoA carboxylase, FAS, citrate lyase, malic enzyme, G6PD**, and **6-PGD**. Newly synthesized fatty acids are esterified and packaged into very-low-density lipoproteins (VLDLs) and secreted. 3) Insulin induces the synthesis of **lipoprotein lipase** found in the capillary bed of adipose tissue. This enzyme releases fatty acids from chylomicron and VLDL triglyceride. The fatty acids are taken up by adipocytes and converted to triglycerides. 4) The uptake of glucose by **GLUT-4** in adipocytes is activated by insulin, resulting in increased glycolysis. Dihydroxyacetone phosphate, an intermediate in glycolysis, is the precursor for the glycerol backbone of triglycerides.

Clinical Significance

Impaired fatty acid synthesis due to an inherited **deficiency in acetyl CoA carboxylase** results in excretion of large amounts of acetic acid in the urine. Other effects are myopathy, brain damage, poor growth, and respiratory difficulties. The respiratory problems are likely due to the inability to synthesize surfactant.

For more information see Coffee C, *Metabolism*. Fence Creek, pp 273–282, 327–332.

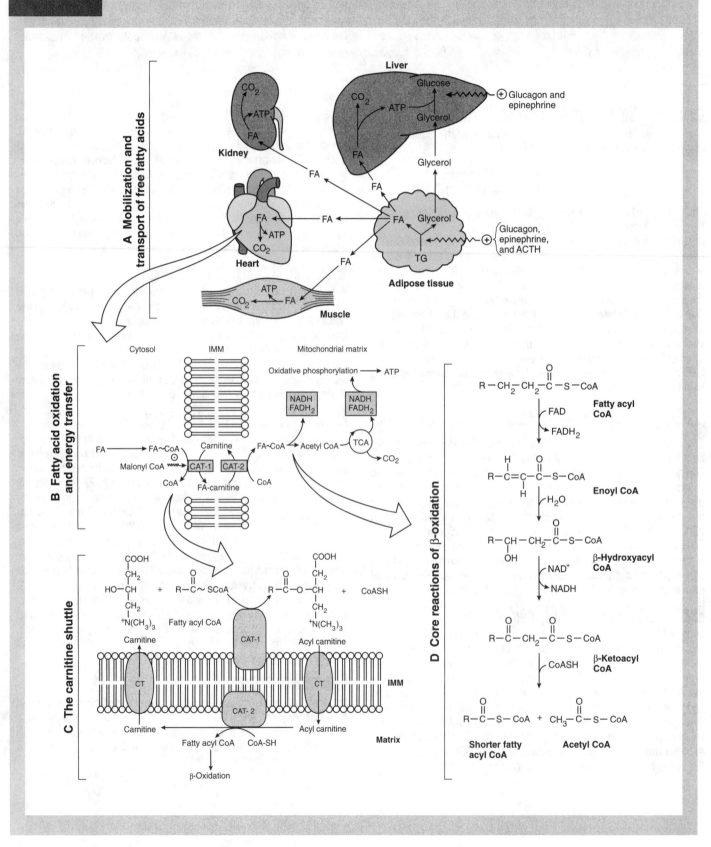

A Mobilization and transport of free fatty acids

B Fatty acid oxidation and energy transfer

C The carnitine shuttle

D Core reactions of β-oxidation

OVERVIEW

The conditions that promote the release of fatty acids from triglyceride stores in adipose tissue are fasting, physical exercise, and stress. In general, free unesterified fatty acids do not exist in solution because of their marked affinity for proteins. Albumin is the major extracellular protein for transporting fatty acids, and after diffusing across the plasma membrane, they bind to an intracellular fatty acid–binding protein. Most of the fatty acids released from adipose tissue are taken up by heart, skeletal muscle, kidney, and liver, where they provide an important source of energy. The carnitine shuttle transports long-chain fatty acyl CoAs into mitochondria, where oxidation occurs. Fatty acid oxidation is regulated primarily by fatty acid availability and the rate at which they enter the mitochondrial matrix.

Mobilization and Transport of Free Fatty Acids

Major hormones stimulating triglyceride degradation in adipose tissue are **glucagon, epinephrine**, and **adrenocorticotropic hormone (ACTH)**, which activate **hormone-sensitive lipase (Part A)**. Circulating levels of glucagon are increased in response to a decrease in blood glucose concentration, whereas epinephrine and ACTH levels are increased by physical exercise and stress. **Cortisol** and **growth hormone** promote a more chronic stimulation of hormone-sensitive lipase. More than 99% of the free fatty acids in plasma are noncovalently bound to **albumin**, which has at least ten binding sites for fatty acids, including three high-affinity sites. Under most conditions, an average of 0.5 to 1.5 fatty acid molecules are bound per molecule of albumin. Free fatty acids diffuse off albumin and across the plasma membrane of cells.

Fatty Acid Oxidation and Energy Transfer

Almost immediately after entering a cell, fatty acids are converted to the corresponding fatty acyl CoA by a family of cytosolic enzymes known as **fatty acyl CoA synthetases (Part B)**. The reaction catalyzed by these enzymes is shown below:

$$\text{Fatty acid} + \text{ATP} \longrightarrow \text{Fatty acid CoA} + \text{AMP} + 2\,P_i$$

Following translocation into the mitochondrial matrix, the fatty acyl CoA is oxidized to acetyl CoA, NADH, and $FADH_2$. The oxidation of palmitoyl CoA, a C_{16} fatty acid, can be described by the following equation:

$$\text{Palmitoyl CoA} + 7\,NAD^+ + 7\,FAD + 7\,CoA \longrightarrow$$
$$8\,\text{Acetyl CoA} + 7\,NADH + 7\,FADH_2$$

ATP is not a direct product of fatty acid oxidation. However, if the products of palmitoyl CoA oxidation are further oxidized to CO_2 and H_2O by the tricarboxylic acid cycle and the electron transport chain, sufficient energy is released to generate 131 mols of ATP per palmitoyl CoA. (This calculation assumes that the complete oxidation of each mol of acetyl CoA will produce 12 mols of ATP.) Since two equivalents of ATP are needed to convert palmitic acid to palmitoyl CoA, the net yield is 129 mols of ATP per mol of palmitic acid oxidized.

The Carnitine Shuttle

A fatty acyl CoA having a length of C_{12} or greater is impermeable to the inner mitochondrial membrane (IMM), and entry into the mitochondrial matrix requires the carnitine shuttle (**Part C**). This shuttle consists of two enzymes and a carnitine transport protein. **Carnitine acyl transferase-1** (CAT-1) is located on the outer surface of the IMM, where it transfers the fatty acid from CoA to carnitine, forming acyl carnitine, which is transported across the membrane by **carnitine transporter** (CT). **Carnitine acyltransferase-2** (CAT-2) is located on the inner surface of the IMM, where it transfers the fatty acid back to CoA as it enters the matrix. Medium- and short-chain fatty acids (C_2–C_{10}) do not require carnitine to be transported across the IMM. Carnitine is not a dietary requirement. It is synthesized from **trimethyllysine**, derived from the degradation of skeletal muscle protein. Synthesis involves sequential reactions that occur in kidney and liver.

Core Reactions of β-Oxidation

β-Oxidation of fatty acids is a cyclic process involving four core reactions that sequentially release acetyl CoA from the carboxyl end of the fatty acid (**Part D**). Each cycle of β-oxidation produces one molecule each of acetyl CoA, $FADH_2$, and NADH. The first reaction introduces a double bond between the α- and β-carbons, producing enoyl CoA and $FADH_2$. This reaction is catalyzed by a family of **fatty acyl CoA dehydrogenases** that are specific for fatty acids of different chain lengths. In the second reaction, water is added across the double bond, producing β-hydroxyacyl CoA. The hydroxyl group is oxidized by an NAD-linked dehydrogenase, producing β-ketoacyl CoA and NADH. The final reaction, catalyzed by **thiolase**, adds CoA across the bond between the α- and β-carbons, releasing acetyl CoA and generating a fatty acyl CoA that is two carbons shorter. The cycle is repeated until the fatty acid has been completely degraded to acetyl CoA. The isozymes of fatty acyl CoA dehydrogenase that catalyze the first step in each cycle are long-chain acyl CoA dehydrogenase (LCAD), medium-chain acyl CoA dehydrogenase (MCAD), and short-chain acyl CoA dehydrogenase (SCAD). The complete oxidation of a long-chain fatty acid requires the participation of all three isozymes. Genetic deficiencies in all three isozymes have been reported.

Clinical Significance

MCAD deficiency is one of the most common inborn errors of metabolism. Its clinical presentation varies widely, and it is believed that as many as 10% of the cases of sudden infant death syndrome may result from MCAD deficiency. Onset frequently occurs in infancy, and common symptoms are episodes of vomiting, lethargy, hypoketonic hypoglycemia, and hyperammonemia. Large quantities of medium-chain fatty acids (C_6–C_{10}) are excreted in the urine. Both **carnitine deficiency** and **CAT-1 deficiency** are also characterized by hypoketonic hypoglycemia, weakness, and hypotonia.

For more information see Coffee C, *Metabolism*. Fence Creek, pp 282–287, 327–331.

44 Ketone Metabolism

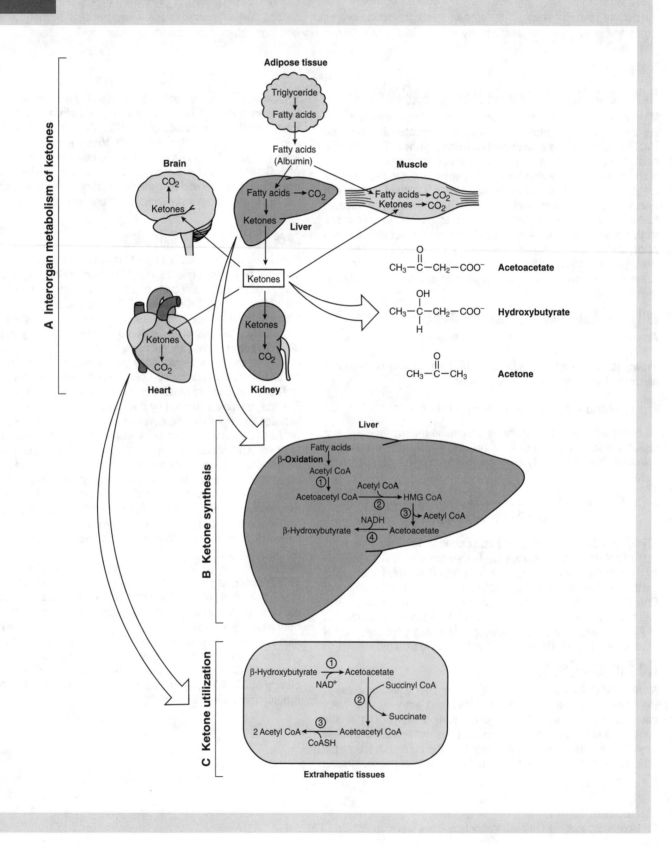

Adipose tissue

Triglyceride → Fatty acids

Fatty acids (Albumin)

A Interorgan metabolism of ketones

Brain
CO_2
Ketones

Liver
Fatty acids → CO_2
Ketones

Muscle
Fatty acids → CO_2
Ketones → CO_2

Ketones

Heart
Ketones → CO_2

Kidney
Ketones → CO_2

CH_3—$\overset{O}{\overset{\|}{C}}$—$CH_2$—$COO^-$ **Acetoacetate**

CH_3—$\overset{OH}{\underset{H}{\overset{|}{C}}}$—$CH_2$—$COO^-$ **Hydroxybutyrate**

CH_3—$\overset{O}{\overset{\|}{C}}$—$CH_3$ **Acetone**

B Ketone synthesis

Liver

Fatty acids
β-Oxidation ↓
Acetyl CoA
① ↓   Acetyl CoA
Acetoacetyl CoA —② → HMG CoA
③ ↓ Acetyl CoA
β-Hydroxybutyrate ← Acetoacetate
NADH ④

C Ketone utilization

β-Hydroxybutyrate —① → Acetoacetate
NAD⁺   Succinyl CoA
②
Succinate
2 Acetyl CoA ← ③ ← Acetoacetyl CoA
CoASH

Extrahepatic tissues

OVERVIEW

The ketone bodies, acetoacetate and β-hydroxybutyrate, are small water-soluble acids that have pK_a values of approximately 3.7 and are completely dissociated at physiologic pH. They play an important role in fuel homeostasis by providing fuel for muscle, brain, and kidney during periods of fasting and starvation. When the circulating concentration of ketones reaches 1 to 3 mM, they begin to be taken up by extrahepatic tissues and oxidized. Although the ketone concentration in the blood is usually less than 0.2 mM, there are several normal states (fasting, late pregnancy, and vigorous exercise) where the concentration can increase to 2 to 3 mM. The ketones play an important role in adaptations that allow blood glucose and tissue protein to be spared during periods of starvation.

Interorgan Metabolism of Ketones

Ketogenesis provides a mechanism for conserving excess acetyl CoA. Ketone synthesis occurs concurrently with fatty acid mobilization and oxidation, and is associated with persistently elevated levels of glucagon (**Part A**). If fatty acids are oxidized more rapidly than acetyl CoA is used, the excess is converted to acetoacetate and β-hydroxybutyrate. Ketone synthesis occurs only in the liver. The liver, however, is unable to oxidize ketones. Therefore, β-hydroxybutyrate and acetoacetate are released into the blood and transported free in solution to extrahepatic tissues. They are readily oxidized to CO_2 by heart, skeletal muscle, and kidney. During prolonged fasting and starvation, the brain acquires the ability to oxidize ketone bodies, although it is unable to oxidize fatty acids. Ketones, however, cannot completely replace the glucose requirement of the brain. A small fraction of acetoacetate is spontaneously decarboxylated to acetone, which is exhaled by the lungs and is responsible for the "fruity breath" sometimes observed in people with uncontrolled diabetes.

Ketone Synthesis

Ketone synthesis occurs when carbohydrate availability is limited and excessive fatty acid oxidation is occurring (**Part B**). Synthesis occurs in the mitochondrial compartment of the liver. The first two reactions, catalyzed by **thiolase** and **3-hydroxy-3-methylglutaryl (HMG) CoA synthase**, involve the sequential condensation of three molecules of acetyl CoA, producing acetoacetyl CoA and HMG CoA, respectively. Cleavage of HMG CoA by **HMG CoA lyase** produces acetoacetate. The NADH-dependent reduction of acetoacetate to β-hydroxybutyrate is catalyzed by **β-hydroxybutyrate dehydrogenase**, an enzyme embedded in the inner mitochondrial membrane (IMM). All of the other enzymes involved in ketone metabolism are located in the mitochondrial matrix. The two initial reactions of ketogenesis that produce HMG CoA also occur in the cytosol, where they participate in the pathway of cholesterol synthesis. Separate isozymes of thiolase and HMG CoA synthase are found in these two cellular compartments.

Ketone Utilization

The uptake and oxidation of ketones by extrahepatic tissues are dependent on the concentration in the blood (**Part C**). Significant uptake does not occur until the blood concentration reaches 1 to 3 mM. The oxidation of ketones involves three sequential reactions catalyzed by **β-hydroxybutyrate dehydrogenase**, **succinyl CoA: acetoacetate CoA transferase, and thiolase**. Following uptake by extrahepatic cells, β-hydroxybutyrate is oxidized to acetoacetate as it crosses the IMM. Acetoacetate acquires CoA in a transfer reaction with succinyl CoA. Thiolytic cleavage of acetoacetyl CoA produces two molecules of acetyl CoA, which can be further oxidized by the tricarboxylic acid cycle. The liver is unable to oxidize ketones because succinyl CoA:acetoacetate CoA transferase, the enzyme that converts acetoacetate to acetoacetyl CoA, is not expressed in the liver. In the well-fed state, this enzyme is also absent in the brain. However, when ketones accumulate to a concentration of 2 to 3 mM, synthesis of the enzyme is induced in the brain.

Clinical Significance

Ketoacidosis is often found in untreated type I diabetes. The lack of insulin in this condition leads to the uncontrolled release of fatty acids from adipose tissue and excessive fatty acid oxidation by the liver, where the excess acetyl CoA is converted to ketones. Extremely high levels of ketones (10 to 20 mM) accumulate in the blood, resulting in ketoacidosis. The pH of the blood can drop from a normal value of about 7.4 to about 6.8. Since acetoacetate and β-hydroxybutyrate are ionized acids, their excretion in the urine requires that they be neutralized by a cation. Excessive excretion of Na^+ and K^+ occurs, which can lead to an electrolyte imbalance. An adaptive increase in NH_4^+ production occurs, providing an expendable cation that can be excreted. The NH_4^+ is produced by **deamination of glutamine** in the kidney. If untreated, ketoacidosis can be fatal. In addition to the overproduction of ketones in untreated type I diabetes, there may also be an impairment of ketone utilization by extrahepatic tissues, accounting for the extremely high levels of ketones that accumulate.

For more information see Coffee C, *Metabolism*. Fence Creek, pp 286–287, 327–331.

Coordinate Regulation of Fatty Acid Metabolism

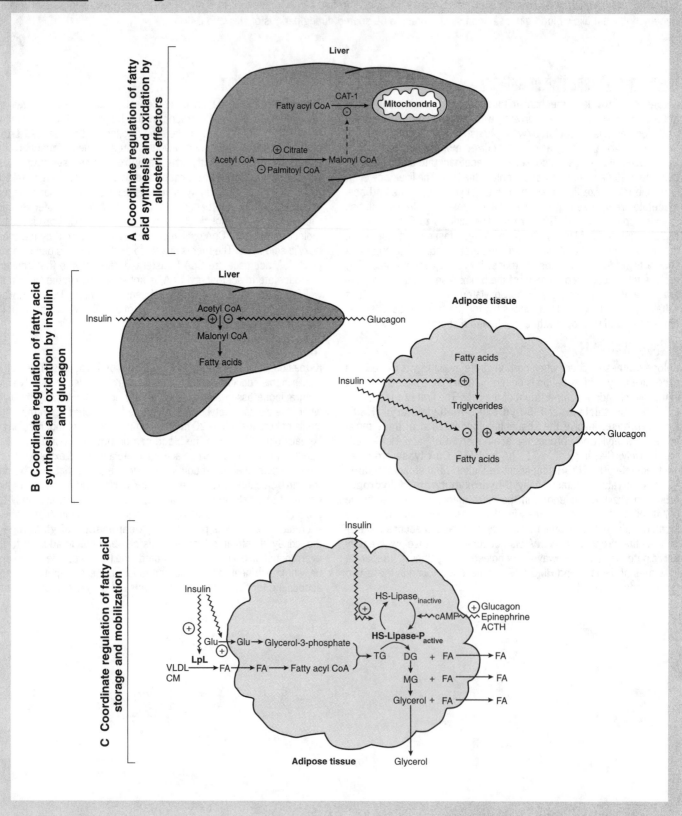

A Coordinate regulation of fatty acid synthesis and oxidation by allosteric effectors

Liver

Fatty acyl CoA — CAT-1 — ⊖ → Mitochondria

Acetyl CoA — ⊕ Citrate → Malonyl CoA
⊖ Palmitoyl CoA

B Coordinate regulation of fatty acid synthesis and oxidation by insulin and glucagon

Liver

Insulin — Acetyl CoA ⊕ ⊖ — Glucagon
Malonyl CoA
Fatty acids

Adipose tissue

Fatty acids
Insulin — ⊕
Triglycerides
⊖ ⊕ — Glucagon
Fatty acids

C Coordinate regulation of fatty acid storage and mobilization

Insulin

Insulin
⊕
⊕
Glu → Glu → Glycerol-3-phosphate
LpL
VLDL → FA → FA → Fatty acyl CoA
CM

HS-Lipase_inactive
⊕
cAMP — ⊕ Glucagon
Epinephrine
ACTH
HS-Lipase-P_active

TG → DG + FA → FA
MG + FA → FA
Glycerol + FA → FA

Glycerol

Adipose tissue

The conditions that promote fatty acid synthesis inhibit fatty acid oxidation, and vice versa, thus preventing futile cycling of energy stores. The coordinate regulation of these opposing pathways is achieved by both allosteric and hormonal regulation. The key enzymes involved in coordinate regulation of fatty acid synthesis and fatty acid oxidation are acetyl CoA carboxylase and carnitine acyltransferase-1 (CAT-1), respectively. The coordinate regulation of triglyceride synthesis and hydrolysis in adipose tissue is hormonally regulated, with insulin and glucagon being the principal hormones involved.

Coordinate Regulation of Fatty Acid Synthesis and Oxidation by Allosteric Effectors

The rate-limiting step in fatty acid oxidation is catalyzed by **CAT-1**, which controls the entry of long-chain fatty acids into the mitochondrial matrix, where they are oxidized (**Part A**). CAT-1 is allosterically inhibited by **malonyl CoA**, the key substrate for fatty acid synthesis. The synthesis of malonyl CoA is stimulated by **insulin**, thereby explaining how insulin inhibits fatty acid oxidation. The rate-limiting step in fatty acid synthesis is catalyzed by **acetyl CoA carboxylase**, which is allosterically activated by the accumulation of **citrate** in the cytosol. Citrate accumulates under conditions that promote fatty acid synthesis. It acts as a carrier of acetyl CoA from the mitochondria, where it is formed, to the cytosol, where fatty acid synthesis occurs. **Palmitoyl CoA**, the end product of fatty acid synthesis in most tissues, allosterically inhibits acetyl CoA carboxylase.

Coordinate Regulation of Fatty Acid Synthesis and Oxidation by Insulin and Glucagon

Insulin, an anabolic hormone, promotes energy storage by activating fatty acid synthesis in liver and triglyceride synthesis in adipose tissue (**Part B**). **Insulin** stimulates fatty acid synthesis by increasing the rate of malonyl CoA synthesis, a reaction catalyzed by acetyl CoA carboxylase. The mechanism involves activation of **protein phosphatase**, which catalyzes the dephosphorylation and the concomitant activation of **acetyl CoA carboxylase**. Conversely, glucagon inhibits the synthesis of malonyl CoA by promoting the cAMP-dependent phosphorylation and inactivation of acetyl CoA carboxylase. The rate of fatty acid oxidation in all tissues is determined by fatty acid availability. **Glucagon** increases fatty acid availability by stimulating **lipolysis** of adipose tissue triglyceride, producing fatty acids that are transported by serum albumin to various tissues for oxidation. Conversely, insulin decreases availability of fatty acids by inhibiting lipolysis in adipose tissue.

Coordinate Regulation of Fatty Acid Storage and Mobilization

Triglyceride synthesis and fatty acid storage in adipose are stimulated by **insulin** (**Part C**). Insulin increases both **fatty acid** and **glucose** uptake by adipose tissue. The synthesis of **lipoprotein lipase (LpL)**, the enzyme that releases fatty acid from lipoprotein triglyceride, is induced by insulin, thereby increasing the uptake of fatty acids into adipose tissue. The number of **GLUT-4 transporters** in the plasma membrane of adipocytes is stimulated by insulin, resulting in increased uptake of glucose. Therefore, insulin stimulates **glycolysis** in adipose tissue. The major function of glycolysis in adipocytes is to provide DHAP, the precursor for the **glycerol backbone** in triglycerides. In addition to promoting triglyceride synthesis, insulin also suppresses triglyceride hydrolysis in adipose tissue by promoting the dephosphorylation and inactivation of **hormone-sensitive lipase**. Conversely, **glucagon, epinephrine**, and **adrenocorticotropic hormone (ACTH)** stimulate the hydrolysis of triglyceride by promoting phosphorylation and activation of hormone-sensitive lipase.

Clinical Significance

Obesity, the accumulation of excess triglyceride in adipose tissue, is the most common nutritional disorder in the United States. The fat cells of adipose tissue are modified fibroblasts that have between 80% and 95% of their cell volume filled with triglyceride. The adipose tissue in obese individuals contains **fewer insulin receptors** than normal individuals. Obesity is associated with an increased number and/or size of fat cells. The rate of fat cell formation is most rapid in early life. In obese children, the number of fat cells is often 2 to 3 times higher than in children of normal weight. However, after adolescence the number of fat cells remains relatively constant. In individuals who become obese in middle age, most of the obesity is associated with an increase in the size of fat cells resulting from increased fat storage. When the adult body weight reaches 170% of the ideal weight, a maximum adipocyte cell size is reached, after which the number of cells and obesity are highly correlated. Obesity due to enlargement of fat cells (**hypertrophy**) appears easier to control than obesity associated with increased number of fat cells (**hyperplasia**). Obesity has been recognized as a risk factor in the development of a number of diseases, including hypertension, diabetes mellitus, coronary artery disease, stroke, and cancer. **The pattern of fat distribution** is often more significant than the amount of fat; visceral or central obesity appears to be more important as a risk factor than subcutaneous or lower body fat.

For more information see Coffee C, *Metabolism*. Fence Creek, pp 273–287, 327–331.

46 Phospholipids

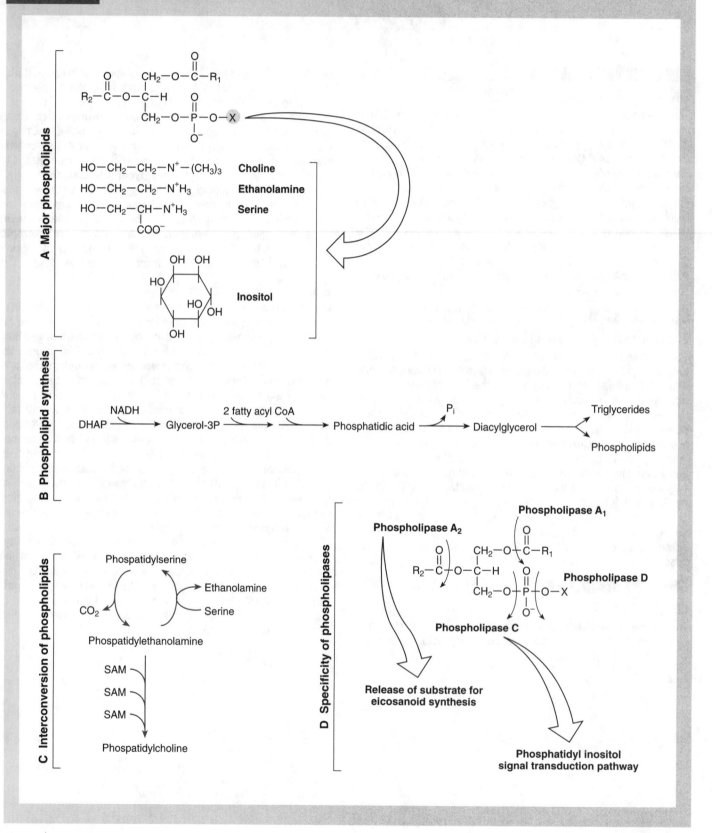

A Major phospholipids

Choline
Ethanolamine
Serine
Inositol

B Phospholipid synthesis

DHAP $\xrightarrow{\text{NADH}}$ Glycerol-3P $\xrightarrow{\text{2 fatty acyl CoA}}$ Phosphatidic acid $\xrightarrow{\text{P}_i}$ Diacylglycerol $\longrightarrow$ Triglycerides / Phospholipids

C Interconversion of phospholipids

Phospatidylserine
CO_2
Ethanolamine
Serine
Phospatidylethanolamine
SAM
SAM
SAM
Phospatidylcholine

D Specificity of phospholipases

Phospholipase A₂
Phospholipase A₁
Phospholipase D
Phospholipase C

Release of substrate for eicosanoid synthesis

Phosphatidyl inositol signal transduction pathway

OVERVIEW

Phospholipids have both structural and dynamic roles in cells. In addition to being the major building blocks of membranes, they are important components of signal transduction pathways, lipoprotein particles, bile, and lung surfactant. Most phospholipids are phosphoglycerides, having a glycerol backbone. The single exception is sphingomyelin, which has a ceramide backbone.

Major Phospholipids

The phosphoglycerides are a diverse family of lipids whose structures are similar to one another (**Part A**). More than 90% of the membrane phospholipids are phosphoglycerides, containing fatty acids esterified to hydroxyl groups on C-1 and C-2 of the glycerol backbone. The fatty acid at C-1 is usually a saturated fatty acid, while that at C-2 is usually unsaturated. The major phospholipids are phosphatidylcholine, phosphatidylethanolamine, phosphatidylserine, and phosphatidylinositol. They contain phosphate that is linked via a phosphodiester bond to two different alcohols, diacylglycerol and either choline, ethanolamine, serine, or inositol. **Phosphatidylcholine** (lecithin) and **phosphatidylethanolamine** (cephalin) are the most abundant phospholipids in the body. They are **neutral phospholipids**, having no net charge at physiologic pH. Phosphatidylcholine serves as a reservoir for arachidonic acid, which can be mobilized and used for eicosanoid synthesis. In contrast, **phosphatidylserine** and **phosphatidylinositol** are **acidic phospholipids** that have a net negative charge at physiologic pH. Phosphatidylserine is enriched in brain, where it constitutes about 15% of the total phospholipid. Although phosphatidylinositol makes up less than 5% of the total lipid in the plasma membrane, it turns over very rapidly and plays an important role in signal transduction. A number of hormones stimulate the degradation of phosphatidylinositol triphosphate, resulting in the release of **diacylglycerol** and **inositol triphosphate**, compounds that have important regulatory roles in cells.

Phospholipid Synthesis

The glycerol backbone in phospholipids, like that in triglycerides, is derived from dihydroxyacetone phosphate (DHAP), an intermediate in glycolysis (**Part B**). DHAP is reduced to glycerol phosphate, and the addition of fatty acids to C-1 and C-2 results in **phosphatidic acid**. The removal of phosphate from phosphatidic acid produces diacylglycerol. Phosphocholine, phosphoethanolamine, and phosphoserine are transferred from their activated carriers (CDP-choline, CDP-ethanolamine, and CDP-serine) to diacylglycerol, producing the corresponding phospholipids. The synthesis of phosphatidylinositol involves the activation of diacylglycerol (CDP-diacylglycerol) rather than inositol. Phosphodiacylglycerol is transferred from CDP-diacylglylcerol to inositol, producing phosphatidylinositol.

Interconversion of Phospholipids

Phosphatidylserine can serve as a precursor for both phosphatidylethanolamine and phosphatidyl choline (**Part C**). Decarboxylation of phosphatidylserine results in phosphatidylethanolamine. Phosphatidylethanolamine can be converted back to phosphatidylserine in a reaction involving a simple exchange of serine for ethanolamine. Phosphatidylethanolamine can be converted to phosphatidylcholine by three successive methylation reactions, each requiring S-adenosylmethionine (SAM) as an activated donor of a methyl group.

Specificity of Phospholipases

The degradation of phospholipids requires four phospholipases: phospholipase A_1, phospholipase A_2, phospholipase C, and phospholipase D (**Part D**). All of these enzymes hydrolyze ester bonds, but each is specific for a particular bond in the phospholipid molecule. **Phospholipase A_2** plays an important role in the **synthesis of eicosanoids**, releasing arachidonic acid from the C-2 carbon of the glycerol backbone. **Phospholipase C** is a key enzyme in the **phosphatidylinositol signal transduction pathway**. This enzyme is activated by several hormones that generate diacylglycerol and inositol triphosphate as intracellular second messengers.

Clinical Significance

Two phospholipids are of particular clinical significance, phosphatidalcholine and dipalmitoyllecithin. **Phosphatidalcholine**, also known as **platelet activation factor (PAF)**, belongs to a minor class of phospholipids known as **plasmalogens**. They are glycerol-based phospholipids that have an **ether**, rather than an ester, linkage at C-1. Thus, the only difference in phosphatid**a**lcholine and phosphatid**y**lcholine is the type of linkage at C-1. PAF is a potent mediator of acute inflammation and anaphylactic shock. Exposure to stimuli such as pollen or bee stings results in the release of PAF from polymorphonuclear leukocytes. Some of the effects of PAF include the aggregation and degranulation of platelets and the dilation of blood vessels.

Dipalmitoyllecithin is the major lipid component of **surfactant**, a surface-active agent that plays an important role in normal lung function. Surfactant lines the walls of alveoli and prevents their collapse at the end of each respiratory cycle. The inability to synthesize surfactant is the cause of acute **respiratory distress syndrome**, which accounts for about 20% of the infant mortality in the United States.

For more information see Coffee C, *Metabolism*. Fence Creek, pp 309–314.

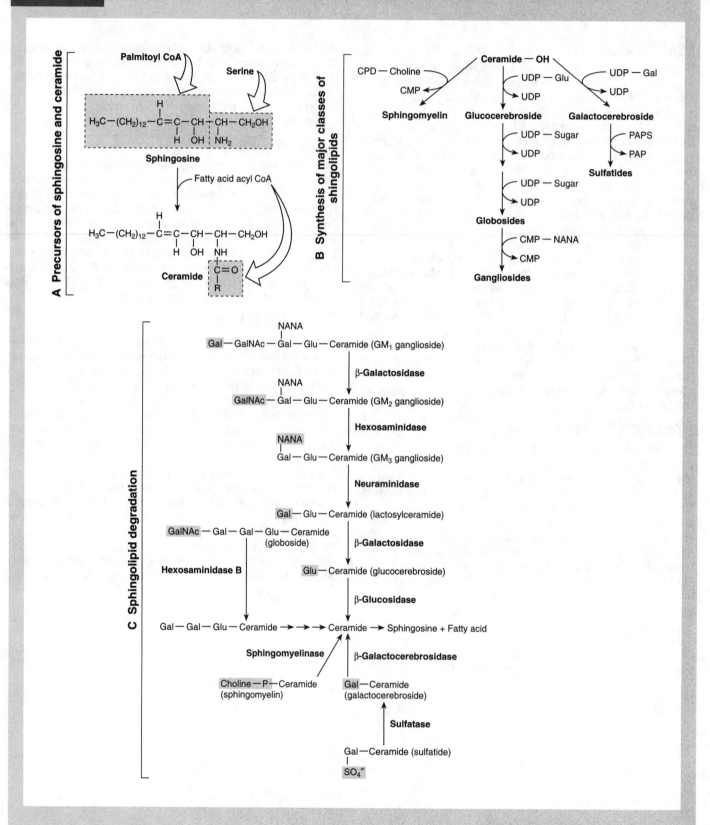

OVERVIEW

Sphingolipids and glycolipids are complex lipids that are found in plasma membrane of cells and the myelin sheath of neurons. There are five classes of sphingolipids: 1) sphingomyelins, 2) cerebrosides, 3) sulfatides, 4) globosides, and 5) gangliosides. All classes, except sphingomyelin, contain one or more monosaccharides and are also classified as glycolipids. The carbohydrate portion of glycolipids has been associated with several functions, including blood group antigens, tumor antigens, and bacterial toxin receptors. The degradation of sphingolipids occurs in lysosomes. Several lysosomal storage diseases result from the inability to degrade sphingolipids.

Precursors of Sphingosine and Ceramide

Sphingosine is a long-chain amino alcohol that is formed from **palmitoyl CoA** and **serine** (Part A). The synthesis of sphingosine involves several reactions and requires three coenzymes: NADPH, FAD, and pyridoxal phosphate. **Ceramide**, also known as N-acylsphingosine, is formed by the attachment of a **long-chain saturated fatty acid** to the amino group of sphingosine. Ceramide has two hydroxyl groups, one attached to C-3 that is never substituted and another attached to C-1 that is always substituted in sphingolipids and glycolipids.

Synthesis of Major Classes of Sphingolipids

Ceramide is the basic structural unit of all sphingolipids and glycolipids. The different classes of sphingolipids are generated by the addition of different groups to the terminal hydroxyl group of ceramide (**Part B**). **Sphingomyelin** is formed by the transfer of phosphocholine from CDP-choline to ceramide. Sphingomyelin is found in high concentrations in the red blood cell membrane and in the myelin sheath that surrounds neurons in the central nervous system. It is the only phospholipid that is not attached to a glycerol backbone. **Cerebrosides** have either glucose or galactose linked to ceramide. **Galactocerebroside** is found in high concentration in nerve tissue, whereas **glucocerebroside** is found primarily in extraneural tissue, where it serves as an intermediate in the synthesis of more complex glycolipids. Synthesis of cerebrosides requires UDP-linked galactose and glucose. **Sulfatides** are cerebrosides in which the monosaccharide contains a sulfate ester. The most common sulfatide is sulfogalactocerebroside, which is found in nerve tissue. The addition of sulfate requires 3′-phosphoadenosine-5′-phosphosulfate (PAPS) as the activated sulfate donor. The sulfatides are acidic lipids, having a negative charge within the physiologic pH range. **Globosides** are synthesized by the addition of galactose and N-acetylglucosamine (GlcNAc) to glucocerebrosides. These glycolipids are important constituents of red blood cell membranes, and they contain the determinants of the ABO blood group system. **Gangliosides** are synthesized from glucocerebrosides by the sequential addition of monosaccharides from their activated donors. Gangliosides contain a variety of oligosaccharides, including glucose, galactose, GalNAc, and sialic acid, also known as N-acetylneuraminic acid (NANA). The gangliosides, like the sulfatides, are acidic lipids due to the presence of NANA. Gangliosides function as receptors for cholera toxin and diphtheria toxin. The nomenclature and classification of gangliosides are based on the number of NANA residues present in the oligosaccharide. The subscript M (mono-), D (di-), and T (tri-) indicate the presence of either one, two, or three residues of NANA. Different members of each class are further identified by a subscript number (GM_1, GM_2, etc.) that indicates a specific sequence of oligosaccharides attached to ceramide.

Sphingolipid Degradation

During the turnover of cells, sphingolipids are degraded by a series of **lysosomal hydrolases** that sequentially remove monosaccharides from the end of the oligosaccharide chain (**Part C**). The failure to remove a particular substituent interferes with subsequent steps in the pathway, resulting in the accumulation of a characteristic intermediate in the pathway.

Clinical Significance

Several inborn errors of metabolism result from deficiencies in the lysosomal hydrolases that degrade sphingolipids, resulting in a family of diseases known as **sphingolipidoses**. The deficient enzyme, the characteristic sphingolipid that accumulates, and the clinical symptoms of these diseases are summarized in the table shown below. The structure of the sphingolipids that accumulate are shown on the previous page. All of these diseases are inherited as autosomal recessive traits, except Fabry disease, which has an X-linked inheritance pattern.

Disease	Enzyme Deficiency	Substance Accumulated	Clinical Symptoms
Tay-Sachs disease	Hexosaminidase A	Ganglioside GM_2	Mental retardation, blindness, cherry-red spot on retina, and death by age 3
Sandhoff disease	Hexosaminidases A and B	Ganglioside GM_2	Same as Tay-Sachs but progresses more rapidly
Gaucher disease	β-Glucocerebrosidase	Glucocerebroside	Enlargement of liver and spleen and erosion of long bones and pelvis
Niemann-Pick disease	Sphingomyelinase	Sphingomyelin	Enlarged liver and spleen, mental retardation, and foam cells in bone marrow
Krabbe disease	Galactocerebrosidase	Galactocerebroside	Mental retardation, demyelination, psychomotor retardation, and death
Metachromatic leukodystrophy	Arylsulfatase	Sulfatide	Demyelination, mental retardation, nerves stain yellow-brown with cresyl-violet dye, and progressive paralysis
Fabry disease	α-Galactosidase A	Ceramide trihexoside	Skin lesions, kidney disease, pain in lower extremities, and X-linked recessive inheritance
Generalized gangliosidosis	β-Galactosidase	Ganglioside GM_1 and proteoglycans	Mental retardation, hepatomegaly, skeletal involvement, and a startle response to sound

48 Essential Fatty Acids and Eicosanoid Metabolism

A Essential fatty acids

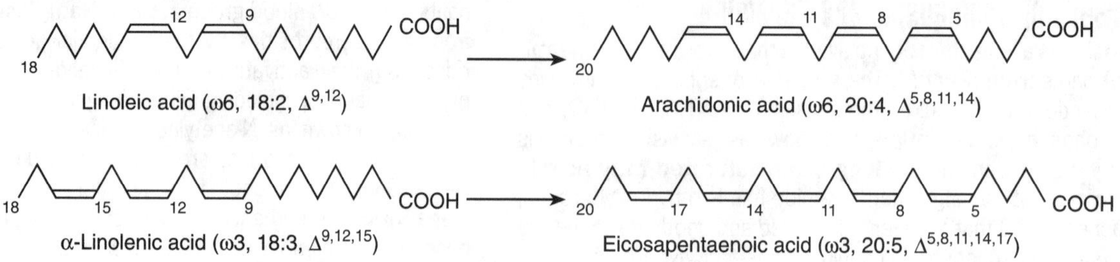

Linoleic acid ($\omega 6$, 18:2, $\Delta^{9,12}$)

Arachidonic acid ($\omega 6$, 20:4, $\Delta^{5,8,11,14}$)

α-Linolenic acid ($\omega 3$, 18:3, $\Delta^{9,12,15}$)

Eicosapentaenoic acid ($\omega 3$, 20:5, $\Delta^{5,8,11,14,17}$)

B Synthesis of eicosanoids

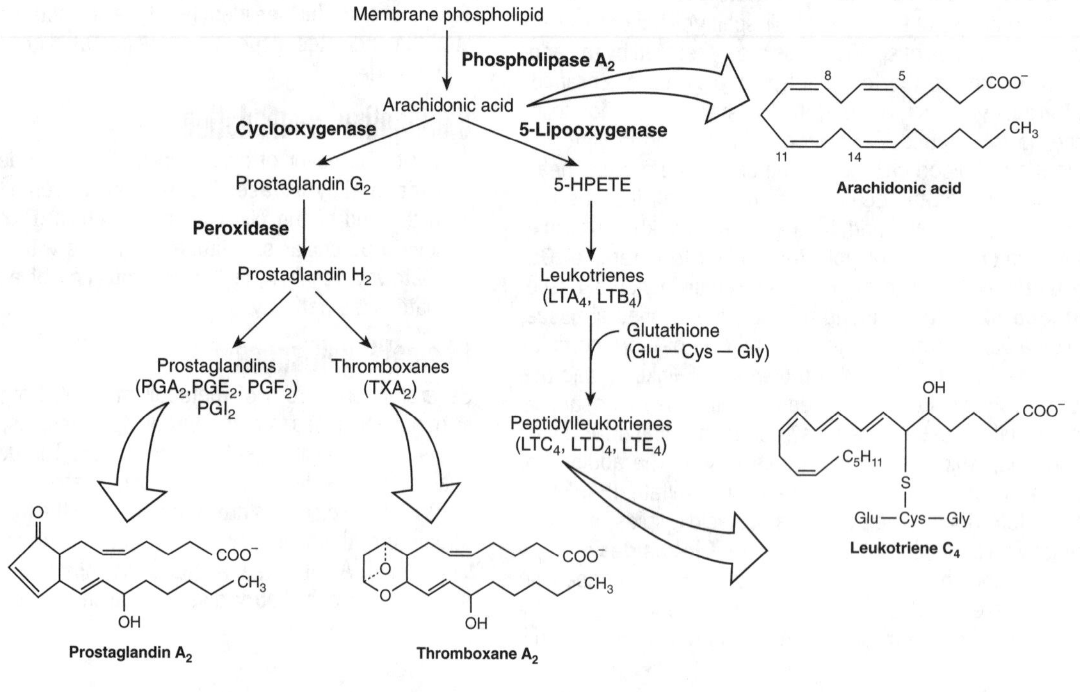

Membrane phospholipid

Phospholipase A$_2$

Arachidonic acid

Cyclooxygenase   **5-Lipooxygenase**

Arachidonic acid

Prostaglandin G$_2$ 5-HPETE

Peroxidase

Prostaglandin H$_2$ Leukotrienes (LTA$_4$, LTB$_4$)

Glutathione (Glu — Cys — Gly)

Prostaglandins (PGA$_2$, PGE$_2$, PGF$_2$) PGI$_2$ Thromboxanes (TXA$_2$)

Peptidylleukotrienes (LTC$_4$, LTD$_4$, LTE$_4$)

Prostaglandin A$_2$ **Thromboxane A$_2$**   **Leukotriene C$_4$**

C Function of eicosanoids

Tissue	Eicosanoid	Biologic effect
Heart	PGE$_2$ and PGF$_2$ PGI$_2$	Contraction Relaxation
Peripheral vasculature	PGE$_2$ and PGI$_2$	Vasodilation and decreased blood pressure in heart, kidney, and skeletal muscle
Gastrointestinal system	PGE$_2$	Suppression of gastric secretion
Lungs	PGE$_2$ PGF$_2$ and TXA$_2$	Relaxation of bronchial smooth muscle Contraction of bronchial smooth muscle
Platelets	PGI$_2$ TXA$_2$	Inhibition of aggregation Stimulation of aggregation

OVERVIEW

The eicosanoids are a group of biologically active C_{20} compounds that include the prostaglandins, thromboxanes, and leukotrienes. One or more eicosanoids are synthesized by all mammalian cells except RBCs. The immediate precursors of the eicosanoids are arachidonic acid and eicosapentanoic acid, which are derived from linoleic and linolenic acids, respectively. The eicosanoids are local hormones that have either **paracrine** or **autocrine** functions, exerting their action on neighboring cells or the cells in which they are synthesized. The eicosanoids are grouped into two major categories: **cyclic eicosanoids**, which include prostaglandins and thromboxanes, and **linear eicosanoids**, which include the leukotrienes. Three major classes of prostaglandins are found in humans: PGA, PGE, and PGF. These classes can be distinguished from one another on the basis of their ring systems. The ring of PGA is the most oxidized ring, containing a double bond and an attached carbonyl oxygen, whereas the ring system of PGF is the most reduced, containing no double bonds and two attached hydroxyl groups. The oxidation state of the ring in PGE is intermediate between that of PGA and PGF. A fourth class, PGI, is a special class of prostaglandin, sometimes referred to as prostacyclin, that has a two member-ring system. Each class of prostaglandins has three different series, designated as 1, 2, and 3 (PGA_1, PGA_2, PGA_3, etc). The 2 series is the most important in humans. All members of the 2 series are derived from arachidonic acid, whereas all members of the 3 series are derived from eicosapentanoic acid.

Essential Fatty Acids

Linoleic acid and linolenic acid are essential fatty acids that cannot be synthesized by human tissues (**Part A**). **Linoleic acid** is an **ω-6 fatty acid**, having 18 carbons and containing two double bonds. **Linolenic acid** is an **ω-3 fatty acid**, having 18 carbons and three double bonds. The ω-numbering system starts at the methyl end of fatty acids. Humans are unable to insert double bonds into fatty acids at either the ω-6 or the ω-3 position thereby making them essential dietary nutrients. The primary source of ω-3 fatty acids is fish oil, whereas the primary sources of ω-6 fatty acids are vegetable oils. Dietary linoleic acid and linolenic acid are converted by human tissues to arachidonic acid and eicosapentanoic acid, respectively. These polyunsaturated fatty acids are stored in membrane phospholipids, primarily at the C-2 position of phosphatidylcholine and phosphatidylinositol.

Synthesis of Eicosanoids

Most of the eicosanoids in humans are derived from arachidonic acid (**Part B**). The synthesis can be considered as occurring in two stages: 1) the release of arachidonic acid from storage sites in membrane phospholipids, and 2) the conversion of arachidonic acid to either prostaglandins, thromboxanes, or leukotrienes. Arachidonic acid is released from cell membranes by the action of **phospholipase A_2**. Cell stimuli such as epinephrine, angiotensin II, and thrombin increase the intracellular concentration of Ca^{2+}, which results in translocation of phospholipase A_2 from the cytosol to the membrane. The step that commits arachidonic acid to the synthesis of cyclic eicosanoids is catalyzed by a multienzyme complex, **prostaglandin synthase**. This complex consists of two enzymes, **cyclooxygenase**, which converts arachidonic acid to PGG_2, and **peroxidase**, which converts PGG_2 to PGH_2. Virtually all cells contain these enzymes and can synthesize PGH_2. Other prostaglandins and thromboxanes are derived by modification of PGH_2. Different types of cells synthesize different eicosanoids, depending on the complement of enzymes present.

The pathway leading to leukotriene synthesis is initiated by **5-lipooxygenase**, an enzyme that catalyzes the addition of O_2 to the double bond between C-5 and C-6 of arachidonic acid. The product of this reaction, **5-HPETE**, is the precursor for all the leukotrienes. LTC_4, LTD_4, and LTE_4 have peptides or amino acids attached. The tripeptide glutathione (Glu-Cys-Gly) is attached to LTC_4, and the sequential removal of glutamate and glycine results in LTD_4 and LTE_4, respectively.

The synthesis of eicosanoids is inhibited by two major classes of drugs. **Glucocorticoids** inhibit phospholipase A_2, thereby decreasing the synthesis of all three classes of eicosanoids. **Nonsteroidal anti-inflammatory drugs** such as aspirin, indomethacin, and phenylbutazone inhibit cyclooxygenase, decreasing the synthesis of prostaglandins and thromboxanes, but having no effect on leukotriene synthesis. The effects of aspirin are irreversible.

Function of Eicosanoids

The eicosanoids are local hormones that exert their action either on the cell that produces them or on neighboring cells. They are synthesized upon demand and not stored. They are present in trace amounts and have a very short half-life, ranging from seconds to minutes. Many of the eicosanoids have opposing effects on different tissues. They initiate their actions by binding to cell-surface receptors and activating signal transduction pathways. Some of the biologic effects of prostaglandins and thromboxanes are summarized in **Part C**. The leukotrienes are potent mediators of inflammatory responses.

Clinical Significance

The antithrombogenic activity of fish oils is due to their high content of the ω-3 fatty acids. Platelets synthesize thromboxane A_3 (TXA_3) from ω-3 fatty acids and TXA_2 from ω-6 fatty acids. **TXA_2 is thrombogenic**, promoting the aggregation of platelets, whereas TXA_3 decreases platelet aggregation in humans. Leukotrienes have been implicated in the pathogenesis of several inflammatory diseases, including asthma, psoriasis, rheumatoid arthritis, and inflammatory bowel disease. Leuketriene D_4 has been identified as the **slow-reacting substance of anaphylaxis**, which causes smooth muscle contraction and constriction of pulmonary airways.

For more information see Coffee C, *Metabolism*. Fence Creek, pp 318–322.

Directions: For each of the following questions, choose the **one best** answer.

1. A patient with pancreatic enzyme deficiency is likely to be deficient in which vitamins?

(A) Folate

(B) Ascorbic acid

(C) Vitamin E

(D) Riboflavin

(E) Niacin

2. Bile salts are effective detergents in the small intestine because

(A) They contain hydrophobic groups

(B) They have an amphipathic structure

(C) They are uncharged at the pH existing in the small intestine

(D) They are zwitterions at the pH existing in the small intestine

(E) They are efficiently recycled by the enterohepatic circulation

3. Which class of lipoproteins has the highest energy content per gram?

(A) High-density lipoprotein (HDL)

(B) Low-density lipoprotein (LDL)

(C) Intermediate-density lipoprotein (IDL)

(D) Very-low-density lipoprotein (VLDL)

(E) Chylomicron

4. The lipoprotein that plays a major role in reverse cholesterol transport from extrahepatic tissues to the liver is

(A) HDL

(B) IDL

(C) LDL

(D) VLDL

(E) Chylomicron

5. An auto mechanic came to the emergency room because of severe epigastric pain. A few hours earlier he had eaten a large meal of pork chops, fried onions, mashed potatoes with gravy, and beer. Analysis of his serum showed a slight elevation in pancreatic amylase and a low level of apo C-II. Which of the following lipoprotein profiles would most likely be seen in this patient?

(A) Decreased chylomicrons and decreased VLDLs

(B) Elevated HDLs and elevated LDLs

(C) Elevated chylomicrons and elevated VLDLs

(D) Decreased chylomicrons and elevated VLDLs

(E) Elevated chylomicrons and decreased VLDLs

6. A patient with hypercholesterolemia is being treated with mevinolin. Which of the following statements describes the most direct effect of this drug?

(A) The activity of HMG CoA reductase is decreased.

(B) The synthesis of LDL receptors is increased.

(C) The activity of acyl-cholesterol acyltransferase (ACAT) is increased.

(D) The synthesis of chylomicrons is increased.

(E) The activity of lecithin-cholesterol acyltransferase (LCAT) is inhibited.

7. Which of the following enzymes and pathways are correctly paired?

(A) Phospholipase C and prostaglandin synthesis

(B) β-Glucocerebrosidase and sphingolipid synthesis

(C) 5-Lipooxygenase and leukotriene synthesis

(D) 7-Hydroxylase and vitamin D synthesis

(E) Phospholipase A_2 and steroid hormone synthesis

8. Which of the following sets of enzymes is required for the synthesis of both aldosterone and cortisol?

(A) 20-22 desmolase, 11-hydroxylase, 17-hydroxylase

(B) 20-22 desmolase, 11-hydroxylase, 21-hydroxylase

(C) 20-22 desmolase, 18-hydroxylase, 3β-hydroxysteroid dehydrogenase

(D) 20-22 desmolase, 21-hydroxylase, 17β-hydroxysteroid dehydrogenase

(E) 20-22 desmolase, 11-hydroxylase, 17-20 lyase

9. Which of the following symptoms is commonly observed in patients with 21-hydroxylase deficiency?

(A) Hypertension with virilization

(B) Hypotension with virilization

(C) Hypertension without virilization

(D) Hypotension without virilization

(E) None of the above

10. During fatty acid synthesis, the presence of acetyl CoA in the cytosol can be attributed directly to the activity of which of the following enzymes?

(A) Citrate synthase

(B) Isocitrate dehydrogenase

(C) Citrate lyase

(D) Malic enzyme

(E) Acetyl CoA carboxylase

11. Which of the following properties is characteristic of acetyl CoA carboxylase?

(A) It is activated by cAMP-dependent phosphorylation

(B) It is allosterically activated by citrate

(C) It is located in the mitochondrial matrix

(D) It catalyzes the synthesis of palmitoyl CoA

(E) It polymerizes into long polymers that have very little catalytic activity

12. The products resulting from β-oxidation of stearic acid (18:0) are

(A) 9 mols acetyl CoA, 18 mols NADH, 9 mols FADH$_2$

(B) 9 mols acetyl CoA, 18 mols NADPH

(C) 9 mols acetyl CoA, 8 mols NADH, 8 mols FADH$_2$

(D) 8 mols malonyl CoA, 1 mol acetyl CoA, 8 mols NADH, 8 mols FADH$_2$

(E) 9 mols malonyl CoA, 8 mols NADPH, 8 mols FADH$_2$

13. The binding of insulin to its receptor on the surface of liver leads to the inhibition of

(A) Acetyl CoA carboxylase

(B) Carnitine acyltransferase-1

(C) Fatty acid synthase

(D) Citrate lyase

(E) Glucose-6-phosphate dehydrogenase

14. Which of the following lipases is most important in mobilizing fatty acids from adipose tissue triglyceride?

(A) Pancreatic lipase

(B) Gastric lipase

(C) Hormone sensitive lipase

(D) Lingual lipase

(E) Lipoprotein lipase

15. Ketone bodies serve as fuel for all of the following cells or tissues **except:**

(A) Skeletal muscle

(B) Brain

(C) Red blood cells

(D) Kidney

(E) Heart

16. Respiratory distress syndrome is associated with a deficiency in which of the following lipids?

(A) Leukotriene C$_4$

(B) Dipalmitoyllecithin

(C) Phosphatidylinositol bisphosphate

(D) Sphingomyelin

(E) β-Glucocerebroside

17. The synthesis of which of the eicosanoids is inhibited by gluco-corticoids?

(A) Prostaglandins

(B) Thromboxanes

(C) Prostacyclins

(D) Leukotrienes

(E) All of the above

18. Which of the following lipids is both a phospholipid and a sphingolipid?

(A) Sulfatide

(B) Globoside

(C) Cerebroside

(D) Sphingomyelin

(E) Ganglioside

Directions: The group of questions below consists of lettered options followed by several numbered items. For each numbered item, select the most appropriate lettered option. Each lettered option can be used once, more than once, or not at all.

Questions 19–21
For each of the lipids listed below, select the compound that is its precursor.

(A) Cholesterol

(B) Linoleic acid

(C) Glycerol

(D) Ceramide

19. Triglyceride

20. Sphingolipid

21. Eicosanoid

Questions 22–24
For each of the functions listed below, select the apoprotein that mediates that function.

(A) Apo A-I

(B) Apo B-100

(C) Apo C-II

(D) Apo E

22. Activates lipoprotein lipase

23. Activates lecithin cholesterol acyltransferase (LCAT)

24. Binds to remnant receptors

Questions 25–26
For each of the clinical conditions listed below, select the most closely associated lipoprotein.

(A) Chylomicron

(B) VLDL

(C) LDL

(D) HDL

25. Familial hypercholesterolemia

26. Tangier's disease

Questions 27–28
For each of the clinical conditions listed below, select the enzyme or cofactor that is deficient.

(A) Medium chain acyl CoA dehydrogenase (MCAD) deficiency

(B) Biotin deficiency

(C) Acetyl CoA carboxylase deficiency

(D) Carnitine deficiency

27. Hypoketonic hypoglycemia with the accumulation of C_6-C_{10} fatty acids

28. Hypoketonic hypoglycemia with the accumulation of C_{16}-C_{20} fatty acids

Questions 29–30
For each of the diseases listed below, select the enzyme deficiency associated with the disease.

(A) Sphingomyelinase

(B) β-Glucocerebrosidase

(C) Hexosaminidase A

(D) Galactocerebrosidase

29. Tay Sachs disease

30. Gaucher disease

PART IV: ANSWERS AND EXPLANATIONS

1. The answer is C.

Pancreatic enzyme insufficiency results in lipid malabsorption. The fat soluble vitamins are normally incorporated into chylomicrons and absorbed with other dietary lipids. Any condition that results in lipid malabsorption can also lead to a deficiency in the fat-soluble vitamins A, D, E, and K.

2. The answer is B.

The detergent properties of bile salts are related to their amphipathic structure. The ring system provides a hydrophobic face that interacts effectively with triglyceride and cholesterol esters, while hydroxyl groups on the sterol ring and negatively charged groups on the side chain provide a hydrophilic face that interacts favorably with the aqueous medium.

3. The answer is E.

Triglycerides make up about 88% of the weight of chylomicrons and the percentage decreases progressively from chylomicrons to VLDL, IDL, LDL, and HDL in that order.

4. The answer is A.

HDL picks up cholesterol from extrahepatic tissues. The cholesterol is esterified by LCAT and then transferred to either chylomicron remnants or VLDL remnants. Most of the remnants are eventually taken up by the liver where the cholesterol is converted to bile salts and secreted into the bile.

5. The answer is C.

A deficiency in apo C-II results in decreased lipoprotein lipase activity. Therefore, the ability to degrade both chylomicron triglyceride and VLDL triglyceride is impaired, resulting in the accumulation of chylomicrons and VLDL and a decreased level of chylomicron remnants, IDLs and LDLs.

6. The answer is A.

Mevinolin inhibits HMG CoA reductase, resulting in decreased synthesis of cholesterol. The cell responds to decreased intracellular cholesterol by increasing the rate of transcription of the LDL receptor gene, which leads to increased LDL receptor synthesis followed by increased uptake of circulating LDL. A decrease in intracellular cholesterol also leads to decreased activity of ACAT. Neither the synthesis of chylomicrons nor the activity of LCAT is affected by mevinolin.

7. The answer is C.

5-Lipooxygenase commits arachidonic acid to the pathway of leukotriene synthesis. Phospholipase C is involved in the phosphatidylinositol signal transduction pathway. β-Glucocerebrosidase participates in the pathway of sphingolipid degradation. 7-Hydroxylase catalyzes the rate-limiting step in the pathway of bile acid synthesis. Phospholipase A_2 releases arachidonic acid from phospholipid stores, providing the substrate for eicosanoid synthesis.

8. The answer is B.

Enzymes common to the pathways of aldosterone and cortisol synthesis include 20-22 desmolase, 3β-hydroxysteroid dehydrogenase, 21-hydroxylase, and 11-hydroxylase. Both 18-hydroxylase and 18-hydroxysteroid dehydrogenase are specific for aldosterone synthesis, while 17-20 lyase is specific for androgen and estrogen synthesis.

9. The answer is B.

Hypotension (secondary to salt wasting) and virilization are commonly seen in patients with 21-hydroxylase deficiency. The major intermediate that accumulates behind the block is 17-hydroxypregnenolone, which is converted to adrenal androgens, leading to virilization. Salt wasting is related to the impaired ability to synthesize aldosterone and the decreased ability to reabsorb sodium.

10. The answer is C.

The citrate shuttle is responsible for the translocation of acetyl CoA from the mitochondrial matrix to the cytosol where fatty acid synthesis occurs. Citrate lyase is present in the cytosol where it cleaves citrate to oxaloacetate and acetyl CoA.

11. The answer is B.

Citrate promotes polymerization of acetyl CoA carboxylase into long polymers that have a high degree of catalytic activity. Phosphorylation of acetyl CoA carboxylase inactivates the enzyme. This enzyme is found in the cytosol where it catalyzes the synthesis of malonyl CoA.

12. The answer is C.

β-Oxidation of fatty acids results in the production of acetyl CoA, NADH, and $FADH_2$. β-Oxidation is a cyclic process involving four sequential reactions: FAD-dependent oxidation, hydration, NAD^+-dependent oxidation, and thiolytic cleavage. Each cycle results in the release of a C_2 fragment (acetyl CoA), $FADH_2$, and NADH. The last cycle results in the oxidation of a C_4 fatty acid that is cleaved, producing two mols of acetyl CoA.

13. The answer is B.

Insulin activates acetyl CoA carboxylase, resulting in increased production of malonyl CoA. The activity of carnitine acyltransferase-1 and the entry of fatty acids into the mitochondria is inhibited by malonyl CoA, thereby ensuring that fatty acid synthesis and oxidation do not occur simultaneously. Insulin also increases the activity of fatty acid synthase, citrate lyase, and glucose-6-phosphate dehydrogenase. All of these enzymes are involved either directly or indirectly in fatty acid synthesis.

14. The answer is C.

Hormone sensitive lipase cleaves fatty acids from the C-1 and C-3 positions of the glycerol backbone of triglycerides. It is located primarily in adipose tissue and is activated by several hormones that increase the intracellular concentration of cAMP. Its activity is inhibited by insulin. Pancreatic lipase, gastric lipase, and lingual lipase are all involved in the hydrolysis of dietary triglyceride in the gastrointestinal tract. Lipoprotein lipase is an extracellular enzyme that hydrolyzes triglyceride associated with lipoproteins.

15. The answer is C.

Oxidation of β-hydroxybutyrate and acetoacetate occurs in the mitochondria, and red blood cells have no mitochondria. Almost all other cells and tissues that have mitochondria can oxidize ketone bodies. The exception is liver, where acetoacetate cannot be converted to acetoacetyl CoA because of the absence of succinyl CoA:acetoacetate CoA transferase.

16. The answer is B.

Dipalmitoyllecithin is a component of surfactant, the surface-active agent that lines the walls of alveoli and prevents their collapse at the end of each respiratory cycle.

17. The answer is E.

Glucocorticoids inhibit phospholipase A_2, the enzyme that releases arachidonic acid from the glycerol backbone of phospholipids. Arachidonic acid is the primary substrate for all classes of eicosanoids.

18. The answer is D.

Sphingomyelin is the only sphingolipid that is also a phospholipid. It is also the only phospholipid that is not a glycerol-based phospholipid.

Sphingomyelin is formed by the addition of phosphocholine to ceramide, and is found in high concentration in the red blood cell membrane and in the myelin sheath that surrounds neurons in the central nervous system.

Questions 19–30:
The answers are 19-C, 20-D, 21-B.

Triglycerides are synthesized by the esterification of fatty acids to a glycerol backbone. All of the sphingolipids contain ceramide as a common structural component. They differ by the groups that are attached to the terminal hydroxyl group in ceramide. The dietary precursor of eicosanoids is linoleic acid, an ω-6 fatty acid that is converted to arachidonic acid.

The answers are 22-C, 23-A, 24-D.

Lipoprotein lipase, an extracellular enzyme attached to luminal surface of capillaries, is activated by apo C-II. Lipoproteins containing apo C-II bind to lipoprotein lipase, allowing triglyceride to be hydrolyzed. The fatty acids that are released are taken up by tissues, where they are either stored or oxidized. Almost all of the apo A-I is found in HDL, where it facilitates the binding of HDL to extrahepatic tissues. Cholesterol diffuses from extraphepatic tissues to the HDL particle, where it is esterified by lecithin cholesterol acyltransferase (LCAT). LCAT is activated by apo A-I. Apo E binds to remnant receptors on the surface of liver and allows chylomicron remnants and VLDL remnants (IDL) to be taken up by receptor-mediated endocytosis.

The answers are 25-C, 26-D.

Familial hypercholesterolemia results from an inherited defect in the LDL receptor, resulting in the accumulation of LDL in the serum. In Tangier's disease the concentrations of apo A-I and HDL are extremely low while the chylomicron and VLDL concentrations are elevated. Normally, HDL donates apo C-II and apo E to chylomicrons and VLDLs. In the absence of apo C-II, chylomicrons and VLDLs cannot be metabolized by lipoprotein lipase, and in the absence of apo E, they cannot be cleared by the liver.

The answers are 27-A, 28-D.

The first step in the oxidation of fatty acids is catalyzed by a family of dehydrogenases that are specific to fatty acids of different chain lengths. A deficiency in medium chain acyl CoA dehydrogenase results in the accumulation of fatty acids that are between C_6 and C_{10} in length. The hypoglycemia can be attributed to an increased reliance of most tissues on glucose for energy and a decreased rate of gluconeogenesis. The energy required to drive gluconeogenesis is normally derived from the oxidation of fatty acids. Hypoketonic hypoglycemia, with the accumulation of fatty acids having a chain length between C_{16} and C_{20}, results from a deficiency in carnitine. Carnitine is required to translocate long chain fatty acids into the mitochondrial matrix where they are oxidized.

The answers are 29-C, 30-B.

Tay Sachs disease results from an inherited deficiency in hexosaminidase A, resulting in the accumulation of ganglioside GM_2. Clinical symptoms of Tay Sachs disease include mental retardation and a cherry-red spot on the macula. Death usually occurs by age 3. Gaucher disease results from an inherited deficiency in β-glucocerebrosidase, resulting in the accumulation of β-glucocerebroside. The infantile form of Gaucher disease shows central nervous system involvement, whereas the adult form is characterized by hepatosplenomegaly and osteoporosis of the long bones.

PART V
Amino Acid and Nitrogen Metabolism

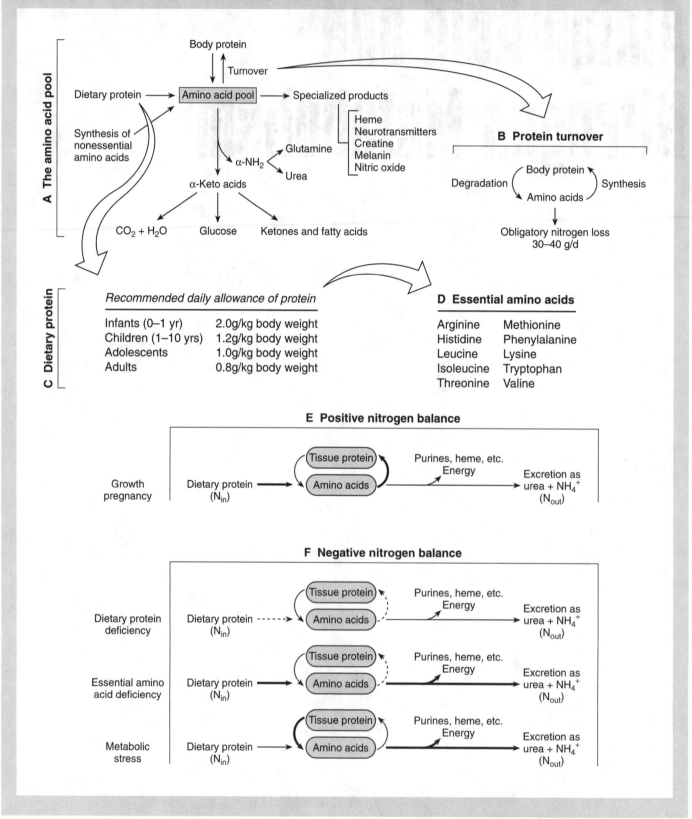

A The amino acid pool

Body protein
Turnover

Dietary protein → Amino acid pool → Specialized products
  Heme
  Neurotransmitters
  Creatine
  Melanin
  Nitric oxide

Synthesis of nonessential amino acids

α-NH₂ → Glutamine
      → Urea

α-Keto acids → CO₂ + H₂O
            → Glucose
            → Ketones and fatty acids

B Protein turnover

Degradation → Body protein → Synthesis
  Amino acids
  → Obligatory nitrogen loss 30–40 g/d

C Dietary protein

Recommended daily allowance of protein

Infants (0–1 yr)	2.0g/kg body weight
Children (1–10 yrs)	1.2g/kg body weight
Adolescents	1.0g/kg body weight
Adults	0.8g/kg body weight

D Essential amino acids

Arginine	Methionine
Histidine	Phenylalanine
Leucine	Lysine
Isoleucine	Tryptophan
Threonine	Valine

E Positive nitrogen balance

Growth pregnancy — Dietary protein (N_in) → Tissue protein / Amino acids → Purines, heme, etc. Energy → Excretion as urea + NH₄⁺ (N_out)

F Negative nitrogen balance

Dietary protein deficiency — Dietary protein (N_in) → Tissue protein / Amino acids → Purines, heme, etc. Energy → Excretion as urea + NH₄⁺ (N_out)

Essential amino acid deficiency — Dietary protein (N_in) → Tissue protein / Amino acids → Purines, heme, etc. Energy → Excretion as urea + NH₄⁺ (N_out)

Metabolic stress — Dietary protein (N_in) → Tissue protein / Amino acids → Purines, heme, etc. Energy → Excretion as urea + NH₄⁺ (N_out)

OVERVIEW

The primary function of dietary protein is to provide amino acids for 1) replacing tissue protein that is broken down during normal metabolism, and 2) synthesizing several specialized products that contain nitrogen. The replacement of tissue protein requires 20 amino acids. Ten of the amino acids are essential components of the diet, whereas the nonessential amino acids can be synthesized from common intermediates in metabolic pathways or from essential amino acids. If the nitrogen intake is equal to the amount of nitrogen excreted, a state of nitrogen balance exists. The concept of nitrogen balance is important in defining the protein nutritional state of an individual.

The Amino Acid Pool

The pool of circulating amino acids is maintained at a relatively constant level under a variety of conditions (**Part A**). The amino acid pool is derived primarily from the turnover of tissue protein. About 75% of the amino acids derived from tissue protein degradation are used for rebuilding tissue protein. The remainder is used for synthesis of glucose, ketones, and a variety of specialized nitrogenous products including heme, neurotransmitters, creatine, melanin, nitric oxide, purines, and pyrimidines. The essential amino acids that are removed from the pool are replaced by dietary protein. Unlike dietary glucose or fatty acids, there is no storage form for amino acids. Excess amino acids are degraded primarily by the liver. Most of the nitrogen is excreted as urea, while a smaller amount is used for glutamine synthesis. The carbon skeletons remaining after removal of the amino groups are either oxidized to CO_2 and H_2O for energy or used as substrates for gluconeogenesis and ketogenesis.

Protein Turnover

Proteins are in a constant state of degradation and resynthesis, with about 1% to 2% of the total body protein turning over each day (**Part B**). Between 30 and 40 g of nitrogen derived from amino acids are excreted daily and are not available for resynthesis of protein. This **obligatory nitrogen loss** results from oxidation of amino acids and excretion of nitrogenous compounds in sweat, urine, and feces. Different proteins are degraded at different rates, each having a characteristic **half-life** ($t_{1/2}$). Some proteins, such as immunoglobulins and collagen, have a very long $t_{1/2}$ (measured in years), while others have a very short $t_{1/2}$ (measured in minutes). Protein turnover occurs in all tissues, but some are more active than others. The proteins of liver, intestine, and kidney turn over much faster than proteins in skeletal muscle.

Dietary Protein

The recommended daily allowance of protein for adults is based on the amount needed to maintain **nitrogen balance (Part C)**. Additional protein is required by women who are pregnant or breast feeding. Throughout pregnancy, an additional 30 g of protein a day is recommended, and during lactation, an additional 20 g per day. The amount of protein required by children is based on the amount needed for **optimal growth**, rather than on the amount needed to maintain nitrogen balance. In all age groups, the protein requirement of a particular individual is increased during catabolic states, such as surgery, sepsis, and trauma. Dietary protein is used efficiently only when adequate calories are included in the diet. When the caloric intake is low, much of the protein is oxidized as a source of energy, thereby increasing the amount needed to maintain nitrogen balance. Excess dietary protein consumed over a long period of time results in increased **loss of urinary calcium**.

Essential Amino Acids

Ten of the amino acids found in proteins cannot be synthesized by humans in an amount sufficient to meet the body needs and are essential components of the diet (**Part D**). The essential amino acids include all the basic amino acids (arginine, histidine, and lysine), all amino acids having a branched side chain (valine, leucine, isoleucine, and threonine), two of the three aromatic amino acids (phenylalanine and tryptophan), and methionine (a sulfur amino acid). Arginine and histidine are essential only in early childhood. If phenylalanine is deficient, tyrosine becomes essential. Similarly, if methionine is deficient, cysteine becomes essential.

Nitrogen Balance

Nitrogen balance is the condition that exists when the amount of nitrogen consumed is equal to the amount excreted from the body. **Positive nitrogen balance (Part E)**, exists when the amount of nitrogen consumed is greater than that excreted. It is associated with periods of growth, pregnancy, lactation, and recovery from metabolic stress. **Negative nitrogen balance (Part F)** occurs when the amount of nitrogen excreted exceeds the nitrogen intake and is associated with several conditions, including 1) inadequate dietary protein; 2) a deficiency in one or more of the essential amino acids, although a large amount of protein is consumed; and 3) metabolic stress, such as uncontrolled diabetes, starvation, sepsis, and trauma.

Clinical Significance

The most common form of malnutrition is **protein-calorie malnutrition**, a condition commonly found in hospitalized patients. The amount of protein required for a hospitalized patient can be calculated from the following formula, which is based on the amount of nitrogen excreted as urea within a 24-hour period:

$$\text{Protein intake (g/24 hr)} = (\text{g urinary urea} + 4) \times 6.25$$

Although the symptoms of malnutrition vary widely among individuals, most cases are classified as either **marasmus** or **kwashiorkor**. The symptoms of these two types of protein-calorie malnutrition are summarized in the following table:

Symptom	Marasmus	Kwashiorkor
Growth failure	Present	Present
Anemia	Present	Present
Edema	Absent	Present
Hepatomegaly	Absent	Present
Depigmentation	Absent	Present
Hypoalbuminemia	Normal/mild	Severe
Muscle wasting	Severe	Absent/mild
Fat reserves	Absent	Normal/mildly diminished

For more information see Coffee C, *Metabolism*. Fence Creek, pp 335–338.

50 Protein Digestion and Amino Acid Absorption

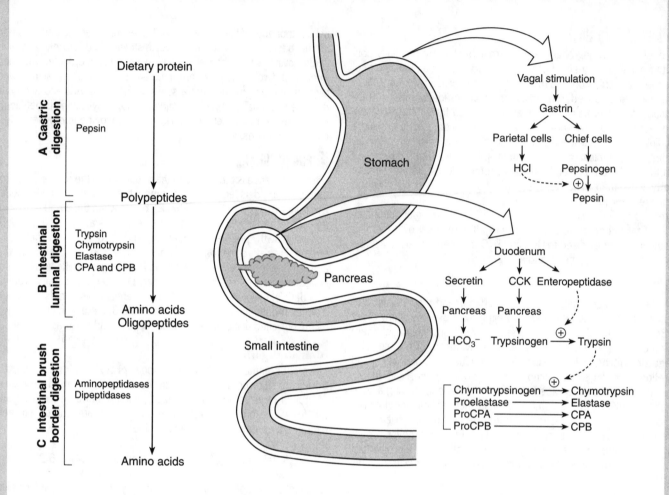

A Gastric digestion

Dietary protein

Pepsin

Polypeptides

B Intestinal luminal digestion

Trypsin
Chymotrypsin
Elastase
CPA and CPB

Amino acids
Oligopeptides

C Intestinal brush border digestion

Aminopeptidases
Dipeptidases

Amino acids

Vagal stimulation

Gastrin

Parietal cells   Chief cells

HCl   Pepsinogen
⊕
Pepsin

Stomach

Pancreas

Small intestine

Duodenum

Secretin   CCK   Enteropeptidase

Pancreas   Pancreas

HCO_3^- Trypsinogen ⊕→ Trypsin

Chymotrypsinogen ⊕→ Chymotrypsin
Proelastase ——→ Elastase
ProCPA ——→ CPA
ProCPB ——→ CPB

D Amino acid absorption

Transport system	Amino acids transported	Genetic disease
Neutral amino acids	Alanine, glycine, serine, threonine, valine, leucine, isoleucine, phenylalanine, tyrosine, tryptophan, histidine, cysteine, methionine, and citrulline	Hartnup disease
Acidic amino acids	Glutamic acid and aspartic acid	Dicarboxylic aminoaciduria
Dibasic amino acids	Lysine, arginine, cystine and ornithine	Cystinuria
Imino acids and glycine	Proline, hydroxyproline and glycine	Joseph syndrome

OVERVIEW

The source of protein to be digested comes from both exogenous and endogenous sources. As much as 50 g of protein a day may be derived from secretions of the gastrointestinal tract and gastrointestinal cells that have been sloughed off. The products of protein digestion are a mixture of amino acids, dipeptides, and tripeptides. Under normal conditions, very little protein is excreted in the feces. Protein digestion is facilitated by three types of secretions elaborated by the stomach, intestine, and pancreas, including 1) aqueous solutions of varying pH and electrolyte composition, which provide the environment required for optimal activity of the digestive enzymes; 2) inactive precursors of the digestive enzymes; and 3) mucoproteins that form highly viscous solutions and act as lubricants to facilitate passage of partially digested food through the gastrointestinal tract. Protein digestion starts in the stomach and is completed in the small intestine, where absorption of amino acids occurs.

Gastric Digestion

The entry of food into the stomach results in the release of **gastrin** from the mucosal cells that line the stomach (**Part A**). Gastrin stimulates the release of **gastric juice** from **parietal cells** and the release of **pepsinogen** from **chief cells**. Gastric juice contains HCl, along with a few other electrolytes, and intrinsic factor, a protein required for absorption of vitamin B_{12}. Gastric juice has a pH of about 1. It denatures dietary protein, making it highly susceptible to proteolysis. The activation of pepsinogen is initiated by the low pH of gastric juice, which results in cleavage of a peptide bond, generating catalytically active **pepsin**. Autocatalytic activation follows, with pepsin rapidly activating other pepsinogen molecules. Pepsin, an **endopeptidase** with broad specificity, hydrolyzes proteins to a mixture of large peptides having C-terminal residues contributed by aromatic amino acids, acidic amino acids, leucine, and methionine.

Intestinal Luminal Digestion

The movement of partially digested chyme through the duodenum stimulates the release of two hormones, secretin and cholecystokinin (CCK) and the release of enteropeptidase (**Part B**). **Secretin** stimulates the release of **pancreatic juice**, an alkaline secretion enriched in HCO_3^-, that neutralizes the acid in the chyme as it enters the small intestine. **CCK** stimulates the release of several **zymogens** from the exocrine pancreas. Some of the zymogens are precursors of endopeptidases (chymotrypsinogen, trypsinogen, and proelastase) and others are precursors of exopeptidases (procarboxypeptidase A and procarboxypeptidase B). **Enteropeptidase** initiates a proteolytic cascade that leads to activation of all the pancreatic zymogens. Enteropeptidase releases a small peptide from trypsinogen, producing catalytically active trypsin. **Trypsin** converts the other pancreatic zymogens to their active forms (**chymotrypsin, elastase, carboxypeptidases A and B**). Each of these proteases has a different specificity, and the products of one enzyme are the substrates for another enzyme. The peptides generated by trypsin have C-terminal residues contributed by lysine and arginine, whereas peptides generated by chymotrypsin have C-terminal residues contributed by aromatic amino acids. The concerted action of the pancreatic enzymes efficiently hydrolyzes the large peptides produced in the stomach to a mixture of **free amino acids** and **small peptides** having 2 to 5 amino acids.

Intestinal Brush Border Digestion

The intestinal mucosal cells contain enzymes that catalyze the terminal steps in protein digestion (**Part C**). There are several **aminopeptidases** and **dipeptidases**, having different specificities, that sequentially remove amino acids from the N-terminus of the peptides. Most of the intestinal enzymes are found both in the brush border membrane and in the cytosol of intestinal cells.

Amino Acid Absorption

Amino acids are transported into intestinal mucosal cells by mechanisms that are analogous to the Na^+-dependent transport of glucose. Several transport proteins are found in the brush border membrane that are specific for groups of structurally similar amino acids (**Part D**). Four amino transporters have been well characterized that are specific for the following groups of amino acids: 1) dibasic amino acids, 2) acidic amino acids, 3) neutral amino acids, and 4) amino acids and glycine. All of the transporters are specific for L-amino acids; the D-amino acids are transported by passive diffusion. These four transporters are also found in the brush border membrane of the kidney, where they reabsorb amino acids from the glomerular filtrate.

Clinical Significance

It is estimated that no more than 10% to 15% of the total protein digestion occurs in the stomach. Individuals whose stomachs have been removed surgically excrete very little protein in the feces and have no difficulty maintaining normal nitrogen balance. Conversely, individuals with impaired intestinal digestion of protein experience negative nitrogen balance and excrete large amounts of protein in the feces.

Several diseases result from inherited defects in amino acid transporters. **Cystinuria**, the most common disease of amino acid transport, results from a deficiency in the **dibasic amino acid transporter**. Patients excrete large amounts of cystine, ornithine, arginine, and lysine in the urine. They frequently suffer from kidney stones that are formed from cystine, which is relatively insoluble at the acidic pH of the urine. **Hartnup disease** results from a deficiency in the neutral amino acid transporter. This disease is characterized by high levels of the neutral amino acids in the urine and low levels in the serum. Mild pellagra-like symptoms are often observed, due to the inability to absorb tryptophan. Tryptophan is a precursor of niacin, providing up to 20% of the daily niacin requirement.

For more information see Coffee C, *Metabolism*. Fence Creek, pp 339–343.

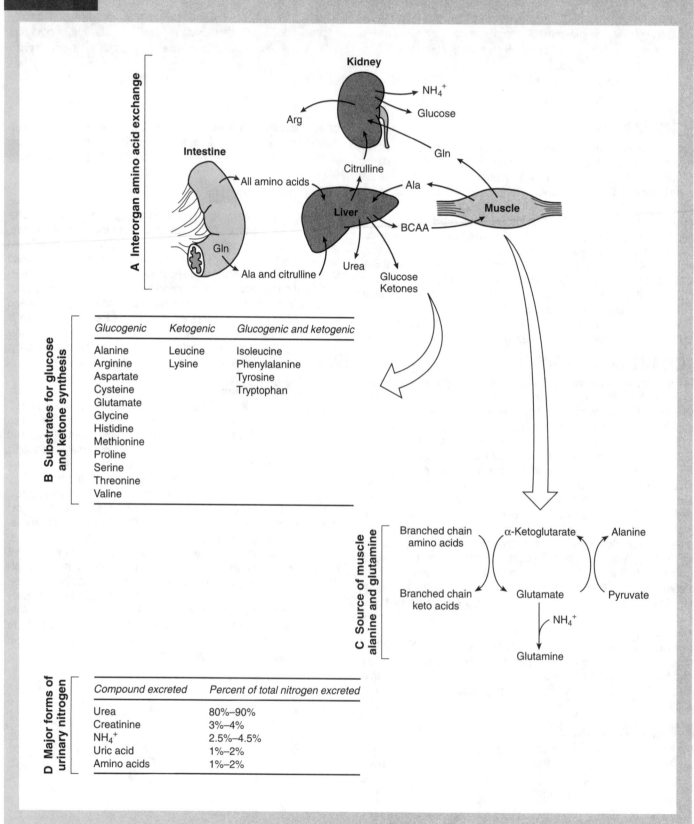

A Interorgan amino acid exchange

Kidney

NH$_4^+$

Glucose

Arg

Gln

Intestine

Citrulline

All amino acids

Ala

Liver

Muscle

BCAA

Gln

Ala and citrulline

Urea

Glucose
Ketones

B Substrates for glucose and ketone synthesis

Glucogenic	Ketogenic	Glucogenic and ketogenic
Alanine	Leucine	Isoleucine
Arginine	Lysine	Phenylalanine
Aspartate		Tyrosine
Cysteine		Tryptophan
Glutamate		
Glycine		
Histidine		
Methionine		
Proline		
Serine		
Threonine		
Valine		

C Source of muscle alanine and glutamine

Branched chain amino acids → α-Ketoglutarate → Alanine

Branched chain keto acids → Glutamate → Pyruvate

NH$_4^+$

Glutamine

D Major forms of urinary nitrogen

Compound excreted	Percent of total nitrogen excreted
Urea	80%–90%
Creatinine	3%–4%
NH$_4^+$	2.5%–4.5%
Uric acid	1%–2%
Amino acids	1%–2%

OVERVIEW

Various organs and tissues play different roles in amino acid metabolism. Each tissue, including the blood, has a pool of free amino acids. The total body pool is equal to about 100 g. Muscle has the largest pool, which makes up 50% to 80% of the total. Interorgan amino acid exchange is essential for maintaining homeostasis. During the fasting state, plasma amino acid levels are maintained by the degradation of tissue protein. In the fed state, tissue protein is rebuilt from amino acids derived from dietary protein. Following absorption, amino acids are carried to the liver by the portal circulation, and from there they are distributed by the general circulation throughout the body.

Intestine

The amino acid composition of dietary protein is altered by intestinal mucosal cells, which oxidize **glutamine** as their major source of energy, producing a mixture of products including CO_2, NH_4^+, and **alanine** (**Part A**). In the fasting state, the intestine oxidizes glutamine, which is released by skeletal muscle. Intestinal cells also synthesize and release **citrulline**, which is converted to arginine by the kidney. Both citrulline and arginine are intermediates in the urea cycle. Although the liver is the only organ that can synthesize urea, intestinal cells have the first two enzymes of the urea cycle which are used to synthesize citrulline. The kidney has the third and fourth enzymes of the cycle, which convert citrulline to arginine. Thus, the intestine and the kidney are responsible for the **interorgan synthesis of arginine**.

Liver

The catabolism of most amino acids starts in the liver, where the amino groups are removed by transamination and deamination and incorporated into **urea** (**Part A**). The carbon skeletons that remain can either be oxidized to CO_2 and H_2O or used as substrates for glucose and ketone synthesis. Amino acids are often classified as **glucogenic** or **ketogenic** amino acids based on whether their carbon skeletons are used for glucose or ketone synthesis (**Part B**). Only leucine and lysine are **strictly ketogenic** amino acids. All others are either glucogenic or both glucogenic and ketogenic. After a meal, the concentration of the amino acid pool leaving the liver is 2 to 3 times higher than in the fasting state, and more than half of the pool is made up of **branched-chain amino acids (BCAAs)**. The catabolism of BCAAs (valine, isoleucine, and leucine) cannot be initiated in the liver because BCAA transaminase is not present in this tissue. The liver does not extract citrulline from the portal blood because the citrulline transport protein is not present in the hepatocyte plasma membrane.

Skeletal Muscle

The catabolism of most BCAAs starts in skeletal muscle (**Part A**), although some of the valine is taken up by brain and used as a carbon source for **myelin** synthesis. In skeletal muscle, the amino groups of BCAAs are transferred via two transamination reactions to pyruvate, forming **alanine** (**Part C**). The amino group is first transferred to α-ketoglutarate, forming glutamate in a reaction catalyzed by **BCAA transaminase**. Glutamate has two fates: 1) the amino group can be transferred from glutamate to pyruvate by **alanine transaminase**, producing alanine; and 2) NH_4^+ can be added to the side chain of glutamate, producing **glutamine**. Glutamine synthesis requires ATP and

is catalyzed by **glutamine synthetase**. Alanine and glutamine make up more than 50% of all the amino acids that leave skeletal muscle. Alanine acts as a **carrier of amino groups** to liver where they can be incorporated into urea and excreted, whereas glutamine is taken up by the kidney and deaminated, producing NH_3 that acts as a sponge for absorbing protons. The synthesis of glutamine occurs in all cells, where it provides a mechanism for detoxifying ammonia.

Kidney

The kidney is an ammoniagenic organ. Most of the NH_4^+ excreted in the urine is derived from glutamine (**Part A**). The release of NH_3 from glutamine occurs in two consecutive reactions that are catalyzed by **glutamate dehydrogenase** and **glutaminase**, respectively. Both enzymes are located in the mitochondria.

$$\text{Glutamine} \xrightarrow{\quad NH_3 \quad} \text{Glutamate} \xrightarrow{\quad NH_3 \quad} \alpha\text{-Ketoglutarate}$$

NH_3 is rapidly converted to NH_4^+ by absorbing a proton (H^+) from the medium. Essentially all of the NH_3 released in the kidney is excreted as NH_4^+. During periods of metabolic acidosis, the activity of glutaminase is increased, thereby providing a mechanism for excreting H^+ in the urine. The α-ketoglutarate produced from glutamine is the major substrate for **renal gluconeogenesis**. The kidney also converts citrulline, released by intestinal cells, to arginine.

Major Forms of Urinary Nitrogen

Most of the end products of nitrogen metabolism are excreted in the urine (**Part D**). Urea is the major excretory form of nitrogen, with small amounts excreted as creatinine, NH_4^+, and uric acid. Less than 2% of the urinary nitrogen is still in the form of amino acids.

Clinical Significance

Hepatic encephalopathy is a neuropsychiatric syndrome associated with advanced liver failure. Several abnormalities in amino acid metabolism occur that are believed to contribute to the neurologic effects. Ammonia is extremely toxic to brain and nerve tissue, and in liver failure, **hyperammonemia** results from a decreased ability to synthesize urea. Plasma levels of **aromatic amino acids** increase, while the levels of **BCAAs** decrease. Normally, most of the aromatic amino acids are catabolized in the liver. However, with impaired liver function, they leave the liver without being degraded. It is believed that high levels of phenylalanine and tyrosine may interfere with dopamine and norepinephrine synthesis in the brain.

For more information see Coffee C, *Metabolism*. Fence Creek, pp 347–360.

52 Removal of Amino Groups and Disposal of Carbon Skeletons

A Pyridoxal phosphate and amino acid metabolism

Pyridoxal phosphate (PLP)

Schiff base between PLP and amino acid

B Removal of amino groups by transamination and deamination

Amino acid → α-Ketoglutarate ← NADH + H$^+$ + NH$_4^+$

α-Keto acid ← Glutamate → NAD$^+$ + H$_2$O

Many transaminases

Glutamate dehydrogenase

C End products of amino acid degradation

Products of glucogenic amino acids	Products of ketogenic amino acids
Pyruvate	Acetyl CoA
Oxaloacetate	Acetoacetyl CoA
Fumarate	
Succinyl CoA	
α-Ketoglutarate	

D Metabolic fate of carbon skeletons

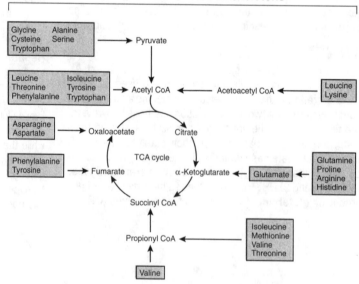

OVERVIEW

The first step in the catabolism of amino acids is the removal of amino groups, which is accomplished by two types of reactions, transamination and deamination. Most transamination reactions channel amino groups into glutamate, which is subsequently deaminated, releasing ammonia. Deamination reactions differ from transamination reactions by directly releasing ammonia from amino acids. Most of the ammonia is excreted as urea. The carbon skeletons of all 20 common amino acids are degraded to seven products, which are intermediates in central pathways of metabolism.

Role of Pyridoxal Phosphate in Amino Acid Metabolism

Pyridoxal phosphate is a cofactor for many enzymes involved in amino acid metabolism (**Part A**). It is derived from two interconvertible forms of **vitamin B_6**, pyridoxal and pyridoxine. The aldehyde group of pyridoxal phosphate forms a **Schiff base** with the α-amino group of an amino acid, resulting in a labile intermediate that is common to many reactions in amino acid metabolism, including reactions catalyzed by **transaminases, decarboxylases, racemases,** and some **deaminases.**

Removal of Amino Groups by Transamination and Deamination Reactions

The catabolism of most amino acids begins with the transfer of the α-amino group to an α-keto acid, usually α-ketoglutarate, pyruvate, or oxaloacetate (**Part B**). These reactions are catalyzed by **transaminases,** also known as aminotransferases. Each transaminase is specific for one or a few amino acid donors, but most transaminases use α-ketoglutarate as a common acceptor of amino groups. This provides a mechanism for channeling amino groups from many different sources into a common product, **glutamate.** Transaminases are usually named by the amino acid that donates the amino group.

$$\text{Alanine} + \alpha\text{-Ketoglutarate} \xrightleftharpoons[]{\text{Alanine transaminase}} \text{Pyruvate} + \text{Glutamate}$$

$$\text{Aspartate} + \alpha\text{-Ketoglutarate} \xrightleftharpoons[]{\text{Aspartate transaminase}} \text{Oxaloacetate} + \text{Glutamate}$$

Transaminase reactions are **reversible**, a property that is particularly important in the reactions catalyzed by alanine transaminase (also known as SGPT) and aspartate transaminase (also known as SGOT). **Alanine transaminase plays a key role in transferring amino groups from skeletal muscle to liver,** where they can be incorporated into urea and excreted. Aspartate transaminase is particularly important in liver, where it acts as an amino donor in the synthesis of urea.

Quantitatively, the most important **deamination reaction** in humans is catalyzed by **glutamate dehydrogenase**, an enzyme found in high concentration in liver mitochondria (**Part B**). Amino groups are released from the common glutamate pool as ammonia, which is used by liver mitochondria to synthesize carbamoyl phosphate, the first intermediate in the urea cycle. Deamination reactions also release ammonia from glutamine, asparagine, histidine, glycine, serine, and threonine.

End Products of Amino Acid Degradation

The degradation of glucogenic amino acids results in five end products, pyruvate, and four intermediates of the tricarboxylic acid (TCA) cycle (**Part C**). All of these end products are substrates for gluconeogenesis. The degradation of ketogenic amino acids produces acetyl CoA or acetoacetyl CoA. These products can be used for the synthesis of ketone bodies or fatty acids, but cannot be converted to glucose.

Metabolic Fate of Carbon Skeletons

The end products derived from each amino acid and the point at which they enter mainstream metabolism is shown in the figure on the opposite page (**Part D**). All or parts of five amino acids (glycine, alanine, cysteine, serine, and tryptophan) enter glycolysis as **pyruvate.** Asparagine and aspartate enter the TCA cycle as **oxaloacetate.** However, all amino acids that are degraded to intermediates in the TCA cycle pass through oxaloacetate, the first intermediate in the pathway of gluconeogenesis. Parts of phenylalanine and tyrosine are converted to **fumarate.** Methionine, threonine, and the branched-chain amino acids, valine and isoleucine, are degraded to **propionyl CoA,** which enters the TCA cycle as **succinyl CoA.** Five amino acids (glutamate, glutamine, proline, arginine, and histidine) enter the TCA cycle as α-**ketoglutarate.** All or parts of six amino acids (leucine, threonine, phenylalanine, isoleucine, tyrosine, tryptophan) are degraded to **acetyl CoA.**

Clinical Significance

The importance of pyridoxal phosphate in amino acid metabolism is illustrated by the consequences of a deficiency in vitamin B_6. The most common deficiency symptoms are changes in the central nervous system and oily dermatitis. Hypochromic microcytic anemia has been observed occasionally. In infants, the most common symptoms are hyperirritability and convulsive seizures, which can be relieved by administration of pyridoxine. The neurological symptoms are believed to result from decreased synthesis of γ-**aminobutyric acid (GABA),** a neurotransmitter derived from glutamate in a pyridoxal phosphate–dependent decarboxylation reaction. Deficiency of vitamin B_6 is most commonly seen in patients with tuberculosis or copper storage disease who are being treated, respectively, with **isoniazid** or **penicillamine.** These drugs combine with pyridoxal and pyridoxal phosphate, depleting the pool unless supplements are provided. Women taking **oral contraceptives** also have an increased requirement for vitamin B_6. Although vitamin B_6 has a low toxicity, daily supplements of 500 mg over an extended period of time may result in a sensory neuropathy. Large supplements also reduce the beneficial effect of L-dopa in patients with Parkinson disease.

For more information see Coffee C, *Metabolism*. Fence Creek, pp 348–357.

53 Detoxification of Ammonia

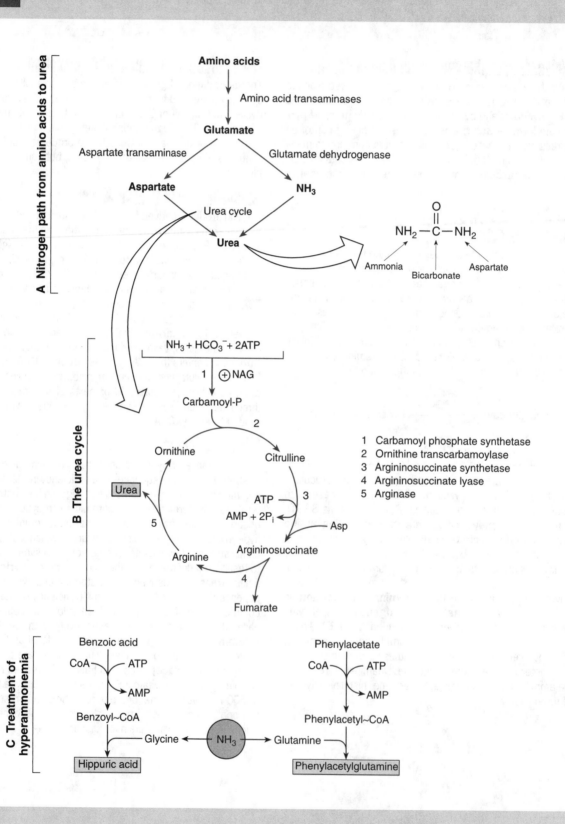

OVERVIEW

Ammonia is extremely toxic to the central nervous system. The body has evolved mechanisms for converting ammonia into two nontoxic compounds, **urea** and **glutamine**. Urea, the major nontoxic product, is formed only in the liver. The rate of the urea cycle is regulated by both short-term and long-term mechanisms. Short-term regulation is determined by the activity of carbamoyl phosphate synthetase-1 (CPS-1), while long-term regulation involves an increase or decrease in all the enzymes in the urea cycle, depending on the amount of protein that is being degraded. Extrahepatic tissues synthesize glutamine as a means of detoxifying ammonia. Glutamine serves as a source of biosynthetic nitrogen, particularly in purine and pyrimidine synthesis. Excess glutamine is taken up by liver and kidney, where it is sequentially deaminated to glutamate and α-ketoglutarate, releasing ammonia in the mitochondria. In liver, the ammonia is incorporated into urea and in kidney it is excreted as NH_4^+.

Flow of Nitrogen from Amino Acids to Urea

The two most important enzymes involved in transferring nitrogen from amino acids to urea are **amino acid transaminases** and **glutamate dehydrogenase (Part A)**. Most transaminases use α-ketoglutarate as an amino acceptor, thereby channeling amino groups into a common glutamate pool. Some of the amino groups in glutamate are transferred to oxaloacetate, producing aspartate, while the remaining amino groups in glutamate are released as ammonia. Urea contains two amino groups, one derived from ammonia and the other from aspartate.

The Urea Cycle

The first two steps in urea synthesis occur in the mitochondria, and all others occur in the cytosol (**Part B**). The formation of urea is described by the following equation:

$$NH_3 + HCO_3^+ + \text{Aspartate} + 3\,ATP \longrightarrow$$
$$\text{Urea} + \text{Fumarate} + 2\,ADP + AMP + 4\,P_i$$

The synthesis of carbamoyl phosphate, the first intermediate in the cycle, is catalyzed by **CPS-1**. The substrates for CPS-1 are ammonia, bicarbonate, and ATP. Two isozymes of CPS exist in cells: CPS-1, a mitochondrial isozyme, is devoted to urea synthesis, while CPS-2, a cytosolic isozyme, is devoted to pyrimidine nucleotide synthesis. The condensation of carbamoyl phosphate with ornithine, producing citrulline, is catalyzed by **ornithine transcarbamoylase (OTC)**, a mitochondrial enzyme. Citrulline is transported to the cytosol, where it condenses with aspartate, producing argininosuccinate. This reaction is catalyzed by **argininosuccinate synthetase** and requires ATP. Cleavage of argininosuccinate by **argininosuccinate lyase**, produces arginine and fumarate. The last step in the cycle is catalyzed by **arginase**, which releases urea from the arginine side chain and regenerates ornithine. Ornithine is transported back into the mitochondria so that a new cycle can begin. Ornithine and citrulline are transported across the mitochondrial membrane by the same transport protein.

The **rate of the urea cycle** is determined by the activity of CPS-1, the rate-limiting enzyme in the cycle. CPS-1 is allosterically activated by **N-acetylglutamate (NAG)**. The synthesis of NAG, as described by the following equation, increases as the concentration of glutamate increases. Therefore, both NAG synthesis and urea synthesis increase as protein degradation and amino acid transamination

increase. The K_m of **NAG synthase** for glutamate is high, and the enzyme is not saturated under physiologic conditions. NAG synthase is allosterically activated by arginine.

$$\text{Glutamate} + \text{Acetyl CoA} \xrightarrow[\oplus \text{ Arginine}]{\text{NAG Synthase}} \text{N-Acetylglutamate} + \text{CoA}$$

An increase in dietary protein over several days results in increased synthesis of all the enzymes in the urea cycle. The process is reversed by a shift to a low-protein diet. During starvation, synthesis of all the urea cycle enzymes also increases. The rate of the urea cycle decreases during metabolic acidosis. The increase in $[H^+]$ shifts the equilibrium between ammonia and ammonium ion, thereby decreasing ammonia, which is the substrate for CPS-1.

Treatment of Hyperammonemia

Treatment of acute hyperammonemia may involve hemodialysis or exchange transfusions to lower the ammonia level rapidly. Management usually involves **decreasing protein intake, avoiding infection**, and **stimulating alternative pathways of nitrogen excretion (Part C)**. **Benzoic acid** and **phenylacetate** activate latent pathways in the liver that conjugate **glycine** and **glutamine** with benzoic acid and phenylacetate, respectively, producing **hippuric acid** and **phenylacetylglutamine**, which are excreted in the urine. This treatment is effective because both glycine and glutamine are in equilibrium with free ammonia in the body. The best indicator of the effectiveness of treatment is the plasma level of glutamine.

Clinical Significance

Genetic deficiencies in the urea cycle enzymes occur at a frequency of about 1 in 25,000 live births. They usually become apparent during the neonatal period. These disorders are associated with mental retardation, convulsions, coma, and death. Because of the high toxicity of ammonia, neonatal hyperammonemia must be treated immediately to avoid brain damage. A summary of diseases resulting from deficiencies in urea cycle enzymes is shown in the table below. Hyperammonemia type II, resulting from an inherited deficiency in ornithine carbamoyltransferase, is the most common disease associated with the urea cycle. It is transmitted as an X-linked trait. Hyperammonemia has been reported for deficiencies in all of the enzymes except arginase.

Disease	Defective Enzyme	Products Accumulated
Hyperammonemia type I	Carbamoyl phosphate synthetase I	Ammonia, glutamine, and alanine
Hyperammonemia type II	Ornithine transcarbamoylase	Ammonia, glutamine, and orotic acid
Citrullinemia	Argininosuccinate synthetase	Citrulline
Argininosuccinic aciduria	Argininosuccinate lyase	Argininosuccinate
Argininemia	Arginase	Arginine

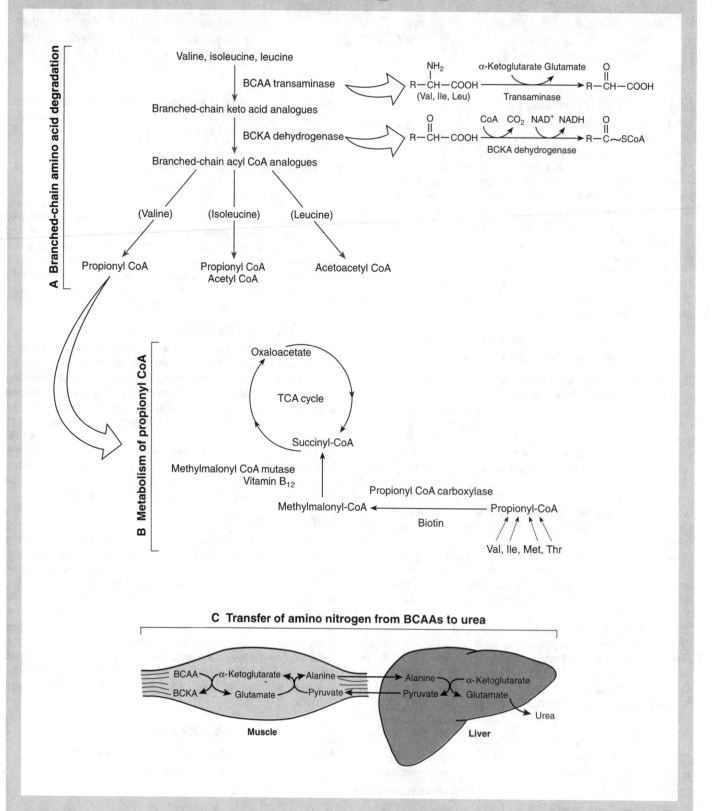

A Branched-chain amino acid degradation

Valine, isoleucine, leucine

BCAA transaminase

Branched-chain keto acid analogues

BCKA dehydrogenase

Branched-chain acyl CoA analogues

(Valine)   (Isoleucine)   (Leucine)

Propionyl CoA

Propionyl CoA
Acetyl CoA

Acetoacetyl CoA

B Metabolism of propionyl CoA

Oxaloacetate

TCA cycle

Succinyl-CoA

Methylmalonyl CoA mutase
Vitamin B$_{12}$

Methylmalonyl-CoA

Propionyl CoA carboxylase

Propionyl-CoA

Biotin

Val, Ile, Met, Thr

C Transfer of amino nitrogen from BCAAs to urea

Muscle

Liver

Urea

The catabolism of valine, leucine, and isoleucine begins in skeletal muscle, where the concentration of branched-chain amino acid (BCAA) transaminase is high. This enzyme is not expressed to a significant extent in the liver, where the catabolism of most amino acids begins. Following a meal, the BCAAs make up more than half of the total amino acid pool leaving the liver. Following transamination in muscle, alanine is the major carrier of amino groups to the liver where they are incorporated into urea and excreted. The branched-chain ketoacids (BCKAs) that result from transamination are oxidized as fuel by muscle, liver, kidney, and brain tissue. Several types of organic acidurias result from inherited defects in the catabolism of the BCAAs.

Branched-Chain Amino Acid Degradation

Catabolism of valine, isoleucine, and leucine share two common reactions, transamination followed by oxidative decarboxylation of the respective BCKAs (**Part A**). A single **BCAA transaminase** catalyzes the transamination of all three amino acids. The three BCKAs resulting from transamination are decarboxylated by the same **BCKA dehydrogenase**. The branched-chain acyl CoA thioesters are further metabolized along separate pathways. The end product of valine degradation is propionyl CoA, while that of leucine is acetoacetyl CoA. Isoleucine is degraded to both propionyl CoA and acetyl CoA.

The **BCKA dehydrogenase** is similar in structure and mechanism to that of the pyruvate dehydrogenase complex and the α-ketoglutarate dehydrogenase complex. All are multienzyme complexes located in the mitochondria, and all catalyze oxidative decarboxylation reactions, requiring five coenzymes (thiamine pyrophosphate, lipoic acid, CoA, NAD^+, and FAD). The **rate-limiting step** in the degradation of the BCAA is catalyzed by BCKA dehydrogenase, which is regulated both allosterically and covalently. NADH and acyl CoA, both products of the reaction, are also allosteric inhibitors of BCKA dehydrogenase. A specific **BCKA dehydrogenase kinase and BCKA dehydrogenase phosphatase** are associated with the multienzyme complex. Phosphorylation of BKCA dehydrogenase results in inhibition. The **BCKA dehydrogenase kinase** is inhibited by the accumulation of BCKAs.

Metabolism of Propionyl CoA

The glucogenic nature of **valine** and **isoleucine** is attributed to the ability of propionyl CoA to be converted to succinyl CoA, an intermediate in the tricarboxylic acid cycle (**Part B**). Propionyl CoA is also derived from the degradation of **methionine** and **threonine**, as well as from the ω-**end of odd-chain fatty acids**. Propionyl CoA is carboxylated to methylmalonyl CoA in the reaction catalyzed by **propionyl CoA carboxylase**, a biotin-requiring enzyme. The reaction is described below:

$$\text{Propionyl CoA} + HCO_3^- + ATP \xrightarrow{\text{biotin}} \text{Methylmalonyl CoA} + ADP + P_i$$

Methylmalonyl CoA undergoes a vitamin B_{12}-dependent rearrangement reaction, resulting in succinyl CoA. The latter reaction is catalyzed by **methylmalonyl CoA mutase**. This is one of the two reactions in human biochemistry that require vitamin B_{12}.

Transfer of Amino Nitrogen from BCAA to Urea

Most of the amino groups of the BCAAs are transported to the liver by alanine (**Part C**). The initial transamination reaction in muscle is catalyzed by **BCAA transaminase**, which uses α-ketoglutarate as an acceptor, producing glutamate. A second transamination, catalyzed by **alanine transaminase**, transfers the amino group from glutamate to pyruvate, producing alanine. Alanine is released by muscle and carried to the liver, where the amino group is transferred from alanine to α-ketoglutarate, producing glutamate. Glutamate is used for the synthesis of aspartate and NH_3, both substrates for urea synthesis.

Clinical Significance

A genetic defect in **BCKA dehydrogenase** is responsible for maple syrup urine disease (MSUD), an **autosomal recessive** disorder. The incidence of MSUD is about 1 in 185,000 newborns throughout the world, although it is particularly prevalent in the Mennonite population in central Pennsylvania, where it occurs in about 1 in 175 newborns. The symptoms appear early in infancy, and death often occurs by 1 year of age. Symptoms include vomiting, lethargy, and severe brain damage. Autopsy shows cerebral edema, lack of myelin, and a reduction in total lipids. Urine has a characteristic odor similar to that of burnt sugar. Urine and plasma contain elevated levels of BCAAs, the corresponding α-ketoacids and α-hydroxyacids. Diagnosis is confirmed by assaying fibroblasts or leukocytes for BCKA dehydrogenase activity.

Defects in **propionyl CoA carboxylase** and **methylmalonyl CoA mutase** result in **propionic acidemia** and **methylmalonic aciduria**, respectively. Defects in either of these enzymes result in metabolic acidosis and the excretion of organic acids in the urine. Some cases of methylmalonic aciduria respond to high doses of vitamin B_{12}.

For more information see Coffee C, *Metabolism*. Fence Creek, pp 357–359.

55 Hepatic Aromatic Amino Acid Metabolism

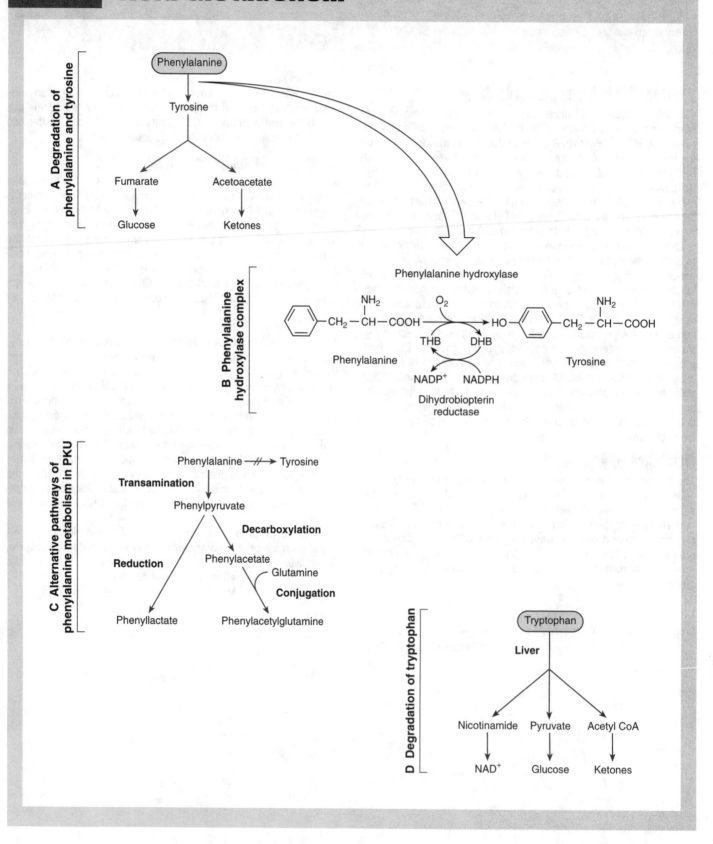

A Degradation of phenylalanine and tyrosine

Phenylalanine → Tyrosine

Tyrosine → Fumarate → Glucose

Tyrosine → Acetoacetate → Ketones

B Phenylalanine hydroxylase complex

Phenylalanine hydroxylase

$$\text{Phenylalanine} + O_2 \xrightarrow{\text{THB} \rightarrow \text{DHB}} \text{Tyrosine}$$

Phenylalanine (structure with NH$_2$, CH$_2$—CH—COOH)

Tyrosine (structure HO— ring —CH$_2$—CH—COOH, NH$_2$)

THB → DHB

NADP$^+$ ← NADPH

Dihydrobiopterin reductase

C Alternative pathways of phenylalanine metabolism in PKU

Phenylalanine —//→ Tyrosine

Transamination

Phenylpyruvate

Decarboxylation

Reduction → Phenylacetate

Glutamine

Conjugation

Phenyllactate

Phenylacetylglutamine

D Degradation of tryptophan

Tryptophan

Liver

Nicotinamide → NAD$^+$

Pyruvate → Glucose

Acetyl CoA → Ketones

The aromatic amino acids are phenylalanine, tyrosine, and tryptophan. Phenylalanine and tryptophan are essential amino acids and must be supplied by the diet. Tyrosine is synthesized from phenylalanine and is nonessential unless there is a dietary deficiency of phenylalanine or a block in the pathway for converting phenylalanine to tyrosine. Although tyrosine and tryptophan are converted to a number of specialized products in extrahepatic tissues, the major site of degradation for all the aromatic amino acids is the liver. Several diseases result from the inability to degrade phenylalanine and tyrosine, the most common being phenylketonuria (PKU).

Degradation of Phenylalanine and Tyrosine

Tyrosine is the first intermediate in the degradation of phenylalanine (**Part A**). It is formed by the addition of a hydroxyl group to the phenylalanine side chain, a reaction catalyzed by **phenylalanine hydroxylase**. Tyrosine undergoes five sequential reactions, resulting in the formation of fumarate and acetoacetate. The five reactions that convert tyrosine to its end products start with **tyrosine transaminase**, which produces hydroxyphenylpyruvate, and end with **fumarylacetoacetate hydrolase**, which generates fumarate and acetoacetate. This sequence of reactions is shown below:

$$\text{Tyrosin} \xrightarrow{1} \text{Hydroxyphenylpyruvate} \xrightarrow{2} \text{Homogentisate} \xrightarrow{3}$$

$$\text{Maleylacetoacetate} \xrightarrow{4} \text{Fumarylacetoacetate} \xrightarrow{5}$$

$$\text{Fumarate + Acetoacetate}$$

Several diseases involving amino acid metabolism result from enzyme deficiencies in this pathway. A deficiency in tyrosine transaminase (enzyme 1) results in **type II tyrosinemia**; a transient deficiency in hydroxyphenylpyruvate oxidase (enzyme 2) is believed to be responsible for **neonatal tyrosinemia**; a deficiency in homogentisate oxidase (enzyme 3) results in **alkaptonuria**, the first disease recognized as an inherited metabolic disorder; a deficiency in fumarylacetoacetate hydrolase (enzyme 5) results in **type I tyrosinemia**.

The Phenylalanine Hydroxylase Complex

The conversion of phenylalanine to tyrosine is an irreversible reaction catalyzed by the phenylalanine hydroxylase complex (**Part B**). This reaction requires O_2 as a substrate; two cofactors, tetrahydrobiopterin (THB) and NADPH; and two enzymes, **phenylalanine hydroxylase** and **dihydrobiopterin (DHB) reductase**. A deficiency in either of these enzymes results in PKU. Although phenylalanine hydroxylase is found only in liver, DHB reductase is also found in brain and adrenal medulla, where it is involved in the synthesis of catecholamines and serotonin. The only known enzymes that use THB as a cofactor are the aromatic amino acid hydroxylases.

Alternative Pathways of Phenylalanine Metabolism in PKU

A deficiency in phenylalanine hydroxylase, DHB reductase, or THB results in the accumulation of phenylalanine, leading to PKU. In patients with PKU, phenylalanine is metabolized by pathways that are normally latent in the liver (**Part C**). The end products of these pathways are phenylpyruvate, phenyllactate, phenylacetate, and phenylacetylglutamine.

Degradation of Tryptophan

Tryptophan is degraded in liver by a complex pathway consisting of several enzymes (**Part D**). The end products are pyruvate and acetyl CoA, accounting for the fact that tryptophan is both a glucogenic and ketogenic amino acid. Tryptophan is also a precursor of niacin, which is used for NAD^+ synthesis. The amount of tryptophan in an average diet, however, will provide only a small fraction of the niacin needed. One of the reactions required to convert tryptophan to niacin requires pyridoxal phosphate. Therefore, a dietary deficiency in vitamin B_6 prevents tryptophan from being used as a source of niacin.

Clinical Significance

The most common inherited disease in amino acid metabolism is PKU, occurring in about 1 in 10,000 live births. Diagnosis can be made within a few days after birth by measuring the level of phenylalanine in the blood. Screening of newborns for PKU is mandated by law. In PKU, the level of phenylalanine in both blood and urine may be increased as much as 30-fold. Phenylpyruvate is normally not detected in either the plasma or urine, but in PKU, the plasma level is between 0.3 and 1.8 mg/dL, and the level in the urine is between 300 and 2000 mg/dL. Phenyllactate, phenylacetate, and phenylacetylglutamine are also excreted in the urine. A distinctive "mousy" odor results from increased levels of phenylacetate. Severe mental retardation occurs unless phenylalanine is restricted in the diet. The dietary goal is to maintain blood phenylalanine between 2 and 6 mg/dL. **Classic PKU** results from an inherited deficiency in phenylalanine hydroxylase. **Atypical PKU**, sometimes called malignant PKU, results from a deficiency in **DHB reductase**. Atypical PKU accounts for about 2% of all cases of PKU. Both forms are inherited as autosomal recessive traits. **Maternal PKU** occurs in unborn children of phenylketonuric mothers whose diets are not restricted in phenylalanine. Phenylketones produced by the mother readily cross the placenta, resulting in brain damage in the unborn child. Nutrasweet, also known as aspartame, is widely used as a synthetic sweetener. It is a dipeptide containing aspartic acid and phenylalanine methyl ester. The use of Nutrasweet by pregnant women who are either heterozygous or homozygous for PKU may cause brain damage in the fetus.

For more information see Coffee C, *Metabolism*. Fence Creek, pp 364, 370–372.

56 Extrahepatic Metabolism of Tyrosine

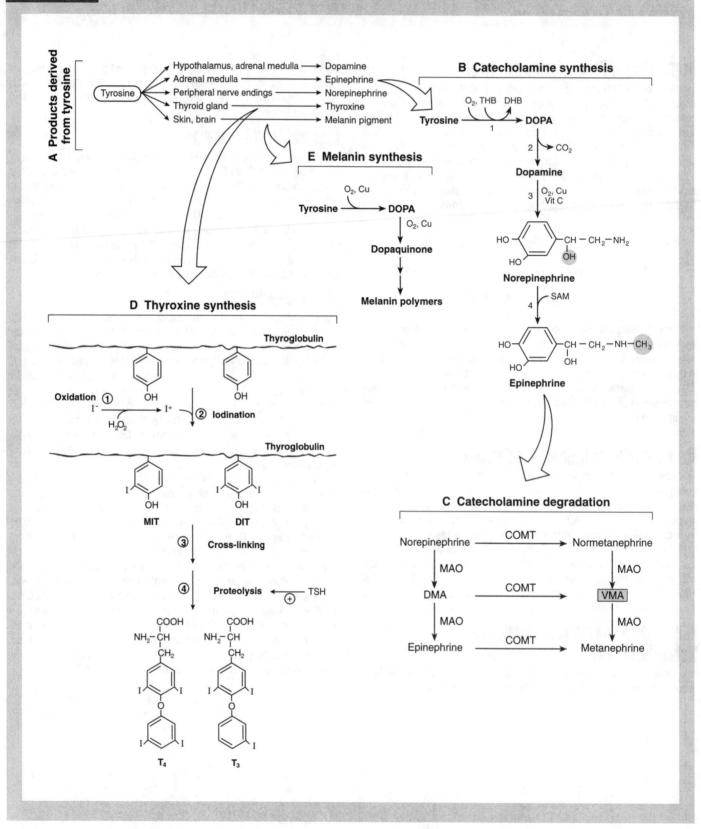

Tyrosine is taken up by extrahepatic tissues and converted to several biologically active compounds including thyroid hormones, melanin and the catecholamines, dopamine, norepinephrine, and epinephrine. Most of the effects of thyroid hormones are mediated by either increasing or decreasing the rate at which specific genes are expressed. The effects are slow in onset and last for several days. The catecholamines act through two major classes of receptors, α-adrenergic and β-adrenergic receptors, each with subclasses. The effects of catecholamines are produced much more rapidly than those of thyroid hormones. Binding to β-receptors stimulates the production of cAMP, whereas binding to α_2-receptors inhibits cAMP production. Binding to α_1-receptors increases cytosolic Ca^{2+}.

Products Derived from Tyrosine

Tyrosine is converted to catecholamines in **chromaffin cells** of the central nervous system (CNS) and the adrenal medulla. The products are different in cell types, depending on the complement of enzymes present (**Part A**). Epinephrine is the major product in the adrenal medulla, while norepinephrine is produced in peripheral nerve endings. Dopamine is an intermediate in the synthesis of both norepinephrine and epinephrine, and is the major end product in the hypothalamus. In skin and brain, tyrosine is converted to melanin.

Catecholamine Synthesis

Three types of reactions are involved in catecholamine synthesis: hydroxylation, decarboxylation, and methylation (**Part B**). **Tyrosine hydroxylase** catalyzes the first step in the pathway, resulting in dopa. This enzyme requires O_2 and tetrahydrobiopterin (THB) as substrates. Dihydrobiopterin (DHB) reductase and NADPH are required to maintain THB in the reduced state. **Dopamine decarboxylase** catalyzes the decarboxylation of dopa to dopamine. This enzyme, also known as aromatic amino acid decarboxylase, requires pyridoxal phosphate as a cofactor. In some cells of the CNS, synthesis stops with dopamine. In other cells, dopamine is hydroxylated by **dopamine-β-hydroxylase**, resulting in norepinephrine. This enzyme requires O_2, ascorbic acid, and copper for activity, and it is found in secretory granules that store norepinephrine and epinephrine. In the adrenal medulla, **phenylethanolamine-N-methyltransferase (PNMT)** catalyzes the S-adenosylmethionine (SAM)-dependent methylation of norepinephrine, producing epinephrine.

Tyrosine hydroxylase catalyzes the **rate-limiting step** in catecholamine synthesis. It is found only in tissues that synthesize catecholamines and is inhibited by both dopamine and norepinephrine. Tyrosine hydroxylase is activated by cAMP-dependent phosphorylation. In the adrenal medulla, the synthesis of **PNMT** is induced by cortisol in response to stress.

Catecholamine Degradation

Catecholamines are rapidly degraded, having half-lives between 15 and 30 seconds (**Part C**). Most tissues contain two enzymes, **catecholamine-O-methyltransferase (COMT)** and **monamine oxidase (MAO)**, which degrade catecholamines, although the reactions can occur in either order. The major end product of epinephrine and norepinephrine degradation is **vanillylmandelic acid (VMA)**, which is excreted in the urine.

Thyroid Hormone Synthesis

The thyroid hormones, T_3 and T_4, are synthesized by modification of protein-bound tyrosine (**Part D**). Synthesis requires three substrates, thyroglobulin, iodine, and hydrogen peroxide. **Thyroglobulin**, a glycoprotein synthesized by the thyroid follicular cells, contains numerous tyrosine residues that can be used for synthesis of T_3 and T_4. The **uptake of I$^-$** occurs against a large gradient and requires energy that is supplied by ATP hydrolysis. The **oxidation of I$^-$ to I$^+$** is an obligatory step in thyroid hormone synthesis. **Incorporation of I$^+$** into the side chains of tyrosine produces monoiodotyrosine (MIT) and diiodotyrosine (DIT). **Crosslinking** of MIT and DIT produces T_3, whereas crosslinking of two residues of DIT produces T_4. **Thyroid peroxidase** catalyzes the oxidation of I$^-$ to I$^+$, the incorporation of I$^+$ into tyrosine, and the crosslinking reactions. The **thioureas** are a class of drugs that inhibit the oxidation of I$^-$ but have no effect on its uptake. The last step in the pathway is the release of T_3 and T_4 from thyroglobulin by proteolysis.

The synthesis of thyroid hormone is regulated by **TSH** (thyroid-stimulating hormone), a pituitary hormone, which stimulates both the uptake of I$^-$ and the release of T_3 and T_4 by proteolysis. The **rate-limiting step** in the pathway is the uptake of I$^-$. Normally, the amount of T_4 released is 20 to 30 times higher than T_3. The biologic activity of T_3, however, is much greater than that of T_4. Most of the T_4 is converted to T_3 in target tissues where these hormones exert their effect. In addition to being required for normal development, T_3 and T_4 affect many pathways in carbohydrate, lipid, and protein metabolism.

Melanin Synthesis

Melanins are insoluble polymers that are synthesized from tyrosine in melanocytes. The color variation in the skin of different people reflects different levels of melanin synthesis. The conversion of tyrosine to melanin is initiated by **tyrosinase**, a copper-containing enzyme that sequentially hydroxylates tyrosine to dopa and dopaquinone (**Part E**). Subsequent reactions involve nonenzymatic oxidation and spontaneous polymerization, leading to the pigment formation. An inherited defect in tyrosinase results in **albinism**.

Clinical Significance

An inadequate supply of dopamine in the brain results in **Parkinson disease**. Dopamine replacement is ineffective because it cannot cross the blood–brain barrier. Replacement therapy uses L-dopa, which enters the brain and is decarboxylated to dopamine. **Pheochromocytomas** are tumors of chromaffin cells that produce large amounts of catecholamines. These tumors are usually not detected until the levels of epinephrine and norepinephrine are high enough to result in severe **hypertension**.

For more information see Coffee C, *Metabolism*. Fence Creek, pp 375–381, 386–387.

57 Biogenic Amines Derived from Amino Acids

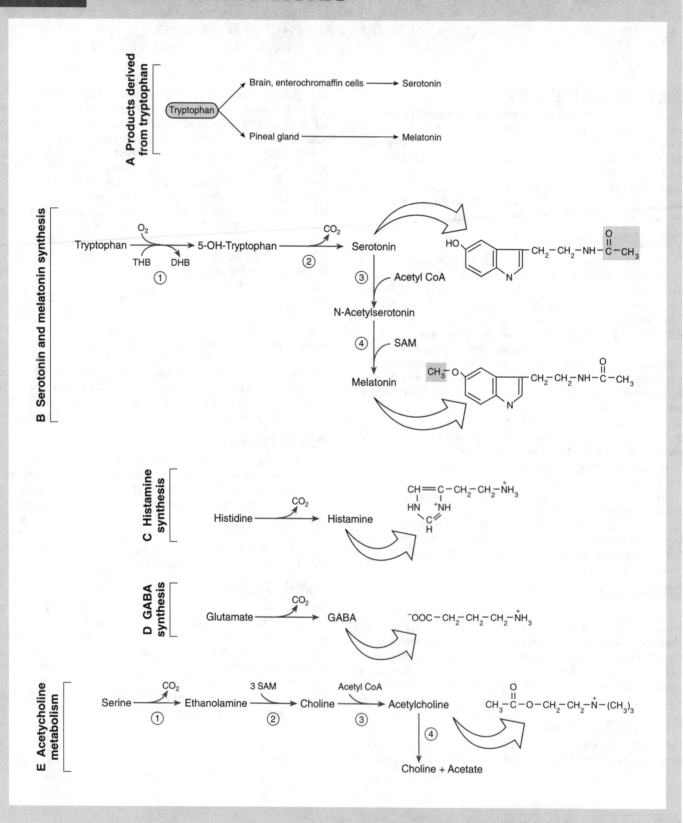

A Products derived from tryptophan

Tryptophan → Brain, enterochromaffin cells → Serotonin

Tryptophan → Pineal gland → Melatonin

B Serotonin and melatonin synthesis

Tryptophan → (O_2; THB → DHB; ①) → 5-OH-Tryptophan → (CO_2; ②) → Serotonin

Serotonin → ③ (Acetyl CoA) → N-Acetylserotonin → ④ (SAM) → Melatonin

C Histamine synthesis

Histidine → (CO_2) → Histamine

D GABA synthesis

Glutamate → (CO_2) → GABA

E Acetycholine metabolism

Serine → (CO_2; ①) → Ethanolamine → (3 SAM; ②) → Choline → (Acetyl CoA; ③) → Acetylcholine → (④) → Choline + Acetate

OVERVIEW

Biogenic amines and some hormones are derived from amino acid precursors. Tryptophan is the precursor of serotonin and melatonin. Histamine, γ-aminobutyric acid (GABA), and acetylcholine are derived from histidine, glutamate, and serine, respectively. Many drugs that are used to treat neurologic, psychiatric, and metabolic disorders alter the metabolism of the biogenic amines.

End Products of Tryptophan in Extrahepatic Tissues

Tryptophan is taken up by some extrahepatic tissues and converted to serotonin and melatonin (**Part A**). The nature of the end product is determined by the enzymes that are present in a particular cell. Serotonin is produced in brain and enterochromaffin cells of the gastrointestinal tract. Melatonin is synthesized by the pineal gland.

Synthesis and Function of Serotonin and Melatonin

The synthesis of serotonin and melatonin is similar to that of the catecholamines, starting with hydroxylation and followed by decarboxylation (**Part B**). **Tryptophan hydroxylase** catalyzes the hydroxylation of the tryptophan ring system, resulting in 5-hydroxytryptophan (5-HTP). Tryptophan hydroxylase requires O_2 and tetrahydrobiopterin (THB). Dihydrobiopterin (DHB) reductase and NADPH are needed to maintain THB in the reduced form. **Aromatic amino acid decarboxylase** catalyzes the conversion of 5-HTP to serotonin, also known as 5-hydroxytryptamine (5-HT). In the pineal gland two additional reactions occur. **Acetylation** of the serotonin amino group, followed by S-adenosylmethionine (SAM)-dependent **methylation** of the ring hydroxyl group convert serotonin to melatonin. The enzymes specific for the pineal gland are **N-acetyltransferase** and **O-methyltransferase**.

Serotonin has several biologic functions, including regulation of sleep, temperature, and blood pressure. It is a powerful **vasoconstrictor** and stimulator of smooth muscle contraction. The action of serotonin is terminated by its reuptake into presynaptic neurons. Once inside the neuron, it is either repackaged into synaptic vesicles or degraded by the sequential action of **monamine oxidase** and a specific **aldehyde dehydrogenase**. The end product of serotonin degradation is **5-hydroxyindoleacetate** (5-HI), which is excreted in the urine. **Carcinoid tumors** arising from neoplastic transformation of enterochromaffin cells secrete excessive serotonin and high levels of 5-HI are excreted in the urine.

The role of melatonin in humans is not well understood, although its synthesis appears to be regulated by the light–dark cycle. It is **secreted only in the dark hours**, and it is believed that melatonin plays a role in establishing circadian rhythms. It may also be involved in normal reproductive functions.

Histamine Synthesis and Function

Histamine, a chemical messenger involved in numerous cellular responses, is formed by the decarboxylation of histidine (**Part C**). This reaction is catalyzed by both **aromatic amino acid decarboxylase** and **histidine decarboxylase**, an enzyme that is found in most cells.

Both enzymes require pyridoxal phosphate as a coenzyme. Histamine plays an important role in mediating allergic and inflammatory reactions. It is stored in mast cells and released during an inflammatory response. It is a powerful **vasodilator**, resulting in the expansion of capillaries, localized edema, and a drop in blood pressure. In the lungs, histamine causes **constriction of the bronchioles**, and in the stomach, it **stimulates HCl secretion**.

GABA Synthesis and Function

GABA is formed by decarboxylation of glutamate (**Part D**). The reaction is catalyzed by **L-glutamate decarboxylase** and requires pyridoxal phosphate. GABA is found in high concentrations in the brain, where it functions as an **inhibitory neurotransmitter**. It is also found in lower concentrations in the kidney and pancreatic islet cells. The underproduction of GABA is associated with **epileptic seizures**. The involuntary movements seen in individuals with Huntington disease is believed to be related to the degeneration of GABAergic neurons and decreased levels of GABA.

Acetylcholine Metabolism and Function

The precursors of acetylcholine are serine, SAM, and acetyl CoA (**Part E**). Serine is decarboxylated, resulting in ethanolamine. The transfer of three methyl groups from SAM to the amino nitrogen of ethanolamine produces choline. Acetylcholine is formed by the condensation of choline and acetyl CoA, a reaction catalyzed by **choline acetyltransferase**. Acetylcholine functions as a neurotransmitter between parasympathetic nerves as well as between nerves and muscle. The action of acetylcholine is initiated by binding to **nicotinic-acetylcholine receptors** in the postsynaptic membrane, and is terminated by the action of **acetylcholinesterase**, which hydrolyzes acetylcholine to choline and acetate. **Myasthenia gravis** is an autoimmune disease in which antibodies against nicotinic-acetylcholine receptors bind to the receptor and inhibit its function.

Clinical Significance

The action of several commonly used drugs interferes with the metabolism of specific biogenic amines. For example, 1) **cimetidine**, a structural analog of histamine, is effective in treating ulcers because it inhibits the secretion of HCl; 2) **valproic acid**, a drug used to treat epilepsy, increases the levels of GABA in brain; 3) the antidepressants **paxil** and **zoloft** inhibit reuptake of serotonin by presynaptic neurons; and 4) **succinylcholine**, an analog of acetylcholine that inhibits the transmission of nerve impulses, is used as a muscle relaxant during surgery.

For more information see Coffee C, *Metabolism*. Fence Creek, pp 375–379.

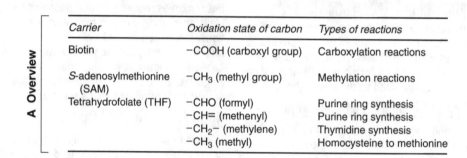

A Overview

Carrier	Oxidation state of carbon	Types of reactions
Biotin	$-COOH$ (carboxyl group)	Carboxylation reactions
S-adenosylmethionine (SAM)	$-CH_3$ (methyl group)	Methylation reactions
Tetrahydrofolate (THF)	$-CHO$ (formyl)	Purine ring synthesis
	$-CH=$ (methenyl)	Purine ring synthesis
	$-CH_2-$ (methylene)	Thymidine synthesis
	$-CH_3$ (methyl)	Homocysteine to methionine

B SAM structure

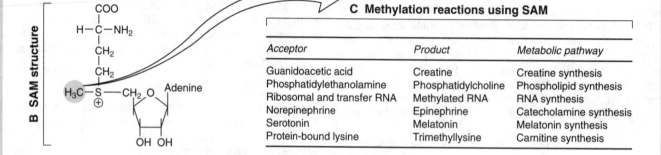

C Methylation reactions using SAM

Acceptor	Product	Metabolic pathway
Guanidoacetic acid	Creatine	Creatine synthesis
Phosphatidylethanolamine	Phosphatidylcholine	Phospholipid synthesis
Ribosomal and transfer RNA	Methylated RNA	RNA synthesis
Norepinephrine	Epinephrine	Catecholamine synthesis
Serotonin	Melatonin	Melatonin synthesis
Protein-bound lysine	Trimethyllysine	Carnitine synthesis

D THF structure

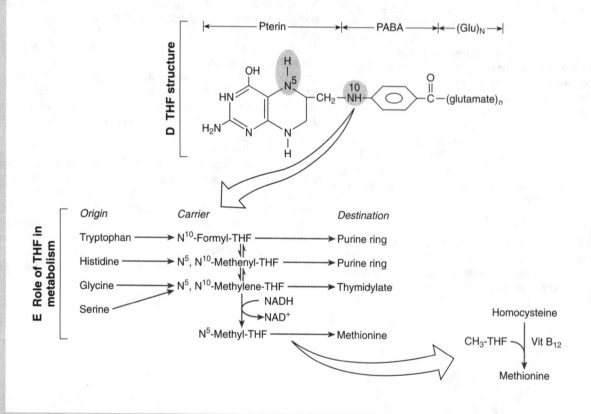

E Role of THF in metabolism

Origin	Carrier	Destination
Tryptophan	N^{10}-Formyl-THF	Purine ring
Histidine	N^5, N^{10}-Methenyl-THF	Purine ring
Glycine	N^5, N^{10}-Methylene-THF	Thymidylate
Serine		
	N^5-Methyl-THF	Methionine

NADH → NAD^+

Homocysteine

CH_3-THF — Vit B_{12}

Methionine

OVERVIEW

Many reactions in metabolism involve the transfer of a single-carbon atom from a donor to an acceptor (**Part A**). Three cofactors serve as carriers of the one-carbon (C_1) units in metabolism: biotin, S-adenosylmethionine (SAM), and tetrahydrofolate (THF). The C_1 units can exist in four oxidation states. Biotin transfers carboxyl groups and is required by three important carboxylases in metabolism: pyruvate carboxylase, acetyl CoA carboxylase, and propionyl CoA carboxylase. SAM transfers methyl groups and participates in numerous methylation reactions. THF transfers formyl, methenyl, methylene, and methyl groups. THF participates in many reactions in the pathways of purine and pyrimidine nucleotide synthesis.

Structure and Formation of SAM

The major carrier of methyl groups in metabolism is SAM, which is formed from methionine and ATP. The following reaction, catalyzed by **methionine adenosyltransferase**, describes the synthesis of SAM:

$$\text{Methionine} + \text{ATP} \longrightarrow \text{SAM} + PP_i + P_i$$

This reaction links the sulfur atom of methionine to the 5′-carbon of adenosine (**Part A**). The bond between the sulfur atom and the methyl group of SAM is a high-energy bond. Cleavage of this bond provides the energy required to drive methyl transfer reactions.

Methylation Reactions Using SAM

A typical methylation reaction that uses SAM as a methyl donor is shown in the equation below. The enzymes catalyzing these reactions are known as **methyltransferases**. The removal of the methyl group from SAM results in S-adenosylhomocysteine, which can be hydrolyzed to adenosine and homocysteine. Homocysteine can be either recycled to methionine or used for cysteine synthesis:

$$\text{Acceptor} + \text{SAM} \longrightarrow \text{acceptor-}CH_3 + \text{S-adenosylhomocysteine}$$

Examples of common acceptors in methylation reactions, together with the product and the corresponding metabolic pathway, are summarized in **Part C** of the figure.

Structure and Formation of THF

THF contains a two-member ring system having one conjugated and one reduced ring (**Part D**). The reduced ring is linked via a methylene group to p-aminobenzoic acid (PABA) which, in turn, is esterified to one or more glutamate residues. The carbon atoms to be transferred are bound to the N^5 and/or N^{10} **atoms** of THF, depending on the oxidation state. In folic acid, the vitamin precursor of THF, both rings are conjugated. Conversion of folic acid to THF involves two sequential **NADPH-dependent reduction** reactions, producing dihydrofolate (DHF) followed by THF. Both reactions are catalyzed by **dihydrofolate reductase**.

Many microorganisms can synthesize folic acid as long as p-aminobenzoic acid is present. **Sulfa drugs**, which are effective in treating many infections, are structural analogs of **p-aminobenzoic acid** that interfere with microbial synthesis of folic acid.

Role of THF in Metabolism

The carbon atoms transferred by THF come from four amino acids: tryptophan, histidine, glycine, and serine (**Part E**). Intermediates in the degradation of these amino acids donate carbon atoms to THF. Most of the acceptors of carbon atoms from THF are intermediates in the synthesis of purine and pyrimidine nucleotides. Therefore, THF integrates several areas of amino acid metabolism with nucleic acid metabolism. All of the THF derivatives except methyl-THF are interconverted by reversible reactions. The only reaction in human biochemistry that uses methyl-THF is the conversion of homocysteine to methionine. This reaction also requires methylcobalamine, a coenzyme derived from vitamin B_{12}. Therefore, a deficiency in vitamin B_{12} traps folate in a form that cannot be used for the synthesis of purine and pyrimidine nucleotides.

Clinical Significance

Megaloblastic anemia results from abnormalities in DNA synthesis, which, in turn, result from abnormalities in the synthesis of purine and pyrimidine nucleotides. Some forms of megaloblastic anemia are responsive to **vitamin B_{12}**. When vitamin B_{12} is deficient, THF is trapped as methyl-THF and is unavailable for purine and pyrimidine nucleotide synthesis. Other forms of megaloblastic anemia are responsive to **folate**. Megaloblastic anemia associated with vitamin B_{12} deficiency is characterized by elevated plasma levels of homocysteine and methylmalonic acid. In contrast, megaloblastic anemia associated with a dietary deficiency of folate is characterized by the accumulation of **formiminoglutamate (FIGLU)**. FIGLU is the intermediate in histidine degradation that donates a C_1 unit to folate. The red blood cell morphology in **pernicious anemia** is indistinguishable from that seen with folate and vitamin B_{12} deficiency. Pernicious anemia results from a deficiency in **intrinsic factor**, a protein required for the absorption of vitamin B_{12}. Intrinsic factor is synthesized by parietal cells of the gastric mucosa. It binds vitamin B_{12} in the ileum; the complex between intrinsic factor and vitamin B_{12} binds to receptors on the intestinal mucosal cells and is taken up by endocytosis.

For more information see Coffee C, *Metabolism*. Fence Creek, pp 68–69, 193, 363–366.

59 Metabolism of Sulfur Amino Acids and Peptides

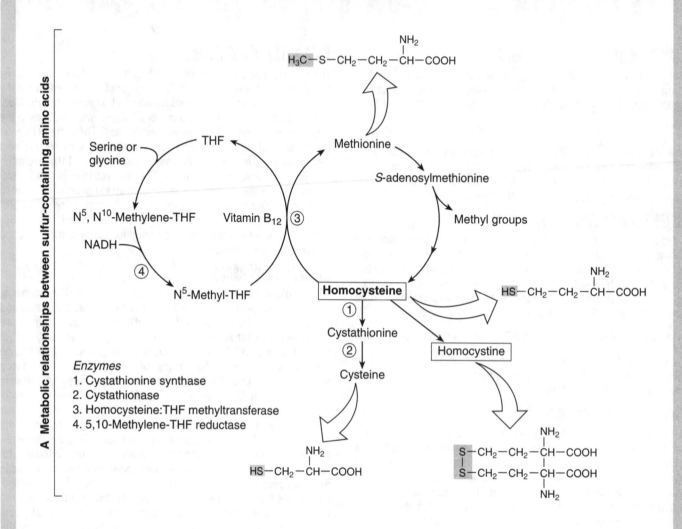

A Metabolic relationships between sulfur-containing amino acids

$H_3C-S-CH_2-CH_2-\overset{\overset{\displaystyle NH_2}{|}}{CH}-COOH$

Serine or glycine

THF

Methionine

S-adenosylmethionine

N^5, N^{10}-Methylene-THF

Vitamin B$_{12}$ ③

Methyl groups

NADH

④

N^5-Methyl-THF

Homocysteine

$HS-CH_2-CH_2-\overset{\overset{\displaystyle NH_2}{|}}{CH}-COOH$

① Cystathionine

② Cysteine

Homocystine

Enzymes
1. Cystathionine synthase
2. Cystathionase
3. Homocysteine:THF methyltransferase
4. 5,10-Methylene-THF reductase

$HS-CH_2-\overset{\overset{\displaystyle NH_2}{|}}{CH}-COOH$

$S-CH_2-CH_2-\overset{\overset{\displaystyle NH_2}{|}}{CH}-COOH$
$S-CH_2-CH_2-\underset{\underset{\displaystyle NH_2}{|}}{CH}-COOH$

B Glutathione structure and function

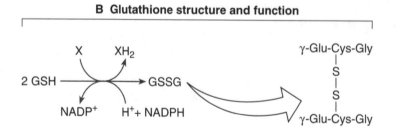

2 GSH ⟶ GSSG

X ⟶ XH$_2$

NADP$^+$ ⟶ H$^+$ + NADPH

γ-Glu-Cys-Gly
|
S
|
S
|
γ-Glu-Cys-Gly

OVERVIEW

Three sulfur-containing amino acids—methionine, cysteine, and cystine—are found in proteins. Methionine, an essential amino acid, is the source of sulfur for cysteine synthesis. The remainder of the cysteine molecule is derived from serine. Therefore, cysteine is a nonessential amino acid unless there is a deficiency in methionine. Homocysteine, another sulfur-containing amino acid, is derived from the metabolism of S-adenosylmethionine (SAM). Cystine and homocystine are dimers of cysteine and homocysteine, respectively, that are linked by a disulfide bond. Glutathione, a tripeptide containing glutamate, cysteine, and glycine, is widely used as a reducing agent.

Structures

The structural relationship between methionine, homocysteine, and cysteine can be seen in the figure on the opposite page. The only difference between methionine and homocysteine is the presence of a methyl group attached to the sulfur atom in methionine. Homocysteine and cysteine differ from one another by the presence of an additional methylene group in the side chain of homocysteine.

Conversion of Methionine to Homocysteine

The synthesis of cysteine requires methionine and serine as substrates, and homocysteine is a key intermediate in the pathway. The metabolic relationships between methionine, homocysteine, and cysteine are shown on the opposite page (**Part A**). Methionine is first converted to SAM, which is used in many reactions as a methylating agent. A by-product of methylation is S-adenosylhomocysteine, which is hydrolyzed to adenosine and homocysteine. Homocysteine can be either used for the synthesis of cysteine or converted back to methionine.

Conversion of Homocysteine to Cysteine

The conversion of homocysteine to cysteine is accomplished by two consecutive reactions (**Part A**). In the first reaction, cystathionine is produced by the condensation of homocysteine and serine. This reaction is catalyzed by **cystathionine synthase**. In the second reaction, cystathionine is cleaved by **cystathioninase**, releasing cysteine. Other products of this reaction are α-ketobutyrate and NH_4^+. The sulfhydryl group of cysteine is derived from homocysteine, and the remainder of the structure comes from serine. Both cystathionine synthase and cystathioninase require **pyridoxal phosphate** as a coenzyme.

Recycling Homocysteine to Methionine

When adequate cysteine is available, excess homocysteine is recycled to methionine in a reaction catalyzed by **homocysteine-THF methyltransferase (Part A)**. This enzyme requires two cofactors, one derived from vitamin B_{12} and the other from folate. As shown in the reaction below, methylcobalamin, the cofactor derived from vitamin B_{12}, acts as a methyl donor, converting homocysteine to methionine. CH_3-THF is used to regenerate methylcobalamin.

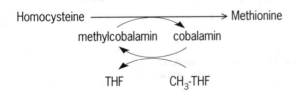

Glutathione Metabolism

Glutathione, a tripeptide containing glutamate (Glu), cysteine (Cys), and glycine (Gly) is the most abundant sulfur-containing compound in cells. Glutathione synthesis involves two consecutive reactions in which peptide bonds are formed. These reactions are catalyzed by **glutathione synthetase**, and they require energy that is supplied by ATP hydrolysis:

$$\text{Glu} + \text{Cys} \xrightarrow[\text{ATP} \quad \text{ADP} + P_i]{} \gamma\text{-Glu-Cys} \xrightarrow[\text{ATP} \quad \text{ADP} + P_i]{} \gamma\text{-Glu-Cys-Gly}$$

Many of the functions of glutathione are dependent on its ability to cycle between its **reduced (GSH)** and **oxidized (GSSG)** forms (**Part B**). Normally the reduced form constitutes about 98% of the total glutathione pool. The free sulfhydryl group in GSH serves as a reducing agent in numerous cellular reactions. The high ratio of reduced/oxidized glutathione is maintained by **glutathione reductase**, which uses NADPH to reduce GSSG back to GSH. One of the most important functions of GSH is to maintain protein sulfhydryl groups in their reduced state. In the red blood cell, GSH prevents oxidative damage by **reducing hydrogen peroxide**. GSH participates in **eicosanoid synthesis**, serving as a reductant in the cyclooxygenase reaction and as a substrate in peptidyl-leukotriene synthesis. It is used by the liver to **detoxify** electrophilic xenobiotics that gain access to the body as food additives, pollutants, or drugs. These compounds conjugate with GSH and are further metabolized to **mercapturic acids**, which are excreted in the urine.

Clinical Significance

The most common abnormality in the metabolism of sulfur-containing amino acids is **homocystinuria**, resulting from a deficiency in **cystathionine synthase**. Homocystine is a dimer of homocysteine. Other enzyme deficiencies that can lead to homocystinuria are **homocysteine-THF methyltransferase** or **5,10-methylene-tetrahydrofolate reductase**. A deficiency of vitamin B_6, folate, or vitamin B_{12} can also result in an increase in plasma homocysteine and excretion of homocystine in the urine. Pathologic findings associated with elevated plasma levels of homocysteine include dislocation of the lens, increased length and decreased thickness of the long bones, curvature of the spine, osteoporosis, and vascular thrombosis. Epidemiologic studies suggest that elevated homocysteine is a risk factor for coronary artery disease that is independent of the risk associated with elevated plasma cholesterol.

For more information see Coffee C, *Metabolism*. Fence Creek, pp 205–206; 321–322; 368–370; 388.

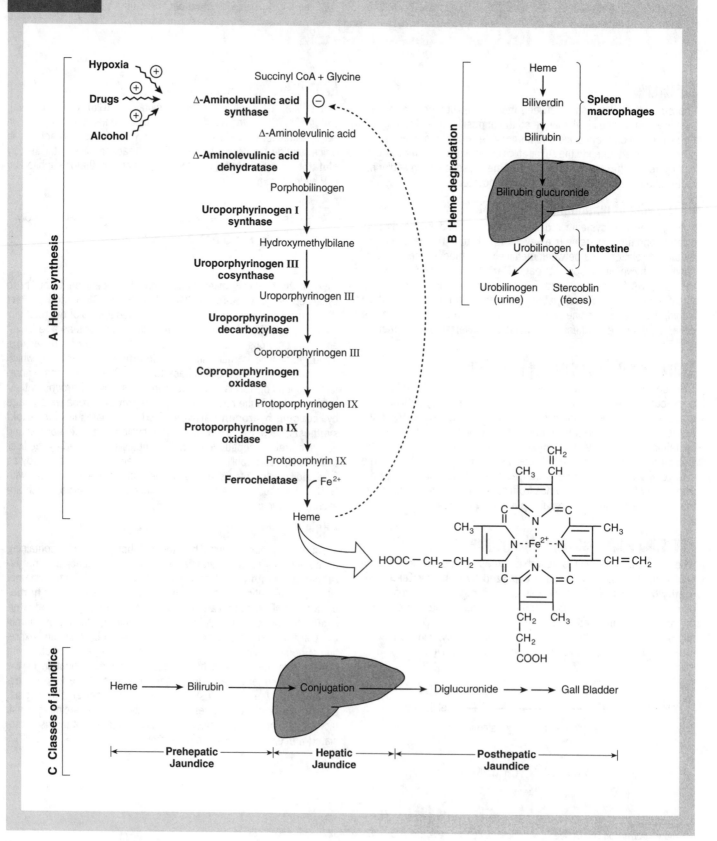

A Heme synthesis

Hypoxia ⊕
Drugs ⊕
Alcohol ⊕

Succinyl CoA + Glycine
→ **Δ-Aminolevulinic acid synthase** ⊖
Δ-Aminolevulinic acid
Δ-Aminolevulinic acid dehydratase
Porphobilinogen
Uroporphyrinogen I synthase
Hydroxymethylbilane
Uroporphyrinogen III cosynthase
Uroporphyrinogen III
Uroporphyrinogen decarboxylase
Coproporphyrinogen III
Coproporphyrinogen oxidase
Protoporphyrinogen IX
Protoporphyrinogen IX oxidase
Protoporphyrin IX
Ferrochelatase Fe²⁺
Heme

B Heme degradation

Heme
↓
Biliverdin } **Spleen macrophages**
↓
Bilirubin
↓
Bilirubin glucuronide
↓
Urobilinogen } **Intestine**
↓   ↓
Urobilinogen   Stercoblin
(urine)   (feces)

C Classes of jaundice

Heme → Bilirubin → Conjugation → Diglucuronide → → Gall Bladder

|← **Prehepatic Jaundice** →|← **Hepatic Jaundice** →|← **Posthepatic Jaundice** →|

OVERVIEW

Porphyrins are cyclic conjugated rings that have a high affinity for metal ions. They contain four pyrrole rings that are linked together by single-carbon bridges. All of the atoms in porphyrins are derived from **glycine** and **succinyl CoA**. Heme is the most common metalloporphyrin in humans, consisting of protoporphyrin IX and Fe^{2+}. The degradation of heme results in bilirubin, which is secreted in the bile. The major excretory products of heme are stercoblin and urobilinogen. Abnormalities in heme synthesis result in a family of diseases known as porphyrias, whereas abnormalities in the degradation and secretion of heme result in jaundice.

Heme Synthesis

Heme synthesis (**Part A**) occurs primarily in the **bone marrow** and **liver**. The first reaction and last three reactions in the pathway occur in the mitochondria, while the other steps are extramitochondrial. The first intermediate, Δ-aminolevulinic acid (Δ-ALA), is formed by condensation of glycine and succinyl CoA. This reaction is catalyzed by **Δ-ALA synthase** and requires pyridoxal phosphate. Two molecules of Δ-ALA are condensed by **Δ-ALA dehydratase**, producing porphobilinogen (PBG). **Uroporphyrinogen I synthase** condenses four molecules of PBG to give a linear tetrapyrrole. In the absence of uroporphyrinogen III cosynthase, the linear tetrapyrrole cyclizes to form uroporphyrinogen I. However, in the presence of **uroporphyrinogen III cosynthase**, the product is uroporphyrinogen III, the isomer required for heme synthesis. The final step in heme synthesis is the insertion of Fe^{2+} into protoporphyrin IX, a reaction catalyzed by **ferrocheletase**. The rate-limiting step is catalyzed by Δ-ALA synthase, a cytochrome P_{-450} enzyme, whose synthesis is induced by hypoxia, alcohol, and drugs, and inhibited by heme.

Heme Degradation

The degradation of heme (**Part B**) starts in the reticuloendothelial cells of liver, spleen, and bone marrow, where **heme oxygenase** oxidizes one of the carbon bridges connecting the pyrrole rings. This reaction releases Fe^{3+}, carbon monoxide, and biliverdin, which is reduced to **bilirubin**. The colors of biliverdin and bilirubin are responsible for the characteristic tones of bruises. Bilirubin, a hydrophobic compound, is transported by albumin to the liver, where it is conjugated with glucuronic acid in a reaction catalyzed by **bilirubin glucuronyltransferase**. Bilirubin glucuronide is secreted into the bile, and following entry into the gastrointestinal tract, bacterial enzymes remove glucuronic acid and the bile pigment is reduced to **urobilinogen**, a colorless compound, which is oxidized to **stercobilin** and excreted in the feces. Stercobilin gives feces their characteristic brown color. A small fraction of the urobilinogen is reabsorbed into the blood, extracted by the kidney and excreted in the urine.

Types of Jaundice

When the serum concentration of bilirubin exceeds 2 to 2.5 mg/dL, it begins to accumulate in the skin, sclera, and other tissues, giving a yellow or blue color. Although jaundice is not a disease, it is an important symptom of some underlying disease that results in either the overproduction or decreased excretion in the bile. Measurement of conjugated (direct), unconjugated (indirect), and total bilirubin in the plasma, along with the urobilinogen in the urine, provides useful information in determining the underlying cause of jaundice (**Part C**). **Prehepatic jaundice** results from excessive red blood cell destruction. The rate at which heme is released exceeds the capacity of the body to process it. A large increase in total serum bilirubin, indirect bilirubin, and urinary urobilinogen is observed. **Hepatic jaundice** results from liver disease, where the ability to extract and/or conjugate bilirubin is impaired. The total bilirubin is elevated and direct bilirubin is decreased. **Posthepatic jaundice**, resulting from bile duct obstruction, is characterized by an elevation in direct bilirubin and decreased urobilinogen excretion. Some of the direct bilirubin that accumulates in the plasma is filtered by the kidney, giving the urine a dark color. The feces are usually pale and chalky.

Clinical Significance

The porphyrias result from a defect in heme synthesis, which may be either inherited or acquired. The most common cause of acquired porphyria is **lead poisoning**, which inactivates Δ-ALA dehydratase and **ferrocheletase**. The inherited porphyrias include: 1) **porphyria cutanea tarda**, the most common porphyria, which results from a defect in urobilinogen decarboxylase; 2) **congenital erythropoietic porphyria**, results from a defect in uroporphyrinogen III cosynthase; and 3) **acute intermittent porphyria**, results from a defect in uroporphyrinogen I synthase. Porphyria cutanea tarda and congenital erythropoietic porphyria are autosomal recessive disorders, while acute intermittent porphyria is an autosomal dominant disorder.

The porphyrias are characterized by the accumulation of intermediates behind the defective enzyme and a decrease in the intermediates beyond the block. Heme production is decreased in all cases of porphyria, resulting in increased activity of Δ-ALA synthase, which exacerbates the condition. Patients with defects that lead to the accumulation of cyclic porphyrins are usually sensitive to light. In contrast, patients with defects that lead to the accumulation of Δ-ALA and PBG experience intermittent bouts of abdominal pain and neuropsychiatric disturbances, but are not photosensitive. Treatment of porphyrias involves administration of hematin, which represses the synthesis of Δ-ALA synthase. Strict avoidance of alcohol, drugs, and anesthetics is urged because they induce the synthesis of Δ-ALA synthase.

For more information see Coffee C, *Metabolism*. Fence Creek, pp 366–367; 381–386; 389.

61 Nitric Oxide Metabolism

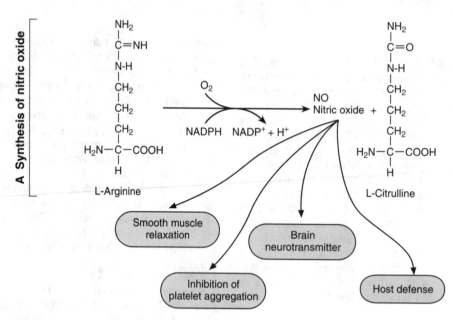

A Synthesis of nitric oxide

L-Arginine

O₂

NADPH → NADP⁺ + H⁺

NO
Nitric oxide + L-Citrulline

- Smooth muscle relaxation
- Inhibition of platelet aggregation
- Brain neurotransmitter
- Host defense

B Effect of NO on cardiovascular system

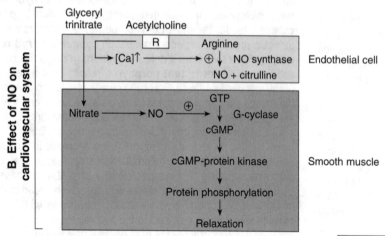

Glyceryl trinitrate

Acetylcholine

R

[Ca]↑ → ⊕ ↓ NO synthase
Arginine
NO + citrulline

Endothelial cell

Nitrate → NO → ⊕ GTP ↓ G-cyclase
cGMP
↓
cGMP-protein kinase
↓
Protein phosphorylation
↓
Relaxation

Smooth muscle

C Biological effects of cGMP

Cell or tissue type	Effect
Cardiac muscle	Relaxation
Vascular smooth muscle	Vasodilation
Kidney	Increased excretion of sodium and water
Platelets	Decreased aggregation

D Role of NO in host defense

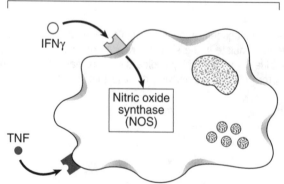

IFNγ

TNF

Nitric oxide synthase (NOS)

OVERVIEW

Nitric oxide (NO) is an important signaling molecule that acts both as an intracellular and intercellular messenger. It elicits a wide spectrum of responses associated with the vascular, immune, and nervous systems. NO is a free radical gas that can rapidly diffuse across membranes into cells. The first physiologic function assigned to NO was that of a vasodilator. It was subsequently identified as **endothelial-derived relaxing factor**. NO is derived from arginine. It has a half-life of about 5 seconds, and its action is terminated either by the sequential oxidation to nitrite and nitrate or by becoming covalently linked to proteins.

Synthesis and Effects of Nitric Oxide

The formation of NO is catalyzed by **nitric oxide synthase (NOS)** (**Part A**). The nitrogen originates in the side chain of **arginine**, and the oxygen donor is O_2. NOS requires NADPH for activity and it contains **FAD, heme**, and **tetrahydrofolate (THF)**. THF appears to play a structural, rather than a catalytic, role in the synthesis of NO. The mechanism of NOS appears to be similar to that of monooxygenation (hydroxylation) reactions catalyzed by cytochrome P-$_{450}$ enzyme complexes. Three distinct **isozymes** have been identified that are responsible for NO synthesis in different tissues. **NOS-I** is found in nerve tissue, **NOS-II** in macrophages, and **NOS-III** in endothelial cells. The endothelial and neuronal isozymes (NOS-I and -III) are synthesized constitutively. These isozymes contain calmodulin, and their activity is regulated by the interaction of Ca^{2+} with calmodulin. Synthesis of the macrophage isozyme (NOS-II) is induced by lipopolysaccharide and cytokines that are released in response to infection. Synthesis of NOS-II is inhibited by glucocorticoids. Biologic effects elicited by NO include smooth muscle relaxation, inhibition of platelet aggregation and adhesion, neural transmission, and destruction of foreign organisms engulfed by macrophages.

Effect of NO on the Cardiovascular System

The production of NO by vascular endothelial cells is stimulated by agents that increase the intracellular concentration of Ca^{2+} (e.g., acetylcholine and bradykinin) (**Part B**). NO that is produced in endothelial cells diffuses into the adjacent vascular smooth muscle cells, where it activates **cytosolic guanylate cyclase**, resulting in increased synthesis of cGMP, which leads to smooth muscle relaxation and vasodilation. Cytosolic guanylate cyclase contains **heme**, which serves as a binding site for NO.

Guanylate cyclase exists as two isozymes, one located in the cytosol and the other in the plasma membrane. The cytosolic isozyme is activated by NO, whereas the plasma membrane isozyme is activated by **atrial natriuretic factor (ANF)**, a family of peptide hormones that regulate cardiovascular function and body fluid homeostasis. The membrane-bound guanylate cyclase is often described as a **catalytic receptor**, having an extracellular domain that binds ANF and a cytosolic domain that synthesizes cGMP. The cytosolic domain is active only when ANF is bound. The membrane-bound isozyme does not contain heme.

Biologic Effects of cGMP

The biologic effects of cGMP (**Part C**) are much more limited in scope than those of cAMP. Most of the known actions of cGMP are linked to processes that regulate **cardiovascular function** and **body fluid homeostasis**, whereas cAMP is involved in regulating many diverse metabolic and cellular functions. Processes affected by cGMP include relaxation of cardiac muscle, vasodilation of vascular smooth muscle, increased excretion of sodium and water, and decreased aggregation and adhesion of platelets. Most, if not all, of these effects are mediated by **cGMP-dependent protein kinase** (protein kinase G), which has both catalytic and regulatory domains on the same polypeptide chain. In the absence of cGMP, the catalytic domain is inactive. The binding of cGMP induces a conformational change that unmasks the active site, allowing the kinase to phosphorylate serine and threonine side chains in target proteins and enzymes. Specific enzymes that are phosphorylated by protein kinase G include myosin light chain kinase in both smooth muscle and platelets.

Role of NO in Host Defense

NO is a potent toxin whose synthesis in macrophages is stimulated by **lipopolysaccharide** and cytokines such as **γ-interferon** (*γ-IFN*) and **tumor necrosis factor-α** (*α-TNF*) (**Part D**). NO contributes to the defense against bacteria, fungi, viruses, and parasites, and it is toxic to tumor cells. NO combines with superoxide in macrophages to form compounds that are more toxic than either NO or superoxide alone.

Clinical Significance

The persistent stimulation of NOS, with concomitant overproduction of NO and cGMP, has been implicated in the onset of **septic shock** following a bacterial infection. Septic shock is characterized by **severe hypotension** that is frequently refractory to conventional treatments, including administration of fluids, vasopressors, and antibiotics. This type of hypotension is commonly seen in patients following abdominal surgery or abdominal trauma complicated by bacterial infection. Development of **NOS inhibitors** that might be useful in treating these patients is being actively explored by the pharmaceutical industry.

The effectiveness of **amyl nitrate** or **glyceryl trinitrate** in treating angina resides in the fact that these compounds spontaneously decompose to NO, resulting in vasodilation of vascular smooth muscle and relaxation of cardiac muscle. **Viagra**, the drug recently marketed to treat impotence, stimulates the production of cGMP and vasodilation in smooth muscle.

For more information see Coffee C, *Metabolism*. Fence Creek, pp 123–124; 388–389.

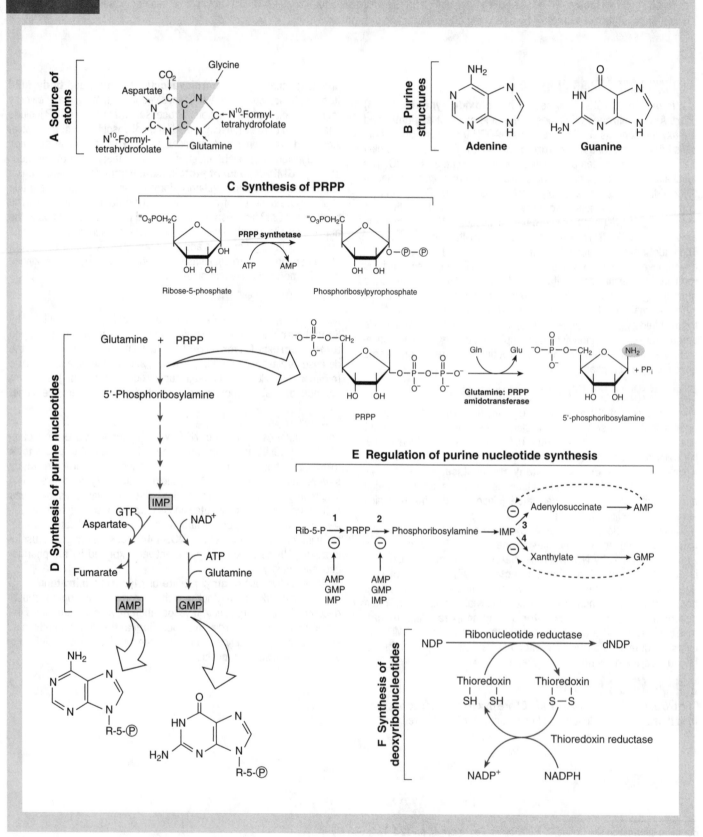

A **Source of atoms**

B **Purine structures**

Adenine

Guanine

C **Synthesis of PRPP**

Ribose-5-phosphate

PRPP synthetase

ATP → AMP

Phosphoribosylpyrophosphate

D **Synthesis of purine nucleotides**

Glutamine + PRPP

5'-Phosphoribosylamine

IMP

GTP
Aspartate

NAD$^+$

Fumarate

ATP
Glutamine

AMP

GMP

Gln → Glu

Glutamine: PRPP amidotransferase

PRPP

5'-phosphoribosylamine

+ PP$_i$

E **Regulation of purine nucleotide synthesis**

Rib-5-P →$_1$ PRPP →$_2$ Phosphoribosylamine → IMP

AMP
GMP
IMP

AMP
GMP
IMP

Adenylosuccinate → AMP

Xanthylate → GMP

F **Synthesis of deoxyribonucleotides**

NDP

Ribonucleotide reductase

dNDP

Thioredoxin
SH   SH

Thioredoxin
S — S

Thioredoxin reductase

NADP$^+$

NADPH

OVERVIEW

Nucleotides have many functions in cells, serving as substrates for nucleic acid synthesis, universal sources of energy, structural components of several coenzymes, and activated carriers of many chemical groups in metabolism. The nucleotides can be synthesized from small molecules or by salvage pathways that recycle the purine and pyrimidine rings. In rapidly dividing cells, most of the nucleotides are synthesized from small precursors. **Nucleosides** contain a nitrogenous base (either a purine or pyrimidine ring) and a pentose (either ribose or deoxyribose). **Nucleotides** contain a nitrogenous base, a pentose, and one or more phosphates. Purine rings are specialized products that are derived from amino acids. The nitrogen atoms are derived from aspartate, glutamine, and glycine, while the carbon atoms are derived from CO_2, glycine, and one-carbon units donated by tetrahydrofolate (THF) that also have their origin in amino acids. All of the intermediates in purine nucleotide synthesis are attached to ribose-5-phosphate by an N-glycosidic linkage.

Structure of Purines

Purines contain two fused rings, each having two nitrogen atoms (**Part A**). The two purines found in nucleic acids are adenine or guanine, which differ only in the substituents attached to the ring (**Part B**). Adenine has an amino group attached to C-6, while guanine has an amino group attached at C-2 and a carbonyl oxygen at C-6.

Synthesis of Phosphoribosylpyrophosphate (PRPP)

The synthesis of all nucleotides uses PRPP as an activated donor of ribose-5-phosphate. PRPP is synthesized from ribose-5-phosphate and ATP (**Part C**). **PRPP synthetase** catalyzes the transfer of pyrophosphate from ATP to the C-1 of ribose-5-phosphate, producing PRPP and AMP. The gene for PRPP synthase is located on the **X-chromosome**. There are several mutations that lead to **superactive forms** of the enzyme, although there are no known mutations that have decreased activity.

Synthesis of Purine Nucleotides

The first step committed to purine nucleotide synthesis is the formation of **5′-phosphoribosylamine**, a reaction catalyzed by **glutamine:PRPP amidotransferase (Part D)**. The amide group from glutamine is transferred to C-1 of PRPP, where it replaces pyrophosphate. The nitrogen atom in 5′-phosphoribosylamine eventually becomes N-9 of the purine ring. Through nine consecutive steps, 5′-phosphoribosylamine is converted to the parent nucleotide, inosine monophosphate (IMP). The pathway branches at IMP, with separate paths for AMP and guanosine monophosphate (GMP) production. The conversion of IMP to both AMP and GMP involves the addition of an amino group to the ring and requires a source of energy. Aspartate is the amino donor for AMP synthesis and the energy is supplied by GTP. Following the addition of the amino group, the remainder of the aspartate structure is released as fumarate. For GMP synthesis, glutamine is the amino donor and the energy is supplied by ATP.

Regulation of Purine Nucleotide Synthesis

The rate-limiting step in purine nucleotide synthesis is the formation of 5′-phosphoribosylamine (**Part E**). The most important factor in regulating **glutamine:PRPP amidotransferse** activity is the cellular concentration of PRPP. The concentration is usually 10 to 100 times lower than the K_m of the enzyme for PRPP. Therefore, small changes in the PRPP concentration result in proportional increases in the rate of 5′-phosphoribosylamine synthesis. This enzyme is also subject to product inhibition by IMP, AMP, and GMP. Secondary targets of product inhibition are **PRPP synthetase**, which is inhibited by IMP, AMP, and GMP; **adenosylsuccinate synthase**, the enzyme at the branch point for AMP synthesis, which is inhibited by AMP; and **IMP dehydrogenase**, the enzyme at the branch point for GMP synthesis, which is inhibited by GMP.

Synthesis of Deoxyribonucleotides

The synthesis of deoxyribonucleotides is catalyzed by **ribonucleotide reductase**, a multienzyme complex containing thioredoxin and thioredoxin reductase (**Part F**). Ribonucleotide reductase converts all four ribonucleoside diphosphates (NDP) to the corresponding deoxyribonucleoside diphosphates (dNDP). **Thioredoxin**, a small protein containing cysteine residues, acts as reducing agent in the reaction. The catalytic cycle is completed by **thioredoxin reductase**, which regenerates the reduced form of thioredoxin. The deoxyribonucleoside diphosphates are subsequently phosphorylated to the corresponding triphosphates for use in DNA synthesis.

Ribonucleotide reductase is subject to a complex pattern of allosteric regulation. The enzyme has two types of regulatory sites, one that controls the overall catalytic activity and another that is responsible for maintaining balance in the cellular pool of dATP, dGTP, dCTP, and dTTP that is required for DNA synthesis. The overall catalytic activity is inhibited by dATP and activated by ATP.

Clinical Significance

Several chemotherapeutic drugs are based on their ability to interfere with the synthesis or utilization of purine nucleotides. **Azaserine**, a structural analog of glutamine, inhibits **amidotransferases** that transfer amide groups from glutamine to intermediates in the pathway of nucleotide synthesis. Azaserine binds to the glutamine site and inactivates these enzymes. **Methotrexate** and **aminopterin** are structural analogs of folic acid that act as competitive inhibitors of dihydrofolate (DHF) reductase. DHF reductase reduces both folate and DHF to the active form, THF. Therefore, methotrexate and aminopterin block steps in nucleotide synthesis that use THF as a one-carbon donor. **6-Mercaptopurine** and **6-thioguanine** are structural analogs of inosine and guanine, respectively. The conversion of IMP to AMP is inhibited by 6-mercaptopurine, while the conversion of IMP to GMP is inhibited by 6-thioguanine. Both of these drugs also inhibit hypoxanthine-guanine phosphoribosyltransferase, the major enzyme involved in salvaging purines.

For more information see Coffee C, *Metabolism*. Fence Creek, pp 393–406.

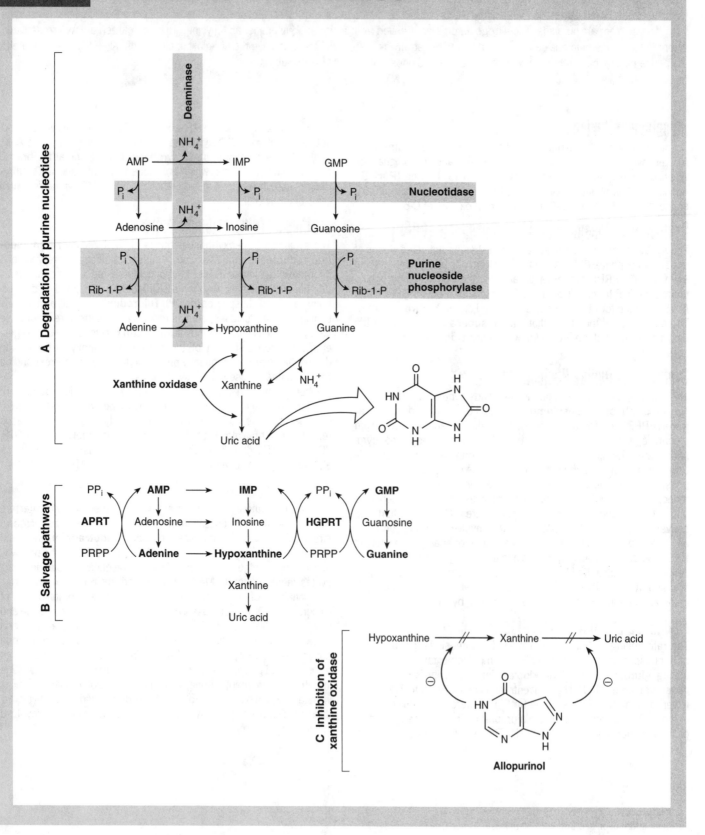

A Degradation of purine nucleotides

B Salvage pathways

C Inhibition of xanthine oxidase

Allopurinol

OVERVIEW

The end product of purine nucleotide degradation is uric acid. There are no enzymes in humans that are capable of opening up the purine ring and degrading it to smaller molecules. Thus, the strategy for degrading purine nucleotides is to remove substituents from the ring system and then either oxidize the ring to uric acid or salvage the ring by converting it back to nucleotides. Several human diseases result from abnormalities in the pathways of degradation and salvaging.

Degradation of Purine Nucleotides

Both ribonucleotides and deoxyribonucleotides are degraded by the same pathway (**Part A**). Substituents attached to the ring of AMP, GMP, and IMP are sequentially removed by parallel pathways. Phosphate groups are removed by **nucleotidase**. Amino groups are removed from adenosine and guanine by **adenosine deaminase** and **guanine deaminase**, respectively. Phosphate is added across the bond linking ribose to the purine ring, releasing ribose-1-phosphate in a reaction catalyzed by **purine nucleoside phosphorylase**. The sum of these reactions converts AMP and IMP to hypoxanthine and GMP to xanthine. The terminal step in purine nucleotide degradation is the sequential oxidation of hypoxanthine and xanthine to uric acid, which is excreted in the urine. Both of these reactions are catalyzed by **xanthine oxidase**, a flavoprotein that requires molybdenum as an essential cofactor.

Salvage Pathways

In most cells, pathways are available that allow hypoxanthine, guanine, and adenine to be recycled (**Part B**). The function of these pathways is to avoid the high-energy demand placed on the cell by de novo synthesis of purine rings. De novo synthesis of each purine nucleoside triphosphate requires nine high-energy phosphate bonds, whereas salvaging a purine base and converting it to the corresponding nucleoside triphosphate requires only four high-energy phosphate bonds. Rapidly dividing cells, particularly liver and placenta, rely heavily on the pathway of de novo synthesis. Other cells, however, derive most of their purine nucleotides from salvage pathways. The purine bases that are salvaged may come from either dietary sources or turnover of intracellular nucleic acids. Two enzymes, **hypoxanthine-guanine phosphoribosyltransferase (HGPRT)** and **adenine phosphoribosyltransferase (APRT)**, are responsible for salvaging purine rings. Both hypoxanthine and guanine are substrates for HGPRT, which transfers ribose-5-phosphate from phosphoribosylpyrophosphate (PRPP) to the purine ring, producing IMP and GMP. APRT transfers ribose-5-phosphate to adenine, producing AMP. The specific activity of APRT in most cells is very low compared to that of HGPRT.

Treatment of Gout with Allopurinol

Allopurinol, one of the drugs used to treat gout, is a structural analog of hypoxanthine (**Part C**). It inhibits **xanthine oxidase**, resulting in the accumulation of hypoxanthine, which is more soluble than uric acid. Allopurinol acts as a **suicide substrate** of xanthine oxidase. Because of its structural similarity to hypoxanthine, it binds to the active site and begins to undergo catalysis. The catalytic cycle, however, cannot be completed.

Gout is a group of metabolic diseases associated with hyperuricemia and the deposition of monosodium urate crystals in tissues. The prevalence of gout is about 3 in 1000, with the incidence being about 10 times higher in men than in women. The symptoms usually appear in the fourth decade in men and after menopause in women. Plasma uric acid levels, however, are usually elevated for several years before the symptoms appear. Only about 5% of the individuals with hyperuricemia develop clinical gout.

Hyperuricemia can result from either the overproduction or underexcretion of uric acid. Lactate inhibits the excretion of uric acid, and conditions that cause lactate accumulation (e.g., acute alcohol intoxication) may precipitate bouts of hyperuricemia and gout. Deficiencies in several enzymes, including HGPRT and **glucose-6-phosphatase**, result in gout. **Superactive mutants of PRPP synthetase** may also result in gout. Some of the PRPP synthetase mutants have an increased V_{max}, while others do not respond to feedback inhibition by purine nucleotides.

Clinical Significance

Lesch-Nyhan syndrome, a severe neurologic disorder, results from an absence of **HGPRT** activity. This disease is characterized by mental retardation, jerky involuntary movements, compulsive self-mutilation, and the overproduction of uric acid. Since hypoxanthine and guanine cannot be salvaged, they are oxidized to uric acid. About one-third of the cases of Lesch-Nyhan result from **spontaneous mutations** in the HGPRT gene. This gene is located on the **X-chromosome** and the disease is transmitted as an X-linked recessive trait. A new mutation may occur in an asymptomatic mother and remain silent until transmitted to a male child.

About 20% of the cases of **severe combined immunodeficiency (SCID)** result from a deficiency in **adenosine deaminase** that leads to impaired function of both T and B cells. The accumulation of dATP that occurs with adenosine deaminase deficiency leads to inhibition of ribonucleotide reductase and DNA synthesis. A deficiency in **purine nucleoside phosphorylase** also results in an immunodeficiency disease that impairs only T cells.

For more information see Coffee C, *Metabolism*. Fence Creek, pp 393–406.

64 Pyrimidine Nucleotide Metabolism

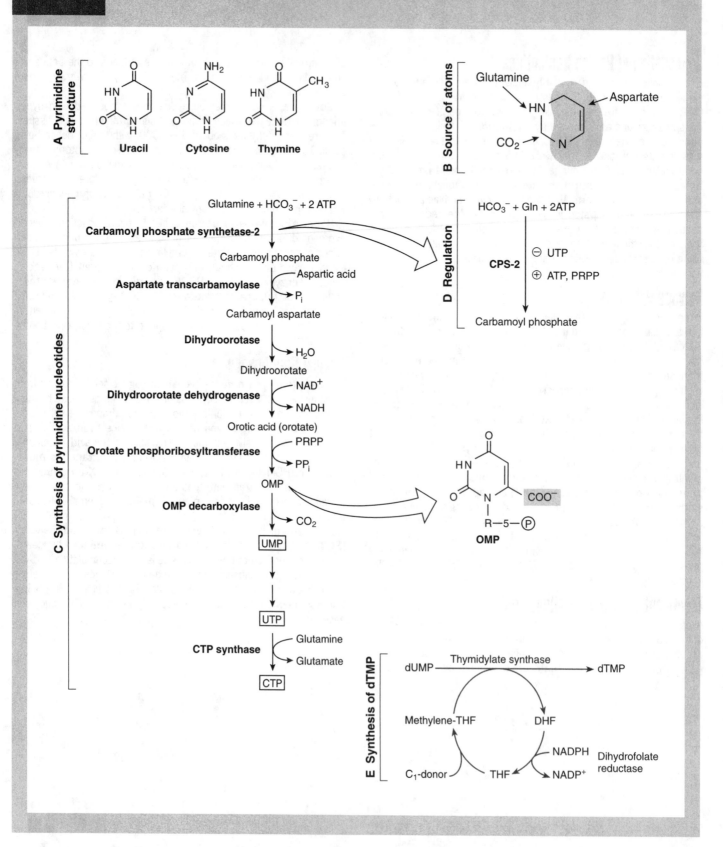

A Pyrimidine structure

Uracil   Cytosine   Thymine

B Source of atoms

Glutamine → HN
Aspartate
CO_2 → N

C Synthesis of pyrimidine nucleotides

Glutamine + HCO_3^- + 2 ATP

Carbamoyl phosphate synthetase-2

Carbamoyl phosphate

Aspartate transcarbamoylase ← Aspartic acid → P_i

Carbamoyl aspartate

Dihydroorotase → H_2O

Dihydroorotate

Dihydroorotate dehydrogenase ← NAD^+ → NADH

Orotic acid (orotate)

Orotate phosphoribosyltransferase ← PRPP → PP_i

OMP

OMP decarboxylase → CO_2

UMP

UTP

CTP synthase ← Glutamine → Glutamate

CTP

D Regulation

HCO_3^- + Gln + 2ATP

CPS-2   ⊖ UTP   ⊕ ATP, PRPP

Carbamoyl phosphate

HN
O   COO⁻
N
R—5—Ⓟ
OMP

E Synthesis of dTMP

dUMP → Thymidylate synthase → dTMP

Methylene-THF   DHF

C_1-donor → THF   NADPH → $NADP^+$ Dihydrofolate reductase

OVERVIEW

Pyrimidine nucleotides consist of a nitrogenous ring attached to ribose phosphate by an N-glycosidic linkage. The nitrogen atoms of the pyrimidine ring come from glutamine and aspartate, and the carbon atoms come from CO_2 and aspartate. Synthesis of the pyrimidine ring is completed before it is attached to ribose-5-phosphate, a strategy that differs from that of purine nucleotide synthesis. Degradation of pyrimidine nucleotides starts by removal of amino groups, phosphate, and ribose from the ring. The ring is then opened up and partially degraded to small soluble molecules, including NH_4^+, CO_2, β-alanine, and β-aminoisobutyrate.

Structure of Pyrimidine Rings

Three pyrimidines are found in nucleic acids: uracil, cytosine, and thymine (**Part A**). Uracil is found only in RNA and thymine only in DNA. The pyrimidine rings contain two nitrogen and four carbon atoms, and they differ from one another only in the substituents attached to the ring. Uracil has two carbonyl oxygens at C-2 and C-4. Cytosine has a carbonyl oxygen at C-2 and an amino group attached to C-4. Thymine differs from uracil by the presence of a methyl group attached to C-5. In pyrimidine nucleotides, ribose phosphate is attached to N-1 of the ring by an N-glycosidic bond. The atoms in the pyrimidine ring are derived from glutamine, aspartate, and CO_2 (**Part B**).

Synthesis of Pyrimidine Nucleotides

Pyrimidine nucleotide synthesis can be described in two stages: 1) synthesis of orotidine monophosphate (OMP), the parent nucleotide; and 2) conversion of OMP to UTP and CTP (**Part C**). Carbamoyl phosphate, the first intermediate in the pathway, is synthesized from glutamine, bicarbonate, and ATP in a reaction catalyzed by **carbamoyl phosphate synthetase-2 (CPS-2)**. CPS-2 is distinct from CPS-1, a mitochondrial enzyme that participates in urea synthesis. In contrast, CPS-2 is a cytosolic enzyme that is used exclusively for pyrimidine synthesis. Carbamoyl phosphate is converted to carbamoyl aspartate by the action of **aspartate transcarbamoylase** (ATCase). The next two reactions convert carbamoyl aspartate to **orotic acid**, the first complete pyrimidine ring. Transfer of ribose-5-phosphate from phosphoribosylpyrophosphate (PRPP) to orotic acid, a reaction catalyzed by **orotate phosphoribosyltransferase (OPRT)** produces OMP, the parent nucleotide. The reactions converting OMP to UTP and CTP start with decarboxylation of OMP to UMP, which is followed by two sequential phosphorylation reactions, producing UTP. **CTP synthase** catalyzes the transfer of an amide group from glutamine to C-4 of the ring, resulting in CTP.

Regulation

The regulation of pyrimidine nucleotide synthesis is markedly different in eukaryotic and prokaryotic cells. In prokaryotes, **ATCase** is the primary site of regulation. It is allosterically inhibited by CTP and activated by PRPP and ATP. In eukaryotic cells, **CPS-2** is the primary regulatory enzyme (**Part D**). CPS-2 is allosterically inhibited by UTP and activated by PRPP and ATP. Additionally, eukaryotic cells have clusters of enzymes in the pathway organized as separate domains on the same **multifunctional protein**, a feature that allows the synthesis of several enzymes to be coordinately controlled. The first three enzymes in the pathway are found on the same **multifunctional protein**, which is known as **CAD** (from the first letter in the names of the enzymes). Similarly, the two enzymes that convert orotic acid to UMP are separate domains on the same multifunctional protein.

Synthesis of Deoxythymidine Monophosphate (dTMP)

Thymine, rather than uracil, is found in DNA. The immediate precursor of dTMP is deoxyuridine monophosphate (dUMP). **Thymidylate synthase** catalyzes the addition of a methyl group to C-5 in the ring of dUMP, resulting in dTMP (**Part E**). The source of the methyl group is methylene-THF. During transfer the methylene group is reduced to a methyl group. This reaction results in the concomitant oxidation of THF to DHF. The catalytic cycle is completed by the reduction of DHF to THF, a reaction catalyzed by **dihydrofolate reductase**, followed by the addition of another one-carbon fragment to THF.

Clinical Significance

Thymidylate synthase and **DHF reductase** provide the only pathway for the synthesis of thymine nucleotides. Therefore, inhibitors of these enzymes decrease the rate of DNA synthesis and cell division, making them desirable **targets for antitumor drugs**. **5-Fluorouracil** is converted by cells to 5-F-dUMP, a compound that irreversibly inhibits thymidylate synthase. **Methotrexate**, a structural analog of folic acid, is a powerful competitive inhibitor of dihydrofolate reductase. The affinity of the enzyme for methotrexate is about 200-fold higher than its affinity for DHF. Although the division of all cells is affected by these drugs, the cancer cells grow and divide more rapidly than normal cells and, therefore are more sensitive to antitumor drugs. **Azidothymidine (AZT)**, also known as zidovudine, is used in the treatment of AIDS. AZT is a structural analog of thymidine. The cell converts AZT to the corresponding nucleoside triphosphate, which binds to **reverse transcriptase** and terminates DNA synthesis in retroviruses.

Orotic aciduria can result from a deficiency in either the OPRT/OMP decarboxylase multifunctional enzyme or a deficiency in orthinine transcarbamoylase, an enzyme in the urea cycle. To establish the cause of orotic aciduria, other symptoms have to be considered. A deficiency in OPRT/OMP decarboxylase results in megaloblastic bone marrow and growth retardation, whereas a deficiency in ornithine transcarbamoyase results in hyperammonemia.

For more information see Coffee C, *Metabolism*. Fence Creek, pp 393–406.

PART V: QUESTIONS

Directions: For each of the following questions, choose the **one best** answer.

1. A deficiency in which of the following amino acids will result in negative nitrogen balance, even though the diet may contain a large amount of protein.

(A) Serine

(B) Glutamate

(C) Tryptophan

(D) Alanine

(E) Asparagine

2. A deficiency in which of the following proteases would most seriously impair the digestion of dietary protein?

(A) Trypsin

(B) Enteropeptidase

(C) Pepsin

(D) Chymotrypsin

(E) Carboxypeptidase A

3. A patient came to the emergency room complaining of severe abdominal pain. Laboratory analysis revealed high concentrations of the dibasic amino acids in the urine. The patient's pain subsided a few hours later after he passed a kidney stone. The most likely diagnosis for this patient is

(A) Cystinuria

(B) Homocystinuria

(C) Hartnup's disease

(D) Hyperammonemia type I

(E) Organic aciduria

4. The two tissues that are most efficient at extracting glutamine from the blood following a protein-rich meal are

(A) Brain and kidney

(B) Muscle and liver

(C) Kidney and liver

(D) Intestine and kidney

(E) Kidney and muscle

5. In humans, arginine that is used for protein synthesis is produced by sequential reactions that occur in which of the following tissues?

(A) Small intestine and liver

(B) Liver and skeletal muscle

(C) Kidney and skeletal muscle

(D) Small intestine and kidney

(E) Brain and liver

6. Amino acid analysis was performed on a sample of blood taken from the blood leaving the liver. Which of the following amino acids is present at a much higher concentration after a meal than in the fasting state?

(A) Phenylalanine

(B) Histidine

(C) Valine

(D) Arginine

(E) Methionine

7. Pyridoxal phosphate is a coenzyme for all of the following enzymes **except**:

(A) Alanine aminotransferase

(B) Methylmalonyl CoA mutase

(C) Glutamate decarboxylase

(D) Serine dehydratase

(E) Branched chain amino acid transaminase

8. A patient with pneumonia is being treated with isoniazid. This patient should also receive supplements of which of the following vitamins?

(A) Pyridoxine

(B) Biotin

(C) Riboflavin

(D) Pantothenic acid

(E) Niacin

9. A newborn boy developed seizures at 4 days of age. Analysis of serum revealed elevated levels of NH_4^+, glutamine, and alanine. Urine analysis showed the presence of orotic acid. These symptoms are consistent with a deficiency in which of the following enzymes?

(A) Orotidine monophosphate decarboxylase

(B) Ornithine transcarbamoylase

(C) Arginase

(D) Carbamoyl phosphate synthetase I

(E) Argininosuccinate lyase

10. Which of the following conditions would decrease the rate of the urea cycle?

(A) Fasting for 24 hours

(B) Increased production of N-acetylglutamate

(C) Eating a protein rich meal

(D) Excessive production of ketone bodies

(E) Depletion of dihydrobiopterin

11. A vitamin B$_{12}$ deficiency can result in all of the following **except**:

(A) Impaired branched chain amino acid metabolism

(B) Impaired oxidation of palmitoyl CoA

(C) Impaired synthesis of DNA

(D) Excretion of methylmalonic acid

(E) Accumulation of homocysteine

12. Maple syrup urine disease results from a deficiency in which of the following enzymes?

(A) Branched chain amino acid transaminase

(B) Propionyl CoA carboxylase

(C) Alanine transaminase

(D) Branched chain ketoacid dehydrogenase

(E) Methylmalonyl CoA mutase

13. The most common inherited disease in amino acid metabolism is

(A) Maple syrup urine disease

(B) Homocystinuria

(C) Propionic aciduria

(D) Phenylketonuria

(E) Hyperammonemia type II

14. All of the following are essential amino acids in a patient with phenylketonuria **except**:

(A) Tyrosine

(B) Phenylalanine

(C) Isoleucine

(D) Alanine

(E) Valine

15. The major end product of catecholamine catabolism is

(A) Vanillylmandelic acid

(B) Hydroxyindoleacetic acid

(C) Dopamine

(D) Dihydroxymandelic acid

(E) None of the above

16. In humans, the major route of nitrogen transfer from amino acids to urea involves which of the following pairs of enzymes?

(A) Glutamine synthetase and urease

(B) Transaminases and glutaminase

(C) Glutamate dehydrogenase and transaminases

(D) Amino acid oxidases and arginase

(E) Glutaminase and amino acid oxidases

17. The thioureas are a class of antithyroid drugs that inhibit

(A) The oxidation of I$^-$ to I$^+$

(B) The uptake of I$^-$ by the thyroid follicle

(C) Cross-linking of monoiodotyrosine and diiodotyrosine residues

(D) The proteolysis of iodinated thyroglobulin

(E) The secretion of thyroid stimulating hormone by the pituitary

18. The synthesis of which of the following biogenic amines involves hydroxylation, decarboxylation, and methylation reactions?

(A) Norepinephrine

(B) Serotonin

(C) Epinephrine

(D) γ-Aminobutyric acid

(E) Histamine

19. A deficiency in dihydrobiopterin reductase involves which of the following conditions?

(A) Increased tyrosine synthesis

(B) Increased serotonin synthesis

(C) Increased vanillylmandelic acid excretion

(D) Increased nitric acid synthesis

(E) Negative nitrogen balance

20. S-adenosylmethionine is required for synthesis of all of the following compounds **except**:

(A) Phosphatidylethanolamine

(B) Surfactant

(C) tRNA

(D) Melatonin

(E) Carnitine

21. Which of the following amino acids contributes most to the buffering capacity of plasma proteins?

(A) Lysine

(B) Histidine

(C) Glutamic acid

(D) Serine

(E) Asparagine

22. All of the following conditions can result in phenylketonuria **except**:

(A) Impaired biopterin absorption

(B) Phenylalanine deficiency

(C) Dihydrobiopterin reductase deficiency

(D) Phenylalanine hydroxylase deficiency

(E) Uncontrolled dietary protein intake by a pregnant woman with phenylketonuria

23. The renal metabolism of glutamine

(A) Produces one molecule of ammonia per molecule of glutamine

(B) Is initiated by a transaminase

(C) Is increased by metabolic acidosis

(D) Occurs in the cytosol

(E) Requires tetrahydrofolate

24. Which of the following combinations of substrates and coenzymes is required for the recycling of methionine in humans?

(A) Homoserine, methyl-tetrahydrofolate (THF), and vitamin B_{12}

(B) Homocysteine, vitamin B_{12}, and methyl-THF

(C) Cysteine, pyridoxine, and methylene-THF

(D) S-Adenosylmethionine, biotin, and vitamin B_{12}

(E) Homocysteine, vitamin B_{12}, and thiamin

25. Which of the following functions can be attributed to glutathione?

(A) It is a coenzyme in the pathway of prostaglandin synthesis.

(B) It is a substrate in the synthesis of the peptidylleukotrienes.

(C) It is a substrate for glutathione peroxidase.

(D) It is involved in the synthesis of mercapturic acids.

(E) All of the above.

26. Which of the following enzymes is inhibited by lead?

(A) Δ-Aminolevulenic acid synthase

(B) Ferrochelatase

(C) Heme oxygenase

(D) Biliverdin reductase

(E) Uroporphyrinogen I synthase

27. A patient presented with high serum levels of indirect bilirubin and elevated urobilinogen in the urine. Direct serum bilirubin was only slightly higher than normal. The most likely diagnosis for this patient is

(A) Crigler-Najjar syndrome

(B) Neonatal jaundice

(C) Bile duct blockage

(D) Hemolytic anemia

(E) Viral hepatitis

28. All of the following statements about nitric oxide are correct **except**:

(A) It is synthesized from the side chain of arginine.

(B) It stimulates the production of cGMP in smooth muscle cells.

(C) Its synthesis is stimulated by γ-interferon in macrophages.

(D) It is spontaneously produced by the decomposition of glyceryl trinitrate.

(E) It is synthesized by smooth muscle and diffuses into endothelial cells.

29. Which of the following amino acids is a direct precursor to the synthesis of both purine and pyrimidine rings?

(A) Glutamate

(B) Aspartate

(C) Glycine

(D) Asparagine

(E) Serine

30. Methotrexate is used as a chemotherapeutic agent. Which of the following enzymes is directly inhibited by this drug?

(A) Xanthine oxidase

(B) Thymidylate synthase

(C) Dihydrofolate reductase

(D) Phosphoribosylpyrophosphate (PRPP) synthetase

(E) Glutamine:PRPP amidotransferase

Questions 31–34
Match each of the diseases listed below with the most appropriate enzyme deficiency. Each letter can be used only once.

(A) OMP decarboxylase

(B) Adenosine deaminase

(C) Xanthine oxidase

(D) Glucose-6-phosphatase

(E) Hypoxanthine-guanine phosphoribosyltransferase (HGPRT)

(F) Purine nucleoside phosphorylase

31. Severe combined immunodeficiency

32. Lesch-Nyhan syndrome

33. Orotic aciduria

34. Gout

PART V: ANSWERS AND EXPLANATIONS

1. **The answer is C.**

A deficiency in a single amino acid will result in negative nitrogen balance if that amino acid is an essential amino acid. The only essential amino acid listed is tryptophan. Some protein sources provide a better balance of the essential amino acids than others. In general, animal protein is a better source of essential amino acids than plant protein, although vegetarians can obtain a balance of essential amino acids by choosing protein sources that complement one another.

2. **The answer is B.**

Enteropeptidase, an enzyme secreted by the duodenum, initiates the proteolytic cascade that activates trypsin, chymotrypsin, elastase, carboxypeptidase A, and carboxypeptidase B. Enteropeptidase cleaves a single peptide bond in trypsinogen, producing active trypsin that then activates all of the other inactive pancreatic zymogens. A deficiency in pepsin does not seriously impair protein digestion.

3. The answer is A.

The dibasic amino acids (arginine, lysine, ornithine, and cystine) are transported across the brush border membrane of intestinal and kidney cells by the same transport protein. A deficiency in the dibasic amino acid transporter results in the inability to absorb dietary amino acids and to reabsorb these amino acids from the urinary filtrate. Cystine is very insoluble and precipitates out of solution at the acidic pH of the urine, forming kidney stones.

4. The answer is C.

Skeletal muscle releases large amounts of glutamine into the blood. The glutamine is formed from glutamate and NH_4^+ and provides a mechanism for detoxification of ammonia that is produced in extrahepatic tissues. Most of the glutamine is taken up by the kidney and liver. The kidney deaminates glutamine, producing ammonia that is excreted in the urine at NH_4^+. The liver also deaminates glutamine, releasing ammonia that is incorporated into urea and excreted in the urine. In the fasting state, the intestine is very effective in extracting glutamine from the blood and using it as its major source of energy. Following a meal, the intestinal cells use glutamine from dietary protein as a fuel.

5. The answer is D.

Although the liver synthesizes arginine as an intermediate in the urea cycle, it is cleaved by arginase as rapidly as it is made and is not available for protein synthesis. The intestinal cells have the first two enzymes in the urea cycle and they synthesize citrulline, which is released into the blood. Citrulline is extracted from the blood by the kidney, which has the third and fourth enzymes of the urea cycle and can convert citrulline to arginine. The kidney has very little arginase and does not further metabolize arginine.

6. The answer is C.

Following a meal, the catabolism of excess amino acids occurs in the liver where catabolism is usually initiated by transaminases. The major exception is the catabolism of the branched chain amino acids (valine, leucine, and isoleucine) that is initiated in skeletal muscle. The transaminase for these amino acids is not present in the liver. Therefore, the branched chain amino acids present in the portal blood following a meal are not extracted by the liver and are enriched in the blood leaving the liver.

7. The answer is B.

Pyridoxal phospate is a coenzyme in many reactions in amino acid metabolism. Pyridoxal phosphate activates the α-carbon atom of amino acids, and reactions that involve the α-carbon atom usually require pyridoxal phosphate as a coenzyme. Examples of enzymes that catalyze these reactions are amino acid transminases, decarboxylases, deaminases, and dehydratases. Methylmalonyl CoA mutase, an enzyme involved in metabolism of propionyl CoA, requires vitamin B_{12} as a coenzyme but does not require pyridoxal phosphate.

8. The answer is A.

Isoniazid forms a complex with pyridoxine (vitamin B_6), thereby decreasing the amount of pyridoxine available for synthesis of pyridoxal phosphate and impairing enzymes in amino acid metabolism that require pyridoxal phosphate. Supplements of pyridoxine should also be given to patients that are being treated with penicillamine for copper storage diseases and to women taking oral contraceptives.

9. The answer is B.

A genetic deficiency in any enzyme in the urea cycle except arginase can result in elevated levels of NH_4^+ and glutamine in the urine. However, the only enzyme deficiency in the urea cycle that results in the accumulation of orotic acid is ornithine transcarbamoylase. A deficiency in orotidine monophosphate decarboxylase, an enzyme in the pathway of pyrimidine synthesis, also leads to the excretion of orotic acid but NH_4^+ and glutamine do not accumulate.

10. The answer is D.

Ketone bodies are organic acids that are completely ionized at physiologic pH. Therefore, excessive production of ketone bodies results in ketoacidosis. The associated increase in H^+ concentration shifts the equilibrium between ammonia (NH_3) toward ammonium ion (NH_4^+) toward NH_4^+ accumulation. Since the substrate for carbamoyl phosphate synthetase I is NH_3, the rate-limiting step in the urea cycle is decreased. Conditions that result in an increase in the rate of urea synthesis are an increase in N-acetylglutamate, eating a protein-rich meal, and a 24-hour fast.

11. The answer is B.

Vitamin B_{12} is required by two reactions in human metabolism, the conversion of methylmalonyl CoA to succinyl CoA and the methylation of homocysteine to methionine. Therefore, a vitamin B_{12} deficiency results in the accumulation of methylmalonic acid which is excreted in the urine, and an accumulation of homocysteine which is accumulates in the plasma and is excreted as the homocystine dimer. Most of the methymalonyl CoA is derived from propionyl CoA that is a product of branched chain amino acid and odd-chain fatty acid oxidation. Therefore, a deficiency in vitamin B_{12} would also impair branched chain amino acid metabolism, but would not alter the oxidation of palmitoyl CoA because it is an even-chain fatty acid. In addition to vitamin B_{12}, the methylation of homocysteine to methionine also requires methyl-tetrahydrofolate. A vitamin B_{12} deficiency traps tetrahydrofolate in a form that cannot be used for synthesis of purine and pyrimidine nucleotides.

12. The answer is D.

Maple syrup urine disease results from an inherited deficiency in branched chain ketoacid dehydrogenase. Symptoms include vomiting and lethargy. Severe brain damage usually leads to death at a very young age. Urine and plasma contain elevated levels of the branched chain amino acids and the corresponding α-ketoacids and α-hydroxyacids.

13. The answer is D.

Phenylketonuria occurs in about 1 in 10,000 live births. Screening of newborns for phenylketonuria is mandated by law.

14. The answer is D.

Alanine is a nonessential amino acid that is readily synthesized by the transamination of pyruvate. Normally tyrosine is synthesized from phenylalanine, an essential amino acid, but in phenylketonuria this reaction is blocked and tyrosine also becomes an essential amino acid. Isoleucine, valine, and phenylalanine cannot be synthesized by human tissues and are essential components of the diet.

15. The answer is A.

Vanillylmandendic acid (VMA) is the major end product of dopamine, norepinephrine, and epinephrine degradation. The amount of VMA excreted is used clinically to access the overproduction of catecholamines. Hydroxyindoleacetic acid is the endproduct of serotonin degradation.

16. The answer is C.

The amino group is removed from most amino acids by transaminases that use α-ketoglutarate as an amino receptor, producing a common pool of glutamate. Some of the glutamate is transaminated with oxaloacetate, producing aspartate. The remainder of the glutamate is deaminated by glutamate dehydrogenase, producing NH_3. Aspartate and NH_3 are the donors of the nitrogen atoms in urea.

17. The answer is A.

Thioureas inhibit the oxidation of I^- to I^+, a reaction that uses hydrogen peroxide as an oxidizing agent.

18. The answer is C.

The three most common types of reactions involved in the synthesis of biogenic amines are decarboxylation, hydroxylation, and methylation reactions. Histamine and γ-aminobutyric acid are formed by decarboxylation of histidine and glutamatic acid, respectively. Serotonin is derived from tryptophan by sequential decarboxylation and hydroxylation reactions. Norepinephrine is derived from tyrosine by hydroxylation and decarboxylation reactions, and epinephrine is formed by the methylation of norepinephrine.

19. The answer is E.

Dihydrobiopterin reductase catalyzes the NADPH-dependent reduction of dihydrobiopterin (DHB) to tetrahydrobiopterin (THB). THB is used as a cofactor in reactions that catalyze the hydroxylation of the aromatic amino acids. Because hydroxylation of phenylalanine is involved in the synthesis of tyrosine and in the synthesis of catecholamines, a deficiency in dihydrobiopterin reductase will impair the synthesis of tyrosine and compounds derived from tyrosine, including the catecholamines and their degradation products. The conversion of tryptophan to serotonin will also be impaired. Tetrahydrobiopterin is also required to maintain the structural integrity of nitric oxide synthase, although it does not act as a cofactor in the synthesis of nitric oxide. Tyrosine becomes an essential amino acid when there is a deficiency in DHB reductase, and negative nitrogen balance will result unless the diet is supplemented with tyrosine.

20. The answer is A.

S-adenosylmethionine acts as a methylating agent in the synthesis of many cellular compounds includinig tRNA, melatonin, carnitine, and phosphatidylcholine (a component of surfactant). Phosphatidylethanolamine is the compound that is methylated to produce phosphatidylcholine.

21. The answer is B.

The protonated nitrogen atom in the side chain of histidine has a pK_a of approximately 7, which is sufficiently close to the physiologic pH to be an effective buffer. The pK_a of the lysine side chain is too high and the pK_a of glutamic acid side chain is too low to contribute significantly to the buffering capacity of proteins. Neither serine nor asparagine side chains act as proton donors or acceptors.

22. The answer is B.

Phenylketonuria results from an excess of phenylalanine that is metabolized by pathways that are normally latent. The classical form of phenylketonuria results from an inherited deficiency in phenylalanine hydroxylase, whereas atypical forms can result from the inability to absorb biopterin or from a deficiency in biopterin reductase, which maintains the cofactor in its reduced form. In women with phenylketonuria it is necessary to control the phenylalanine intake during pregnancy to prevent the development of phenylketonuria in the unborn fetus.

23. The answer is C.

The renal metabolism of glutamine occurs in the mitochondria where ammonia is released in two sequential reactions catalyzed by glutaminase and glutamate dehydrogenase. The only coenzyme involved in this reaction sequence is NAD^+, which is a coenzyme for glutamate dehydrogenase. The activity of glutaminase is significantly increased during periods of metabolic acidosis. The ammonia produced by the catabolism of glutamine absorbs protons to form ammonium ions that are excreted in the urine.

24. The answer is B.

Homocysteine is converted to methionine in a reaction that requires both methylcobalamin (a vitamin B_{12} derivative) and methyl-THF as coenzymes. Methylcobalamin methylates homocysteine, and methyl-THF is used to regenerate methylcobalamin. The conversion of homocysteine to cysteine requires pyridoxine. Thiamine and homoserine are not involved in methionine and homocysteine metabolism.

25. The answer is E.

Glutathione is a tripeptide consisting of glutamate, cysteine, and glycine that performs many functions in cells. The sulfhydryl group is very reactive and can form conjugates with several compounds. It also undergoes oxidation-reduction reactions, making glutathione the most important sulfhydryl buffering system in cells.

26. The answer is B.

Two enzymes in the pathway of heme synthesis are very sensitive to lead, ferrochelatase and Δ-aminolevulenic acid dehydratase. Inhibition of either of these enzymes can result in acquired porphyria. Δ-Aminolevulenic acid synthase catalyzes the first step in the pathway of heme synthesis, which is also the rate-limiting step in the pathway. Heme oxygenase and biliverdin reductase are involved in the degradation of heme. A genetic deficiency in uroporphyrinogen I synthase results in acute intermittent porphyria.

27. The answer is D.

Hemolysis of red cells is producing more bilirubin than can be handled by the liver, resulting in high levels of indirect (unconjugated) bilirubin. The appearance of elevated urobilinogen in the urine indicates that neither the conjugation of bilirubin nor the secretion into the bile is impaired.

28. The answer is E.

Nitric oxide is a potent vasodilator that is synthesized in endothelial cells and diffuses into smooth muscle cells where it stimulates the synthesis of cGMP. In macrophages, nitric oxide is a part of the host defense mechanism that kills bacteria, fungi, viruses, and parasites, and it is toxic to tumor cells. Its precursor is arginine, and its synthesis is stimulated by Ca^{2+} in brain and endothelial cells and by γ-interferon in macrophages. The treatment of angina with glyceryl trinitrate is based on the fact that it spontaneously decomposes, releasing nitric oxide that stimulates smooth muscle relaxation.

29. The answer is B.

Aspartate contributes a nitrogen atom to the six-member ring of purines, and it contributes three carbon atoms and one nitrogen atom to the pyrimidine ring. All of the atoms in glycine are incorporated into the purine ring system, but glycine is not used for the synthesis of the pyrimidine ring. Asparagine and serine are not used in the synthesis of either the purine or pyrimidine ring systems.

30. The answer is C.

Methotrexate is a structural analog of folate and a competitive inhibitor of dihydrofolate (DHF) reductase. Thymidylate synthase catalyzes the methylation of dUMP to dTMP, a reaction that requires methylene-tetrahydrofolate (THF) as a carbon donor. The reduction of the meth-ylene group to a methyl group results in the simultaneous oxidation of THF to DHF. DHF reductase catalyzes the NADPH-dependent reduction of DHF to THF, thereby completing the catalytic cycle for dTMP synthesis.

Questions 31–34. The answers are: 31-B, 32-E, 33-A, 34-D.

A deficiency in adenosine deaminase results in severe combined immunodeficiency. Both T and B cell functions are impaired. A deficiency in HGPRT results in Lesch-Nyhan syndrome, which is characterized by gout, neuropsychiatric dysfunction, and self-mutilating behavior. Orotic aciduria results from a deficiency in OMP decarboxylase, an enzyme in the pathway of pyrimidine biosynthesis. The accumulation of uric acid (resulting in gout) results from a deficiency in either HGPRT or glucose-6-phosphatase. Each answer can be used only once, and Lesch-Nyhan results only from a deficiency in HGPRT. Therefore, by elimination, the answer to question 34 is glucose-6-phosphatase.

PART VI
Integration of Metabolism

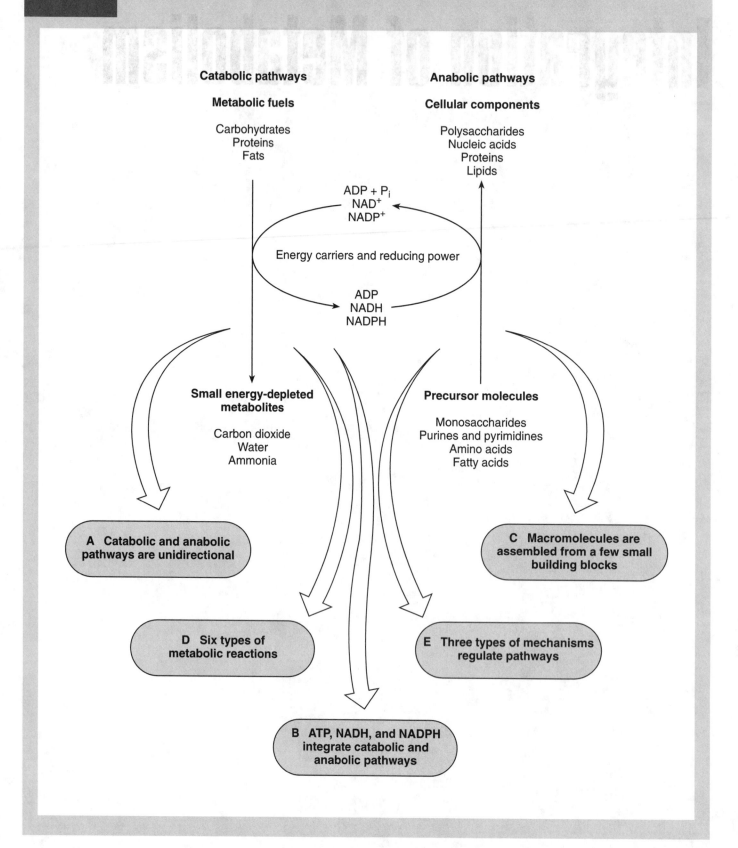

Catabolic pathways

Metabolic fuels

Carbohydrates
Proteins
Fats

Anabolic pathways

Cellular components

Polysaccharides
Nucleic acids
Proteins
Lipids

$ADP + P_i$
NAD^+
$NADP^+$

Energy carriers and reducing power

ADP
NADH
NADPH

Small energy-depleted
metabolites

Carbon dioxide
Water
Ammonia

Precursor molecules

Monosaccharides
Purines and pyrimidines
Amino acids
Fatty acids

A   Catabolic and anabolic
pathways are unidirectional

C   Macromolecules are
assembled from a few small
building blocks

D   Six types of
metabolic reactions

E   Three types of mechanisms
regulate pathways

B   ATP, NADH, and NADPH
integrate catabolic and
anabolic pathways

An apparent paradox in metabolism is that thousands of different enzyme-catalyzed reactions occur in cells, yet both the intracellular and extracellular environments of the cell stay remarkably constant. The thousands of reactions are organized into a few functional pathways that are connected with one another. The rate at which any particular pathway operates in a cell is carefully regulated, and it is coordinated with the rates at which other pathways operate. A few **recurrent themes** and **patterns** exist that provide a framework for the simplification and organization of metabolism.

Catabolic and Anabolic Pathways Are Unidirectional

Pathways that degrade and synthesize metabolic fuels are unidirectional (**Theme A**). For example, fatty acid oxidation and fatty acid synthesis are opposing pathways, having no enzymes in common and occurring in different subcellular compartments. Other opposing pathways may occur in the same subcellular compartment and share some of the same enzymes, but there are always one or more enzymes that are specific for each pathway and render the pathway irreversible. For example, glycolysis and gluconeogenesis are opposing pathways that are irreversible under the conditions found in the cell, although they share many of the same enzymes. Having distinctive synthetic and degradative steps in opposing pathways allows each pathway to operate independently of the other. A futile cycle would occur if uncontrolled glycolysis and gluconeogenesis occurred simultaneously. Other opposing pathways in cells include glycogen synthesis and glycogen degradation, triglyceride synthesis and degradation, protein synthesis and degradation, nucleic acid synthesis and degradation, and amino acid synthesis and degradation. In each case, the opposing pathways are unidirectional.

ATP, NADH, and NADPH Integrate Catabolic and Anabolic Pathways

Many connections between catabolism and anabolism are provided by ATP, NADH, and NADPH that are carriers of energy and electrons (**Theme B**). ATP, a universal carrier of chemical energy, is an end product of catabolic pathways and a substrate for anabolic pathways. Similarly, NAD^+ and $NADP^+$ are universal carriers of electrons in metabolism. NAD^+ and $NADP^+$ are oxidizing agents that serve as electron acceptors in catabolic pathways, whereas NADPH is a universal reducing agent that is used in numerous biosynthetic pathways.

Macromolecules Are Assembled from a Small Number of Building Blocks

Cells synthesize a large and diverse group of unique macromolecules from a small number of simple building blocks (**Theme C**). For example, millions of different proteins are synthesized from 20 common amino acids, all of the nucleic acids are synthesized from five common nucleoside triphosphates, and polysaccharides are assembled from a few monosaccharides. Catabolic pathways provide metabolic intermediates and energy needed for the de novo synthesis and polymerization of these building blocks.

Metabolism Uses Only Six Types of Reactions

Although thousands of different enzymes are found in cells, each having a different substrate and product, only six types of reactions are catalyzed by enzymes (**Theme D**). The types of reactions are: 1) oxidation-reduction, 2) group transfer, 3) hydrolysis, 4) nonhydrolytic cleavage, 5) isomerization, and 6) ATP-dependent formation of bonds. Different enzymes that catalyze the same types of reactions may use the same coenzyme or cofactor. For example, CoA is used by all enzymes that transfer acyl groups. This type of reaction occurs in many pathways, including the tricarboxylic acid cycle, fatty acid synthesis, fatty acid oxidation, phospholipid synthesis, and cholesterol synthesis. Similarly, biotin transfers CO_2 groups in carboxylation reactions, but is not involved in decarboxylation reactions. All enzymes that catalyze group transfer reactions require a coenzyme that acts as a carrier of the chemical group.

Metabolic Pathways Are Regulated by Three Types of Mechanisms

The rates at which metabolic pathways are regulated and coordinated with one another involve only three types of mechanisms: allosteric regulation, covalent modification, and induction and repression of enzyme synthesis (**Theme E**). Each metabolic pathway is regulated by one or more of these mechanisms. Each pathway has one enzyme that is always the primary target of regulation. This enzyme catalyzes the **rate-limiting step** in the pathway. Some pathways have secondary sites of regulation, which are usually enzymes that catalyze reactions that are irreversible under cellular conditions. The activity of some regulatory enzymes may be controlled by all three types of mechanisms. For example, acetyl CoA carboxylase catalyzes the rate-limiting step in fatty acid synthesis. Its activity responds almost instantly to changes in the intracellular concentration of citrate (an allosteric activator) and palmitoyl CoA (an allosteric inhibitor). Covalent regulation of acetyl CoA carboxylase is mediated by protein kinases and protein phosphatases that are activated by the second messengers of glucagon and insulin, respectively. This type of regulation is slower than allosteric regulation, occurring within a time interval of seconds to minutes. Synthesis of acetyl CoA carboxylase is induced by insulin, a mechanism that involves increased synthesis of mRNA and protein synthesis. This mechanism is an adaptive change that takes longer to achieve but persists for a longer period of time.

Clinical Significance

Health and homeostasis are based on the ability of an organism to organize thousands of individual reactions into a few basic pathways, and to coordinate and regulate the rate at which each of the pathways operates. The clinical significance of the multilayered organization and regulatory themes is readily appreciated by examining the myriad metabolic consequences resulting from the deficiency of a single protein (e.g., diabetes) or the metabolic consequences of a single point mutation in a particular protein (e.g., sickle cell anemia).

For more information see Coffee C, *Metabolism*. Fence Creek, pp 101–107.

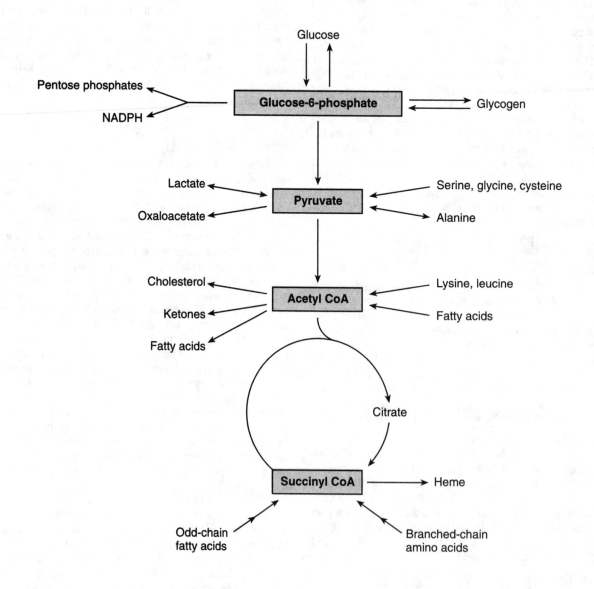

OVERVIEW

Metabolic pathways are connected with one another by a small number of branch points that can be considered as the crossroads in metabolism. Branch points are created by metabolites that are substrates or products of more than one enzyme. Four of the most important branch points in metabolic pathways are created by **glucose-6-phosphate, pyruvate, acetyl CoA**, and **succinyl CoA**. Each of these compounds has several metabolic fates, a common theme that is used to link together numerous pathways in carbohydrate, lipid, and amino acid metabolism.

Glucose-6-Phosphate

Immediately after entering the cell glucose is converted to glucose-6-phosphate, which forms a branch point for several pathways of carbohydrate metabolism. The isomerization of glucose-6-phosphate to glucose-1-phosphate initiates the pathway of **glycogen synthesis** and glucose storage. Isomerization of glucose to fructose-6-phosphate initiates the pathway of **glycolysis**, resulting in the production of pyruvate and ATP. Oxidation of glucose-6-phosphate to 6-phosphogluconate initiates the **pentose phosphate pathway**, resulting in NADPH and pentose phosphates. The pentose phosphates are used almost exclusively for purine and pyrimidine nucleotide synthesis, and NADPH is used as a reducing agent in many biosynthetic pathways. Glucose-6-phosphate can be formed by either **glycogenolysis** or **gluconeogenesis**. The hydrolysis of glucose-6-phosphate to glucose allows glucose to be transported across the plasma membrane into the blood where it can be distributed to other tissues. The direction in which glucose-6-phosphate proceeds at this crossroad in metabolism is determined largely by the nutritional state of the organism.

Pyruvate

Pyruvate is derived from glucose, lactate, alanine, and other glucogenic amino acids, and it can be converted to lactate, alanine, acetyl CoA, or oxaloacetate. Under anaerobic conditions, reduction of pyruvate produces **lactate**, a reaction that allows NAD^+ to be regenerated and glycolysis to supply the cell with ATP under conditions where mitochondrial ATP synthesis is inhibited. Rapidly contracting skeletal muscle and red blood cells release lactate into the blood, which transports it to other tissues where it can be oxidized. Transamination of pyruvate results in **alanine**. Alanine acts as a vehicle for transporting amino groups from skeletal muscle to liver, where it is transaminated back to pyruvate and the amino groups are incorporated into urea. Therefore, alanine provides an important connection between amino acid and carbohydrate metabolism. Carboxylation of pyruvate to **oxaloacetate** initiates the pathway of gluconeogenesis and provides a mechanism for replenishing intermediates in the tricarboxylic acid (TCA) cycle. Oxaloacetate is used for gluconeogenesis when there is an abundance of ATP and the TCA cycle is inhibited. Pyruvate can be converted to **acetyl CoA** by oxidative decarboxylation, a reaction catalyzed by **pyruvate dehydrogenase**. This reaction is irreversible, and it commits carbon from carbohydrate and glucogenic amino acids to the TCA cycle and pathways of lipid synthesis. **Pyruvate dehydrogenase** is tightly regulated by allosteric effectors and covalent modification. These regulatory mechanisms ensure that carbohydrate

is converted to acetyl CoA only when there is excess dietary glucose that can be used for fatty acid synthesis or when there is a need for ATP that cannot be met by the oxidation of other fuels.

Acetyl CoA

Most of the acetyl CoA is derived either from the oxidative decarboxylation of pyruvate or from β-oxidation of fatty acids, with a small contribution coming from the ketogenic amino acids. Both the source and fate of acetyl CoA are determined primarily by the nutritional and/or hormonal state of the organism. Most of the acetyl CoA derived from pyruvate is used for either **fatty acid** or **cholesterol synthesis**. An elevation of insulin, which occurs in the well-fed state, stimulates both the conversion of carbohydrate to acetyl CoA and the pathways of fatty acid and cholesterol synthesis; simultaneously, insulin inhibits β-oxidation of fatty acids. Acetyl CoA that is used for **ketone synthesis** is derived from the oxidation of fatty acids, a condition that is stimulated by glucagon. 3-Hydroxy-3-methylglutaryl (HMG) CoA is a common intermediate in the pathways of cholesterol and ketone synthesis. However, there are two separate pools of HMG CoA: a mitochondrial pool that is used for ketone synthesis and a cytosolic pool that is used for cholesterol synthesis. Synthesis of cytosolic HMG CoA is stimulated by insulin, whereas mitochondrial HMG CoA synthesis is stimulated by glucagon.

Succinyl CoA

Succinyl CoA, a C_4 intermediate in the TCA cycle, is used for synthesis of heme. The primary source of succinyl CoA is propionyl CoA, a product derived from the oxidation of branched-chain amino acids and odd-chain fatty acids.

Clinical Significance

The significance of these organizational and regulatory strategies can be appreciated by considering the mechanism that spares glucose and proteins from terminal oxidation during prolonged fasting and starvation. An increase in plasma glucagon increases fatty acid mobilization and oxidation, producing excess acetyl CoA. The acetyl CoA has multiple fates: 1) it is oxidized by the TCA cycle for the purpose of generating ATP; 2) surplus acetyl CoA is converted to ketones that can be oxidized by brain, thereby reducing the dependence of the brain on glucose; and 3) acetyl CoA inhibits the conversion of pyruvate to acetyl CoA by pyruvate dehydrogenase, thereby sparing glucose and glucogenic amino acids.

For more information see Coffee C, *Metabolism*. Fence Creek, pp 101–107.

67 Tissue and Subcellular Specialization

A Function and fuels of major tissues

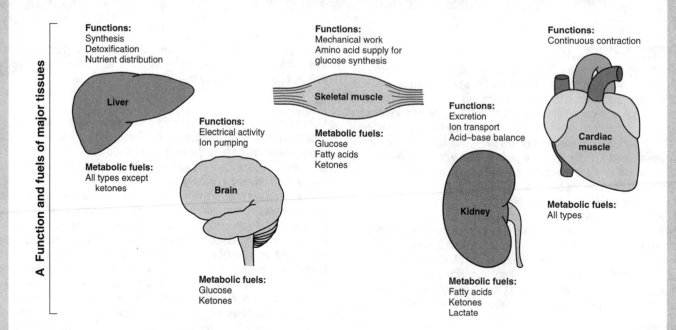

Functions:
Synthesis
Detoxification
Nutrient distribution

Liver

Metabolic fuels:
All types except ketones

Functions:
Electrical activity
Ion pumping

Brain

Metabolic fuels:
Glucose
Ketones

Functions:
Mechanical work
Amino acid supply for glucose synthesis

Skeletal muscle

Metabolic fuels:
Glucose
Fatty acids
Ketones

Functions:
Excretion
Ion transport
Acid–base balance

Kidney

Metabolic fuels:
Fatty acids
Ketones
Lactate

Functions:
Continuous contraction

Cardiac muscle

Metabolic fuels:
All types

B Metabolic pathways in major tissues

Pathway	Liver	Muscle	Brain	Kidney	Adipocyte	RBC
TCA cycle	+++	+++	+++	+++	+	−
Fatty acid oxidation	+++	+++	−	+++	−	−
Ketone synthesis	+++	−	−	−	−	−
Ketone oxidation	−	+++	+++[a]	++	+	−
Pentose phosphate	+++	+	+	+	++	+++
Glucose synthesis	+++	−	−	++[b]	−	−
Fatty acid synthesis	+++	−	−	−	+	−
Lactate synthesis	+	+++[c]	−	+	+	+++
Glycogen metabolism	+++	+++	+/−	+	+	−
Urea synthesis	+++	−	−	−	−	−

[a] Ketones are oxidized only in the fasted state.
[b] Glucose synthesis is maximum during metabolic acidosis when glutamine is being converted to ammonia and α-ketoglutarate.
[c] Lactate is formed under anaerobic conditions that exist during prolonged exercise.

C Subcellular localization of pathways

Cytosol	Mitochondria	Cytosol and mitochondria	Smooth endoplasmic reticulum
Glycolysis	TCA cycle	Gluconeogenesis	Triglyceride synthesis
Pentose phosphate pathway	Ketogenesis	Urea synthesis	Phospholipid synthesis
Fatty acid synthesis	Fatty acid oxidation	Heme synthesis	Cholesterol synthesis
Nucleotide synthesis	Ketone oxidation		Detoxification reactions
Protein synthesis	Oxidative phosphorylation		

OVERVIEW

The metabolic pathways that operate in an organ, tissue, or cell are closely correlated with the function of the cell or tissue (**Parts A** and **B**). Some metabolic pathways, such as glycolysis and the pentose phosphate pathway, are found in all cells, whereas other pathways may occur only in certain tissues or within specific types of cells within a particular tissue.

Liver

The major functions of the liver include numerous synthetic and detoxification reactions. The liver is the major site of glucose, fatty acid, and cholesterol synthesis and is the only site of urea, bile acid, and ketone synthesis. These synthetic pathways require ATP and NADPH. The liver has a high density of mitochondria and a large capacity for oxidative metabolism. It can oxidize all of the metabolic fuels except ketones. Detoxification functions include **hydroxylation** and **conjugation** reactions that occur in the smooth endoplasmic reticulum.

Skeletal Muscle

The major function of skeletal muscle is to perform mechanical work. The major pathways in skeletal muscle are those that oxidize fuels for ATP synthesis. **White muscle fibers** can store large amounts of glycogen and are dependent on glycogenolysis and glycolysis for ATP synthesis. These fibers have fewer mitochondria than red fibers, and they have a limited capacity to generate ATP by oxidative phosphorylation. **Red muscle fibers** have a high content of mitochondria and derive their energy from the oxidation of glucose, fatty acid, and ketones. During fasting and starvation, muscle protein is degraded so that amino acids can be used by the liver as a carbon source for gluconeogenesis.

Cardiac Muscle

The heart is constantly contracting and requires a continuous supply of ATP. It is rich in mitochondria and has a high capacity for oxidation of glucose, pyruvate, lactate, fatty acids, and ketones. The synthetic capacity of the heart is limited.

Brain and Nerve

Brain and nerve cells specialize in ion pumping and generation of electrical signals. A constant supply of ATP is need for active transport of ions. Most of the ATP is derived from oxidation of glucose and amino acids. Fatty acids cannot be oxidized by the brain because of the impermeability of the blood–brain barrier. During prolonged fasting, ketone oxidation can supply some of the ATP. The pathways of glycolysis, tricarboxylic acid cycle, oxidative phosphorylation, and neurotransmitter synthesis are particularly enriched in brain.

Kidney

The kidney has several highly specialized functions, including active transport of ions and regulation of acid-base balance. The high rate of active transport requires a large supply of ATP, which is derived primarily from oxidation of fatty acids, lactate, and ketones. The kidney is the only organ, other than the liver, where gluconeogenesis occurs. The excretion of NH_4^+ contributes to acid-base balance. Most of the NH_4^+ is derived from deamination of glutamine. Glutamine releases NH_3 that absorbs a proton, forming NH_4^+. α-Ketoglutarate, the carbon skeleton derived from deamination of glutamine, is the major carbon source for renal gluconeogenesis.

Adipocyte

Adipose tissue specializes in the synthesis and degradation of triglycerides. Fatty acids that are used for triglyceride synthesis are derived from both dietary sources and the liver, where they are synthesized from excess glucose. The glycerol backbone for triglyceride synthesis is derived from dihydroxyacetone phosphate, an intermediate in glycolysis.

Red Blood Cell

The major function of the red blood cell is to transport oxygen and carbon dioxide. The maintenance of the characteristic shape of the red blood cell requires ATP, which is derived solely from anaerobic glycolysis. The release of oxygen from hemoglobin is regulated by 2,3-bisphosphoglycerate, which is synthesized from an intermediate in glycolysis. The end product of glycolysis in the red blood cell is lactate. There are no mitochondria in the red blood cell and, therefore, no oxidative metabolism. The lactate is released by the red blood cell and used by liver for gluconeogenesis.

Subcellular Compartmentation of Major Metabolic Pathways

Metabolic pathways occur within characteristic subcellular compartments in eukaryotic cells. The localization of a pathway is always determined by the localization of the enzymes in that pathway. The major pathways in metabolism, together with the subcellular compartments that house the pathways, are summarized in **Part C** of the figure. Some pathways have enzymes that are located in more than one cellular compartment. In these cases, intermediates must be transported back and forth across the membranes that segregate the compartments.

Clinical Significance

A knowledge of the relationship between function and metabolism of a particular cell, tissue, or organ provides a cornerstone that is essential for understanding how alterations in metabolism lead to aberrant function and disease.

For more information see Coffee C, *Metabolism*. Fence Creek, pp 105–107.

Liver: The Nutrient Clearing Center

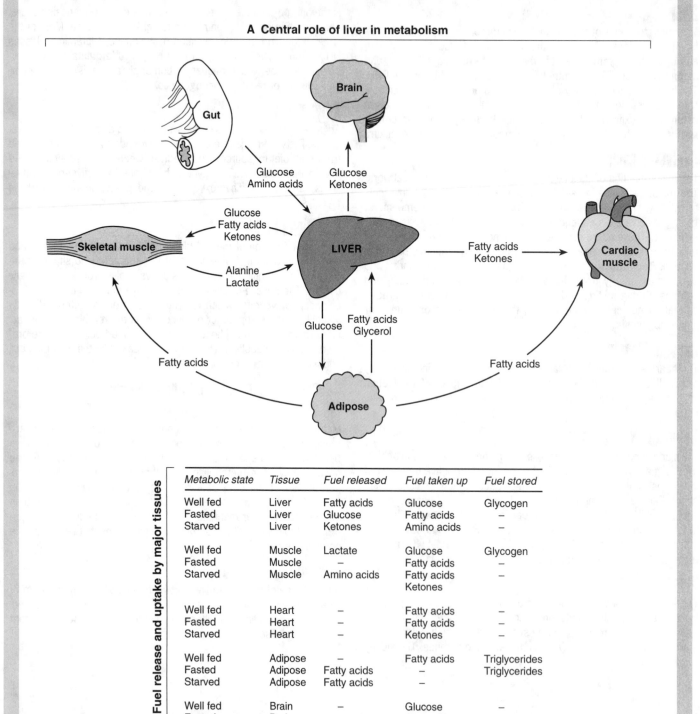

A Central role of liver in metabolism

Gut

Brain

Glucose
Amino acids

Glucose
Ketones

Glucose
Fatty acids
Ketones

LIVER

Skeletal muscle

Alanine
Lactate

Fatty acids
Ketones

Cardiac
muscle

Glucose

Fatty acids
Glycerol

Fatty acids

Fatty acids

Adipose

B Fuel release and uptake by major tissues

Metabolic state	Tissue	Fuel released	Fuel taken up	Fuel stored
Well fed	Liver	Fatty acids	Glucose	Glycogen
Fasted	Liver	Glucose	Fatty acids	–
Starved	Liver	Ketones	Amino acids	–
Well fed	Muscle	Lactate	Glucose	Glycogen
Fasted	Muscle	–	Fatty acids	–
Starved	Muscle	Amino acids	Fatty acids Ketones	–
Well fed	Heart	–	Fatty acids	–
Fasted	Heart	–	Fatty acids	–
Starved	Heart	–	Ketones	–
Well fed	Adipose	–	Fatty acids	Triglycerides
Fasted	Adipose	Fatty acids	–	Triglycerides
Starved	Adipose	Fatty acids	–	
Well fed	Brain	–	Glucose	–
Fasted	Brain	–	Glucose	–
Starved	Brain	–	Ketones	–

Anatomically, the liver is ideally suited for processing dietary nutrients (**Part A**). The portal blood that drains the gut and the pancreas enters the liver before going into the general circulation. Therefore, after a meal, the blood entering the liver contains both insulin from the pancreatic β-cells and nutrients derived from the digestion of dietary protein and carbohydrate. The liver either oxidizes these nutrients, converts them into storage forms, or distributes them to extrahepatic tissues. In contrast, dietary lipids are packaged into chylomicrons and absorbed from the gut into the lymphatic system, thereby bypassing the liver. A table is provided that summarizes the various fuels that are taken up, stored, and released by the major organs during the well-fed state and during periods of fasting and starvation (**Part B**).

Central Role of Liver in Metabolism

During the **well-fed state**, the major nutrients taken up by the liver are glucose and amino acids (**Part A**). About half of the absorbed **glucose** is used by the liver for synthesis of glycogen and fatty acids, and the remainder is distributed among the extrahepatic tissues. The fatty acids that are synthesized by the liver are esterified and packaged into very-low-density lipoproteins (VLDLs), which transport them primarily to skeletal muscle and heart. The dietary **amino acids** are used by the liver for synthesis of plasma proteins and replacement of liver proteins. Surplus amino acids are distributed to other tissues for protein synthesis or are oxidized by the liver as a source of energy. The preferred fuel for the liver in the well-fed state is amino acids. Unlike glucose and fatty acids, there is no specific protein that acts as a storage form for amino acids. Therefore, excess amino acids are oxidized by the liver for energy.

During periods of **fasting and starvation**, the liver supplies other tissues with glucose and ketones. The liver takes up fatty acids and glycerol that are released by adipose tissue and amino acids that are released by skeletal muscle. The liver oxidizes fatty acids for energy and uses amino acids and glycerol as substrates for gluconeogenesis.

Fuel Exchange Between Skeletal Muscle and Liver

Skeletal muscle, which makes up about 50% of the normal body weight, consumes more metabolic fuel than other tissues. In the **well-fed state**, large amounts of glucose and fatty acids are taken up by muscle (**Part A**). Fatty acids are the preferred fuel as long as oxygen is available. In the well-fed state, the fatty acids are derived from hydrolysis of VLDL and chylomicron triglyceride. The glucose taken up by skeletal muscle is converted to glycogen. During periods of intense exercise, when oxygen is limiting, glycogen is degraded and glucose is oxidized by anaerobic glycolysis for ATP synthesis. Lactate, the end product of this pathway, is released from muscle and taken up by the liver where it is converted back to glucose. In periods of **fasting and starvation**, fatty acids and ketones are taken up and oxidized by skeletal muscle. The fatty acids are supplied by adipose tissue, and ketones are supplied by the liver. During the first few days of fasting, skeletal muscle releases a large amount of alanine, which is taken up by the liver and used for glucose synthesis. The alanine is produced in muscle by transamination of pyruvate, where the major amino donors are the branched-chain amino acids.

Fuel Exchange Between Adipose Tissue and Other Organs

The primary function of adipose tissue is the storage of triglycerides. In the **well-fed state**, the major pathways operating in adipose tissue are glycolysis and triglyceride synthesis. Most of the fatty acids used for triglyceride synthesis are derived from dietary fat, and they are delivered to adipose tissue by chylomicrons. The major function of glycolysis in adipose tissue is to provide the glycerol backbone for triglyceride synthesis. In periods of **fasting and starvation**, triglycerides are degraded to fatty acids and glycerol. The fatty acids are transported by albumin to the liver, heart, and skeletal muscle. Glycerol is taken up by the liver where it is converted to glucose.

Cardiac Muscle

Cardiac muscle differs from skeletal muscle in two important ways: it does not store metabolic fuel, and it is totally dependent on oxidative metabolism for its energy. Therefore, the heart must be continually supplied with fuel. In both the **well-fed and fasting states**, the preferred fuel is fatty acids. However, ketones are also oxidized when they are available. In the well-fed state, the fatty acids are derived from hydrolysis of VLDL and chylomicron triglyceride, and in the fasting state fatty acids are supplied by adipose tissue. Ketones are supplied by the liver.

Brain

Brain is normally dependent on glucose for almost all of its energy. Since there is no storage form of energy in the brain, all of the glucose is taken up from the blood. During the **well-fed state**, the normal blood glucose level is maintained by dietary sources. During **early fasting**, the liver releases glucose into the blood. During **prolonged fasting and starvation**, the amount of glucose released by the liver is decreased, primarily because the brain begins to oxidize ketones.

Clinical Significance

The liver plays a central role in integrating carbohydrate, lipid, and amino acid metabolism. It is the organ primarily responsible for maintenance of blood glucose. In a typical healthy adult, the liver releases about 180 g of glucose, 100 g of triglyceride, and 14 g of albumin into the blood each day. It has more metabolic flexibility than any other organ and undergoes significant changes in size, glycogen content, and metabolic profile, depending on the availability of nutrients.

For more information see Coffee C, *Metabolism*. Fence Creek, pp 106–107, 130–132, 176–183, 188–193, 327–330.

Glucose Homeostasis During Fasting

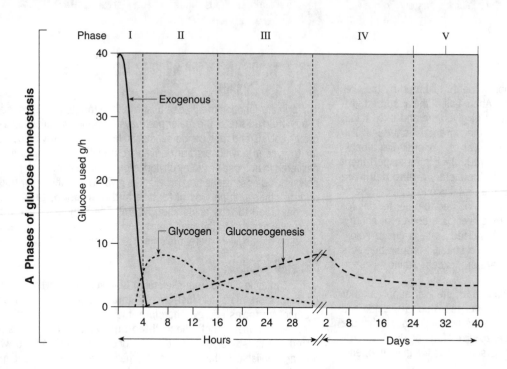

A Phases of glucose homeostasis

B Plasma concentration of fuels

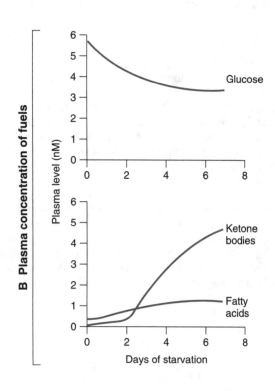

C Plasma hormone and fuel levels

	Fed	12 hours	3 days	3 weeks
Insulin/glucagon	0.5	0.15	0.05	0.05
Blood glucose (mM)	6.1	4.8	3.8	3.6
Amino acids (mM)	4.5	4.5	4.5	3.1
Fatty acids (mM)	0.14	0.6	1.2	1.4
Ketones (mM)	0.1	0.2	2.0	10.0

D Protein sparing

	3-day fast	40-day fast
Fuel used by brain (g/24 hr)		
Glucose	100	40
Ketones	50	100
Glucose used by all other tissues (g/24 hr)	50	40
Fuel released by liver (g/24 hr)		
Glucose	150	80
Ketones	150	150
Fuel released (g/24 hr)		
Adipose tissue fatty acids	180	180
Muscle amino acids	75	20

OVERVIEW

Glucose is usually an obligate fuel for the brain and always an obligate fuel for RBCs. In contrast, most other tissues can use any one of several fuels. The plasma concentration of glucose is sufficient to supply the brain and RBCs with glucose for 24 to 36 hours of fasting. During this period, the glucose used by the brain and RBCs is replenished by hepatic glycogenolysis and gluconeogenesis. After 3 days of fasting, most tissues are using fatty acids for fuel, and ketones begin to accumulate in the plasma. The brain can oxidize ketones, although it is unable to oxidize fatty acids. After 3 days of fasting, the brain derives about 30% of its energy from ketones, thereby sparing glucose for RBCs. The shift in the major type of fuel from glucose to fat marks the progression from fasting to starvation. By 40 days of starvation, ketones supply about 75% of the fuel for the brain. The progressive transitions from the well-fed state to fasting and starvation are orchestrated by the capacity of the liver for glycogenolysis, gluconeogenesis, and ketogenesis.

Phases of Glucose Homeostasis

Glucose homeostasis has five phases that are illustrated in the figure (**Part A**). The figure shows the source and amount of glucose used per hour in an individual who was fed 100 g of glucose and then fasted for 40 days. **Phase I** is the well-fed phase where exogenous glucose is available for about 4 hours. All tissues use glucose during this phase. **Phase II** begins when exogenous glucose is exhausted and continues until 16 hours of fasting. At the onset of phase II, the liver ceases to use glucose and begins to supply glucose to other tissues. The major source of glucose is glycogenolysis, with gluconeogenesis progressively becoming a more important source. Substrates for gluconeogenesis are lactate, glycerol, and alanine. **Phase III** begins at 16 hours and extends to 32 hours. During this time, glycogenolysis continues to diminish and gluconeogenesis becomes the major source of glucose. **Phase IV** extends from 32 hours to 24 days, a period when all of the glucose comes from hepatic and renal gluconeogenesis. Glycerol and amino acids are the glucogenic substrates. At the beginning of phase IV, all tissues except the RBCs are using fatty acids and/or ketones as their primary fuel, thereby reducing the need for glucose. **Phase V** occurs after prolonged starvation and is characterized by a further decrease in the dependence of the brain on glucose.

Plasma Levels of Fuels and Hormones

During the transition from feasting to fasting, the concentration of **plasma glucose decreases** as exogenous glucose diminishes (**Parts B** and **C**). When plasma glucose reaches a concentration of about 80 mg/dL (4.5 mM), the **plasma insulin decreases**, resulting in reduced uptake of glucose by muscle and adipose, an effect that allows the brain and RBCs to compete more effectively for the available glucose. A further decline in plasma glucose to about 40 mg/dL results in **glucagon secretion**, which stimulates glycogenolysis, gluconeogenesis, and lipolysis. The effect of these hormonal changes is a transition from exogenous glucose to endogenous glucose sources, resulting in a **stabilization of plasma glucose** and an **increase in plasma fatty acids**. This state, known as the postabsorptive state, usually prevails after an overnight fast of 10 to 12 hours.

With decreased uptake of glucose and increased availability of fatty acids, the liver, muscle, heart, and kidney become increasingly dependent on fatty acids for energy. The most significant change that occurs between 2 and 3 days of fasting is an **increase in plasma ketones**, providing the brain with an alternative fuel (**Part C**). The **plasma amino acid concentration** remains remarkably constant during the first few days, but by 3 weeks the circulating concentration is significantly decreased, reflecting a decreased dependence of the brain on glucose and a corresponding decrease in gluconeogenesis.

Adaptations During Starvation and Protein Sparing

The major adaptation that occurs during starvation is a shift in fuel consumption from glucose to fatty acids and ketones. This differs significantly from the adaptation seen in early fasting, where a shift from exogenous to endogenous sources of glucose occurs. After about 32 hours of fasting (the onset of phase IV), the sole source of glucose is gluconeogenesis, and the precursors are amino acids and glycerol. During this time, the **shift in fuel** from glucose to fatty acids and ketones **spares tissue protein degradation**. This shift and its consequences are illustrated in **Part D** of the figure where the fuels consumed and released by various tissues are compared after 3 days of fasting and 40 days of starvation. The following changes were observed: 1) use of glucose by the brain decreased from 100 to 40 g/24 hr; 2) use of ketones by the brain increased from 50 to 100 g/24 hr; 3) glucose release by the liver decreased from 150 to 80 g/24 hr; and 4) amino acid release by muscle decreased from 75 to 20 g/24 hr. In contrast, the amount of fatty acids released by adipose tissue and ketones released by the liver remain constant.

Clinical Significance

During starvation, the energy stores of the body are depleted at different rates. Carbohydrate stores are depleted within 12 to 24 hours. Fat is depleted at a constant rate. In early starvation, protein is degraded rapidly, but degradation decreases when ketones are available and the need for glucose decreases. However, when almost all the fat stores are depleted, protein degradation increases again because it is the only remaining source of energy. Continued hydrolysis of muscle protein leads to **loss of diaphragm and intercostal muscle**, resulting in impaired **respiration**, which leads to **pneumonia** and **death**. Death usually occurs when about half of the total body protein has been depleted.

For more information see Coffee C, *Metabolism*. Fence Creek, pp 130–132, 174–183, 188–197, 233–239, 273–287, 329–330.

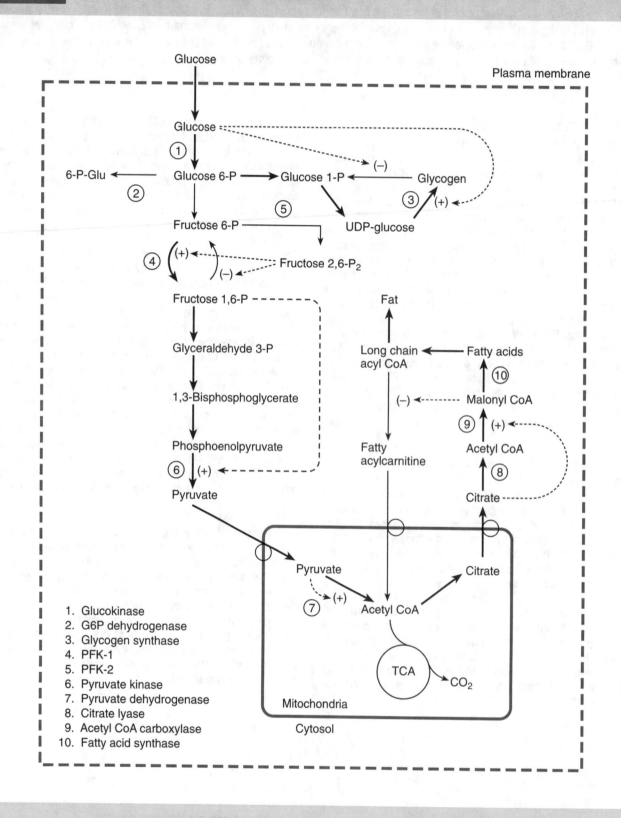

1. Glucokinase
2. G6P dehydrogenase
3. Glycogen synthase
4. PFK-1
5. PFK-2
6. Pyruvate kinase
7. Pyruvate dehydrogenase
8. Citrate lyase
9. Acetyl CoA carboxylase
10. Fatty acid synthase

In the preceding section, the transitions in fuel metabolism that occur between the well-fed and fasting states were reviewed at the organ level. The liver, with its capacity for glycogenolysis and gluconeogenesis, was identified as having a central role in orchestrating this transition. In this section, the molecular basis of hepatic fuel metabolism in the well-fed state will be reviewed. Emphasis will be placed on the major pathways that are operative in the well-fed state, and how homeostasis is maintained by the regulation of a few key enzymes.

Major Patterns of Metabolism in the Well-Fed State

Following a meal, the liver is presented with portal blood that has drained the small intestine and pancreas and is enriched in amino acids, glucose, and insulin. Surplus amino acids are the preferred fuel for the liver in the well-fed state. The major pathways of fuel storage that are operative under these conditions are **glycogen synthesis, glycolysis, fatty acid synthesis**, and the **pentose phosphate pathway**, which supplies NADPH for fatty acid synthesis. All of these pathways are activated by insulin. Simultaneously, glycogenolysis, gluconeogenesis, and fatty acid oxidation, the opposing pathways of energy utilization, are inhibited by insulin. Key enzymes that are activated in the well-fed state are **glucokinase, G6P dehydrogenase, glycogen synthase, PFK-1, PFK-2, pyruvate kinase, pyruvate dehydrogenase, citrate lyase, acetyl CoA carboxylase**, and **fatty acid synthase**. Enzymes that are inhibited in the well-fed state are G6Pase, glycogen phosphorylase, FBPase-1, and carnitine acyltransferase-1. Mechanisms of regulation include allosteric and covalent regulation, as well as induction and repression of enzyme synthesis. Different enzymes are regulated by different mechanisms, and some enzymes are regulated by more than one of these mechanisms.

Allosteric Regulation

Allosteric regulation in the well-fed state can be described in terms of **enzyme pairs** that catalyze reactions in opposing pathways. The members of each enzyme pair are **coordinately regulated** by allosteric mechanisms. For example, 1) **glycogen synthase** and **glycogen phosphorylase** catalyze the rate-limiting steps in glycogen synthesis and degradation, respectively. Glucose activates glycogen synthase and inhibits glycogen phosphorylase. 2) **PFK-1** and **FBPase-1** catalyze the rate-limiting steps in glycolysis and gluconeogenesis, respectively. $F-2,6-P_2$ activates PFK-1 and inhibits FBPase-1. The cellular concentration of $F-2,6-P_2$ is elevated when the plasma level of insulin is elevated. 3) **Acetyl CoA carboxylase** and **carnitine acyltransferase-1** catalyze the rate-limiting steps in fatty acid synthesis and fatty acid oxidation, respectively. Acetyl CoA carboxylase is activated by citrate, which acts as a carrier of acetyl CoA groups from the mitochondria to the cytosol; carnitine acyltransferase-1 is inhibited by malonyl CoA, the product of the acetyl CoA carboxylase reaction. Other enzymes that are allosterically activated in the well-fed state are **pyruvate kinase**, the last enzyme in glycolysis, and **pyruvate dehydrogenase**, the enzyme that converts pyruvate to acetyl CoA for use in fatty acid synthesis. Pyruvate kinase is activated by $F-1,6-P_2$, and pyruvate dehydrogenase is activated by the entry of pyruvate into the mitochondria. The overall effect of the allosteric mechanism is to direct glucose into pathways leading to synthesis of glycogen and fatty acids, while inhibiting pathways that use glycogen and fatty acids as fuels.

Covalent Regulation

Energy storage in the well-fed state is mediated by insulin. **Insulin activates a protein phosphatase**, leading to dephosphorylation of several enzymes. The key enzymes in fuel storage pathways that are active in the **dephosphorylated** form are glycogen synthase, PFK-2 (the enzyme that synthesizes $F-2,6-P_2$), pyruvate kinase, pyruvate dehydrogenase, and acetyl CoA carboxylase. The active forms of these enzymes direct glucose into the pathways of glycogen synthesis, glycolysis, and fatty acid synthesis. Simultaneously, insulin inhibits pathways of fuel mobilization and oxidation. Glycogen phosphorylase and hormone-sensitive lipase in adipose tissue are both inactivated by insulin, which promotes dephosphorylation of these enzymes.

Changes in Enzyme Concentration

Insulin induces the synthesis of several enzymes in liver that promote uptake of glucose and conversion to fatty acids. These enzymes include glucokinase, G6P dehydrogenase (which provides NADPH for fatty acid synthesis), citrate lyase, acetyl CoA carboxylase, and fatty acid synthase. Simultaneously, the synthesis of G6Pase, which opposes the action of glucokinase, is repressed by insulin.

Clinical Significance

The uptake and storage of glucose by the liver is an important mechanism for avoiding hyperglycemia following a meal. The high glucose concentration in the portal blood that drains the gut is lowered by the liver. **GLUT-2**, the glucose transporter in the hepatocyte plasma membrane, and **glucokinase** are responsible for the uptake of glucose and its conversion to G6P. Both GLUT-2 and glucokinase have a high K_m for glucose and are never saturated under physiologic conditions, a property that is responsible for the glucose buffering properties of the liver.

For more information see Coffee C, *Metabolism*. Fence Creek, pp 130–131, 156–166, 173–178, 202–205, 233–239, 262–265, 274–280.

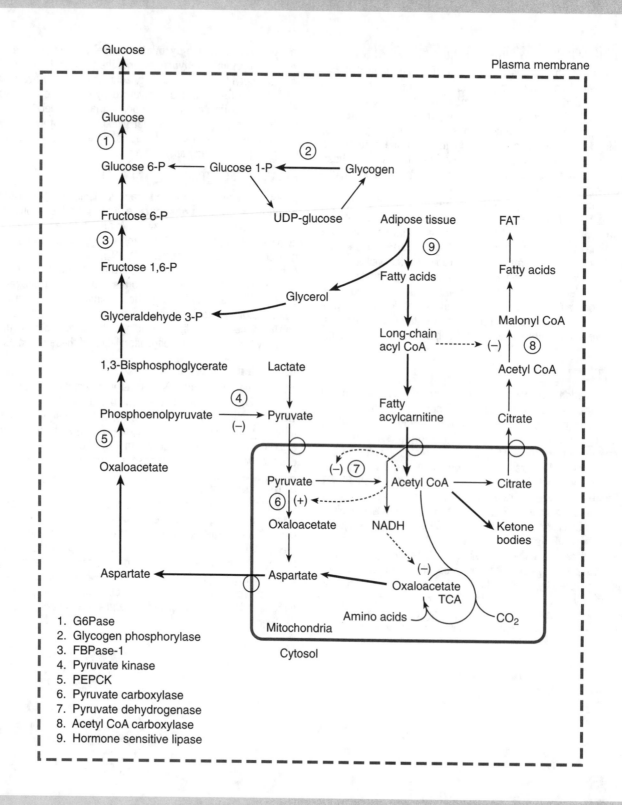

1. G6Pase
2. Glycogen phosphorylase
3. FBPase-1
4. Pyruvate kinase
5. PEPCK
6. Pyruvate carboxylase
7. Pyruvate dehydrogenase
8. Acetyl CoA carboxylase
9. Hormone sensitive lipase

OVERVIEW

In preceding sections, the transitions in fuel metabolism that occur between the well-fed and fasting states were reviewed at the organ level. The pivotal role of the liver in orchestrating this transition has been established, and the molecular basis of hepatic fuel metabolism in the well-fed state has been reviewed. In the current section, the molecular basis of hepatic fuel metabolism in the fasting state will be reviewed. Emphasis will be placed on the major pathways that are operating in the fasting state, and how homeostasis is maintained by the regulation of a few key enzymes.

Major Patterns of Metabolism

In the transition from the fed to the fasting state, the decrease in plasma glucose results in **glucagon release** by the pancreatic α-cells. The liver ceases to use glucose and begins to release glucose into the blood for use by other tissues. The major pathways of fuel metabolism that are operating under these conditions are **glycogenolysis, gluconeogenesis**, and **fatty acid oxidation**, and **ketogenesis**. The substrates for gluconeogenesis are lactate, glycerol, and amino acids, which are supplied by red blood cells (RBCs), adipose tissue, and skeletal muscle respectively. Most of the amino acids are degraded to intermediates in the tricarboxylic acid (TCA) cycle, which get converted to oxaloacetate, the first intermediate in gluconeogenesis. Oxaloacetate is transported to the cytosol as aspartate. Glucagon activates glycogenolysis and gluconeogenesis in the liver and lipolysis in adipose tissue, resulting in increased availability of fatty acids, which serve as fuel for the liver during fasting. These pathways are also activated by epinephrine. Fatty acid oxidation by the liver leads to surplus acetyl CoA, which is converted to ketones. Key enzymes that are activated in the fasting state are **glucose-6-phosphatase (G6Pase), glycogen phosphorylase, fructose bisphosphatase-1 (FBPase-1), phosphoenolpyruvate carboxykinase (PEPCK), pyruvate carboxylase**, and **hormone-sensitive lipase**. Enzymes that are inhibited include pyruvate kinase, pyruvate dehydrogenase, and acetyl CoA carboxylase, thereby ensuring that the flow of metabolites is in the direction of glucose production rather than glucose utilization. Mechanisms of regulation include allosteric and covalent regulation as well as induction and repression of enzyme synthesis.

Allosteric Regulation

The most important sites of allosteric regulation in the fasting state are the following enzymes:

1. **FBPase-1**, the rate-limiting enzyme in gluconeogenesis, is activated by ATP, which is supplied by fatty acid oxidation and oxidative phosphorylation. Additionally, the cellular concentration of $F-2,6-P_2$ is low during fasting, which has two effects: a) the **inhibition** imposed by $F-2,6-P_2$ on FBPase-1 in the fed state **is relieved**, and b) the activation imposed by $F-2,6-P_2$ on PFK-1 in the fed state is relieved. Therefore, the net effect of decreased $F-2,6-P_2$ in the fasting state is to stimulate the flux of intermediates in the direction of glucose synthesis.

2. **Pyruvate dehydrogenase** and **pyruvate carboxylase** are coordinately regulated by acetyl CoA, which accumulates from fatty acid oxidation. Acetyl CoA inhibits pyruvate dehydrogenase, thereby preventing the irreversible oxidation of carbon sources that can be used for gluconeogenesis. Acetyl CoA simultaneously activates pyruvate carboxylase, the first enzyme in gluconeogenesis.

3. **Citrate synthase**, the first enzyme in the TCA cycle, is inhibited by NADH, acetyl CoA, and ATP which accumulate as a result of fatty acid oxidation. The decreased rate of citrate synthesis allows oxaloacetate to accumulate and be directed toward gluconeogenesis.

4. **Acetyl CoA carboxylase**, the rate-limiting enzyme in fatty acid synthesis, is inhibited by the accumulation of long-chain acyl CoA, thereby preventing simultaneous synthesis and oxidation of fatty acids.

Covalent Regulation

The release of glucose from the liver in the fasting state is stimulated by both glucagon and epinephrine. These hormones stimulate the production of cAMP, resulting in activation of protein kinase A, which catalyzes the **phosphorylation** of several enzymes. Enzymes that are **activated by phosphorylation** are **glycogen phosphorylase, FBPase-2**, and **hormone-sensitive lipase**. The function of FBPase-2 is to decrease the cellular concentration of $F-2,6-P_2$. Phosphorylation simultaneously results in the inhibition of several enzymes in opposing pathways, thereby ensuring that glucose production and release by the liver is a unidirectional process. Enzymes that are inhibited by phosphorylation are glycogen synthase, PFK-2, and acetyl CoA carboxylase.

Changes in Enzyme Concentration

Glucagon induces the synthesis of **PEPCK** and **G6Pase**, resulting in an increase in hepatic gluconeogenesis and glucose release, respectively. In prolonged fasting and starvation, the primary adaptation that spares protein is the acquired ability of the brain to oxidize ketones, which decreases the dependence of the brain on glucose. This adaptation corresponds to the synthesis of **succinyl CoA : acetoacetate CoA transferase**, an enzyme essential for ketone oxidation. Normally the gene for this enzyme is not expressed in the brain. However, after about 3 days of fasting, synthesis of the enzyme is induced and the brain is able to oxidize ketones. The absence of this enzyme in the liver accounts for the fact that the liver cannot use ketones as a fuel.

Clinical Significance

The ability of the liver to release glucose into the blood is an important mechanism for combating hypoglycemia. The transient hypoglycemia that occurs during fasting is corrected by glucose release from the liver. Inherited deficiencies in several enzymes, including G6Pase, FBPase-1, and glycogen phosphorylase, are characterized by hypoglycemia. von Gierke disease, a glycogen storage disease, resulting from a deficiency in G6Pase is characterized by severe hypoglycemia. Neither glycogenolysis nor gluconeogenesis can be completed in the absence of G6Pase.

For more information see Coffee C, *Metabolism*. Fence Creek, pp 130–131, 174–183, 187–197, 233–239, 282–287, 327–332, 356–357.

A Metabolic patterns

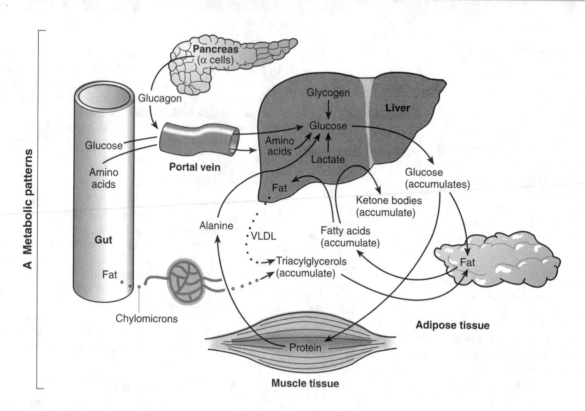

B Glucose Tolerance Test

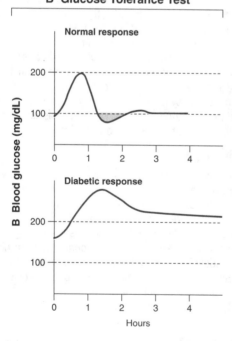

Normal response

Diabetic response

Hours

B Blood glucose (mg/dL)

C Glucose toxicity

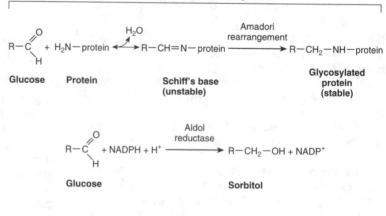

$$R-\overset{O}{\underset{H}{C}} + H_2N-protein \underset{H_2O}{\rightleftharpoons} R-CH=N-protein \xrightarrow{\text{Amadori rearrangement}} R-CH_2-NH-protein$$

Glucose   Protein   Schiff's base (unstable)   Glycosylated protein (stable)

$$R-\overset{O}{\underset{H}{C}} + NADPH + H^+ \xrightarrow{\text{Aldol reductase}} R-CH_2-OH + NADP^+$$

Glucose   Sorbitol

OVERVIEW

The word *diabetes* is derived from the Greek word meaning "to pass through" or "to siphon," referring to the observation that individuals with diabetes mellitus drink lots of water and excrete large volumes of urine. Insulin-dependent (juvenile-onset) diabetes is frequently caused by an autoimmune disease that destroys the pancreatic β-cells. Metabolically, this disease can be described as a **multiorgan catabolic response** to a lack of insulin (**Part A**). The hallmark symptom of diabetes is **sustained hyperglycemia**, which results from both the over-production and underutilization of glucose. When the blood glucose concentration exceeds the renal threshold for reabsorption (>180 mg/dL), glucose is excreted in the urine. The need to maintain osmolality results in increased excretion of water, accounting for the excessive thirst and urination. Other symptoms include **elevated plasma triglycerides, fatty acids,** and **ketones**. The inability of the pancreas to release insulin into the nutrient-rich portal blood results in **metabolic profiles** in liver, muscle, and adipose tissue that are characteristic of the fasting state.

Muscle

Normally, insulin stimulates glucose uptake by increasing the number of GLUT-4 transporters in the plasma membrane. In the absence of insulin, the uptake of glucose by muscle is impaired, and muscle experiences a fasting state (**Part A**). **Protein degradation** and the release of amino acids provides liver with carbon skeletons for glucose synthesis. More than half of the amino acids released by muscle are **alanine** and **glutamine**, which act as carriers of amino groups from muscle to liver and kidney, respectively. Muscle wasting and **negative nitrogen balance** are seen in untreated diabetes.

Adipose Tissue

Adipose tissue, like muscle, is dependent on insulin for glucose uptake, and in the absence of insulin, the metabolic profile is that of fasting (**Part A**). **Uncontrolled lipolysis** leads to the accumulation of fatty acids in plasma and accelerated uptake and oxidation by the liver. The absence of insulin results in decreased uptake of both glucose and fatty acids by adipose tissue, and the inability to synthesize triglycerides. Very-low-density lipoproteins (VLDLs) and chylomicrons accumulate in the absence of insulin, accounting for the elevated plasma triglycerides. The **lipoprotein lipase** isozyme found in the capillary bed of adipose tissue is synthesized at a very low level in the absence of insulin.

Liver

Normally after eating, the liver shifts from a fasting to a well-fed state, and energy storage pathways are activated. However, in the absence of insulin, the liver remains in the fasting state, and the pathways of **gluconeogenesis, fatty acid oxidation, ketogenesis,** and **VLDL synthesis** continue to operate (**Part A**). Amino acids, derived from skeletal muscle protein, are taken up and used as substrate for gluconeogenesis. Quantitatively, alanine is the most important glucogenic amino acid. Fatty acids, released from adipose, are used as the primary fuel for liver. As plasma levels of fatty acids increase, accelerated uptake and oxidation by the liver produce excess acetyl CoA that is used for ketone synthesis. Ketones are released into the blood and, in cases of uncontrolled diabetes, the ketone concentration can reach 10 to 20 mM, resulting in ketoacidosis. When the uptake of fatty acids by the liver exceeds the rate of oxidation, the surplus is esterified and packaged into VLDLs, which are secreted into the blood.

Kidney

Ketones are excreted in the urine when the plasma concentration exceeds the renal threshold for reabsorption. The ketones are small organic acids that exist as anions at physiologic pH, and excretion must be accompanied by a cation. To conserve Na^+ and K^+, the kidney undergoes an adaptation that allows NH_4^+ to be excreted. Most of the NH_4^+ is derived from glutamine, which is released from skeletal muscle and taken up by the kidney. The sequential action of **glutaminase** and **glutamate dehydrogenase** releases two molecules of NH_3, which absorb protons to become NH_4^+. The **synthesis of glutaminase** in the kidney is induced by metabolic acidosis.

Glucose Tolerance Test

The ability to dispose of glucose can be assessed by the glucose tolerance test (**Part B**). Following an overnight fast, glucose is ingested and the plasma glucose concentration is measured over the next 4 hours. In a normal response, the plasma glucose peaks between 30 and 60 minutes and then declines with a slight "overshoot" below the baseline concentration before establishing the fasting glucose concentration. The "overshoot" follows a pulse of insulin secretion and is missing in the diabetic response.

Clinical Significance

Glucose **toxicity**, resulting from persistently elevated plasma glucose levels, poses a threat to the diabetic (**Part C**). In many tissues, such as nerve, retina, lens, kidney, and small blood vessels, the uptake of glucose is insulin independent. These tissues are very susceptible to the chronic complications of diabetes. Two types of reactions have been implicated in the pathologic changes that occur in these tissues, protein glycosylation and sorbitol formation. **Protein glycosylation** occurs when the aldehyde group of glucose reacts with amino groups of proteins producing a stable glycosylated protein that may have altered properties. This reaction is nonenzymatic and is driven by the concentration of glucose. **Sorbitol** is formed in tissues that contain **aldol reductase**, an enzyme that reduces glucose to sorbitol. Sorbitol cannot diffuse through membranes and has been shown to accumulate in human lens, resulting in osmotic shifts that lead to cataract formation. Both the accumulation of sorbitol and the formation of cataracts in diabetics can be retarded by inhibitors of aldol reductase.

For more information see Coffee C, *Metabolism*. Fence Creek, pp 132–137.

Effect of Ethanol on Metabolism

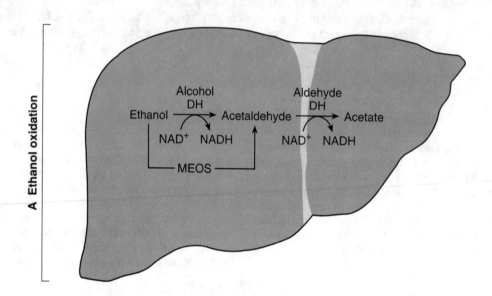

A Ethanol oxidation

Ethanol → (Alcohol DH, NAD^+ → NADH) → Acetaldehyde → (Aldehyde DH, NAD^+ → NADH) → Acetate

MEOS

B Manifestations of alcohol consumption

Hypoglycemia
Lactic acidosis
Ketoacidosis
Fatty liver
Cirrhosis

C Metabolic changes resulting from ethanol ingestion

Carbohydrate metabolism	Nitrogen metabolism	Lipid metabolism	Vitamin deficiencies
Gluconeogenesis	Protein synthesis	Fatty acid synthesis	Thiamin
Glycolysis	Protein glycosylation	Fatty acid oxidation	Folate
Plasma lactate	Protein secretion	Adipose lipolysis	Vitamin B_6
TCA cycle	Plasma uric acid	Hepatic fatty acid uptake	Vitamin A
		Lipoprotein synthesis	
		Plasma triglyceride	
		Ketogenesis	

OVERVIEW

Excess consumption of ethanol is a major health problem in most societies. When consumed in significant amounts, ethanol and its metabolites can produce toxic effects in all organs and tissues of the body. It is rapidly absorbed from the stomach and intestine and can be detected in the blood within minutes of ingestion. It diffuses across biologic membranes and distributes to all cells and compartments in the body. Normally, about 80% of the metabolism of ethanol occurs in the liver; the remainder is broken down by the gastrointestinal epithelium. Some of the metabolic effects are due to the direct action of ethanol and its metabolites, whereas others result from changes in the NADH/NAD$^+$ ratio that occurs during ethanol metabolism.

Ethanol Oxidation by Liver

The major route of ethanol metabolism in the liver involves two steps (**Part A**). The first step occurs in the cytosol, where ethanol is oxidized to acetaldehyde by **alcohol dehydrogenase**. The K_m of alcohol dehydrogenase for ethanol is about 1 mM, and the enzyme is essentially saturated after moderate alcohol consumption. Acetaldehyde is further oxidized to acetate by the action of **aldehyde dehydrogenase**, which is found in both the cytosol and mitochondria. These reactions use NAD$^+$ and produce NADH, resulting in an increase in the **NADH/NAD$^+$** ratio. A second mechanism for converting ethanol to acetaldehyde is the **microsomal ethanol oxidizing system (MEOS)**, a member of the cytochrome P-$_{450}$ family of enzymes. Although MEOS normally plays a minor role in ethanol oxidation, the activity is increased in chronic alcoholism. Acetate, the end product of ethanol metabolism, is converted to acetyl CoA by both liver and extrahepatic tissues. In liver, it is used for fatty acid and ketone synthesis; in extrahepatic tissues it is oxidized to CO_2 and H_2O.

Manifestations of Alcohol Consumption

The consumption of moderate amounts of ethanol (one to two drinks) results in the production of more NADH than can be oxidized by the mitochondrial electron transport chain, accounting for the increased NADH/NAD$^+$ ratio. The ratios of other pairs of metabolites that are related by NAD$^+$-dependent oxidation or NADH-dependent reduction are also altered. For example, the ratios of lactate/pyruvate, malate/oxaloacetate, and β-hydroxybutyrate/acetoacetate are all increased by ethanol metabolism. Many clinical manifestations of alcohol consumption can be accounted for by these changes (**Part B**). **Hypoglycemia** results from impaired gluconeogenesis due to decreased pyruvate. The high ratio of lactate/pyruvate also accounts for **lactic acidosis**. Other pathways that operate at a reduced rate in the liver are glycolysis, fatty acid oxidation, and the tricarboxylic acid (TCA) cycle. All of these pathways have one or more reactions that require NAD$^+$. The appearance of a **fatty liver** results from several metabolic changes caused by the alcohol. Increased release of fatty acids from adipose tissue results in increased uptake by the liver. Additionally, decreased fatty acid oxidation and increased fatty acid synthesis occur. Elevated concentrations of acetyl CoA and NADPH are responsible for increased fatty acid synthesis. Increased NADPH results from transfer of reducing equivalents from NADH to NADP$^+$. Acetyl CoA accumulates because the TCA cycle is operating at a reduced rate. Acetate, the end product of ethanol oxidation, also contributes to the acetyl CoA pool.

Metabolic Changes Induced by Ethanol Consumption

Essentially every area of metabolism is affected by ethanol (**Part C**). In **carbohydrate metabolism**, the rates of hepatic gluconeogenesis, glycolysis, and the TCA cycle are all decreased. In **nitrogen metabolism**, protein synthesis, glycosylation, and secretion are inhibited in the liver. These effects appear to be due to toxic effects of acetaldehyde, which inhibits several microsomal enzymes. An increase in plasma uric acid is associated with the accumulation of lactate, which inhibits excretion of uric acid by the kidney. Increased turnover of adenine nucleotides may also contribute to hyperuricemia. In patients with gout, the ingestion of alcohol can precipitate a bout of gouty arthritis. In **lipid metabolism**, increased plasma triglyceride is associated with increased VLDLs. The elevation in VLDLs is associated with increased synthesis rather than decreased clearance. Increased HDLs and decreased LDLs are also seen. **Vitamin deficiencies** associated with ethanol consumption result from several factors, including decreased consumption, impaired absorption, and alterations in cellular vitamin metabolism. For example, absorption of thiamin and folate is inhibited by ethanol; degradation of pyridoxal phosphate is accelerated by acetaldehyde; and oxidation of retinol to retinal is impaired by the high NADH/NAD$^+$ ratio.

Clinical Significance

Many of the toxic effects of ethanol have been attributed to acetaldehyde, a reactive compound that forms covalent bonds with amino and sulfhydryl groups on proteins. Acetaldehyde has been shown to inactivate enzymes, decrease DNA repair, and change the morphology of mitochondrial and plasma membranes. These modified proteins provide a useful marker for the drinking history of an individual. Acetaldehyde also depletes cellular glutathione, resulting in increased damage by free radicals. It is believed that the transition from a fatty liver to **cirrhosis** is mediated by acetaldehyde. **Disulfiram**, a drug used to treat chronic alcoholism, inhibits acetaldehyde dehydrogenase. The accumulation of acetaldehyde produces nausea, vomiting, abdominal pain, and tachycardia. The rationale underlying this treatment is that the unpleasant side effects will discourage the patient from drinking.

74 Inheritance Patterns of Metabolic Diseases

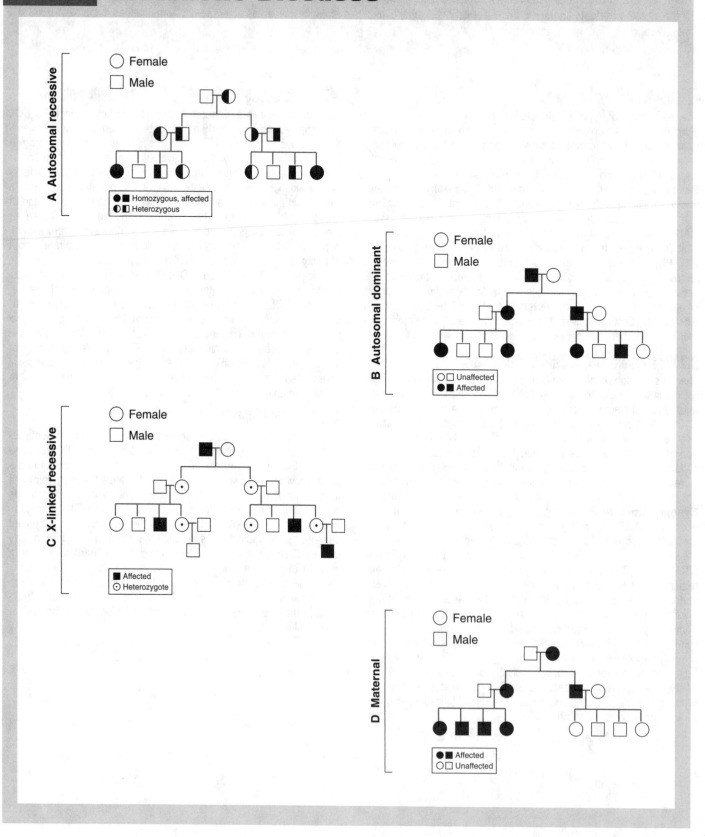

OVERVIEW

Inborn errors of metabolism are genetically determined disorders that affect metabolic pathways in the body. A mutation in a structural gene may affect the corresponding protein, resulting in a deficiency in enzyme activity or in the transport of metabolites across membranes. An inborn error of metabolism produces a block in a metabolic pathway that leads to accumulation of intermediates behind the block and impaired synthesis of products ahead of the block. The clinical findings are usually related to the metabolites that accumulate or to the products that are deficient. Conditions that are caused by a mutation in a single gene of nuclear DNA are inherited in a defined pattern, referred to as a Mendelian pattern. The three Mendelian patterns of inheritance most often seen in metabolic diseases are autosomal dominant, autosomal recessive, and X-linked recessive. Mutations in mitochondrial DNA show a maternal inheritance pattern.

Autosomal Recessive Inheritance

Autosomal recessive diseases require two copies of the mutant gene in order to be expressed. Heterozygotes are carriers of the disease, but they do not express the disease (**Part A**). The transmission of autosomal recessive diseases shows the following characteristics: 1) both parents of an affected child must have a mutant gene; 2) males and females are affected in equal numbers; 3) each child has a 25% chance of being affected if both parents are heterozygotes; 4) each child has a 50% chance of being affected if one parent is homozygous and the other heterozygous; 5) the rarer the disease, the greater the chance that the affected individual is a product of consanguineous parents.

Commonly occurring autosomal recessive diseases include phenylketonuria (PKU), Tay-Sachs disease, cystic fibrosis, von Gierke disease, galactosemia, homocystinuria, maple syrup urine disease, sickle-cell disease, Gaucher disease, and the various forms of congenital adrenal hyperplasia.

Autosomal Dominant Inheritance

Autosomal dominant diseases require only one mutant gene in order to be expressed (**Part B**). The transmission of these diseases shows the following characteristics: 1) only one parent has to have the disease in order for it to be transmitted to the offspring; 2) affected individuals are usually heterozygotes, having only one mutant gene; homozygotes with two mutant genes usually die in utero; 3) each child of an affected parent has a 50% chance of inheriting the mutant gene; 4) both males and females can inherit and transmit the disease; 5) normal children of affected parents have normal offspring.

Commonly occurring autosomal dominant diseases include familial hypercholesterolemia, Huntington disease, acute intermittent porphyria, congenital spherocytosis, and neurofibromatosis.

X-Linked Recessive Inheritance

Diseases that show X-linked recessive inheritance patterns (**Part C**) show the following characteristics: 1) only males are affected; 2) affected males transmit the mutant gene to all of their daughters, who are asymptomatic carriers; 3) affected males cannot transmit the disease to their sons; 4) each child of an asymptomatic mother has a 50% chance of inheriting the mutant gene; 5) occasionally, female carriers exhibit symptoms of the disease. This is related to the fact that females are genetic mosaics because of the random inactivation of one of the X chromosomes in each cell. Usually a structurally abnormal X chromosome is preferentially inactivated. However, if the normal X chromosome is inactivated, the female carriers will exhibit symptoms of the disease. The symptoms of glucose-6-phosphate dehydrogenase (G6PD) deficiency are seen in female carriers because the normal X chromosome has been inactivated.

Commonly occurring X-linked recessive diseases include Lesch-Nyhan syndrome, Duchenne muscular dystrophy, type II hyperammonemia (ornithine transcarbamoylase deficiency), hemophilia A, Hurler syndrome, and G6PD deficiency.

Maternal Inheritance

Mutations in mitochondrial DNA are always inherited from the mother (**Part D**). During fertilization, the mitochondria from sperm do not enter the fertilized egg. A mutation in mitochondrial DNA is transmitted from a mother to all her children. The daughters, in turn, transmit the mutant gene to all of their children. However, a son having the mutant gene cannot transmit it to any of his children.

Commonly occurring diseases showing maternal inheritance include Leber hereditary optic neuropathy (LHON), mitochondrial encephalomyopathy with lactic acidosis and stroke-like episodes (MELAS), and myoclonic epilepsy and ragged-red fibers (MERRF).

Clinical Significance

All inherited diseases are due to changes in DNA. However, the pathologic consequences may be expressed at different levels of gene expression. For example, in some cases of thalassemia, the mutation in DNA leads to altered splicing sites in RNA. However, most DNA mutations that result in metabolic diseases are expressed as changes in protein structure. These diseases have classically been considered as disorders of children; however, delayed onset or milder presentation of any of these diseases can occur during the late teens or in adulthood. Newborn screening is routinely performed for some of the more common metabolic diseases, including phenylketonuria (PKU), maple syrup urine disease, homocystinuria, and galactosemia.

Directions for Questions 1-20: for each of the following questions, choose the **one best** answer.

1. A hormone-stimulated increase in cAMP synthesis by hepatocytes results in

(A) Decreased glycogenolysis

(B) Increased glycolysis

(C) Increased fructose-2,6-bisphosphate synthesis

(D) Increased gluconeogenesis

(E) Increased fatty acid synthesis

2. UDP-glucose participates in the metabolism of all of the following compounds **except**

(A) Glycoproteins

(B) Lactose

(C) Glycogen

(D) Fructose

(E) Glycolipids

3. Which of the following processes is stimulated by insulin?

(A) Glycogen degradation

(B) Malonyl CoA synthesis

(C) Gluconeogenesis

(D) Fructose-2,6-phosphate degradation

(E) Lipolysis

4. Which of the following processes is accelerated in a person with type I diabetes who is not being treated?

(A) Synthesis of glucose from fatty acids

(B) Synthesis of muscle glycogen

(C) Synthesis of skeletal muscle protein

(D) Synthesis of fatty acids from glucose

(E) Synthesis of ketone bodies

5. Which of the following pairs of enzymes are required for the bactericidal function of phagocytic cells?

(A) Methemoglobin reductase and glucose-6-phosphate dehydrogenase

(B) Glucose-6-phosphate dehydrogenase and NADPH oxidase

(C) Malic enzyme and NADPH oxidase

(D) Glutathione reductase and malic enzyme

(E) 6-Phosphogluconate dehydrogenase and glucokinase

6. In an overnight fast, the efficient breakdown of liver glycogen and the release of glucose into the blood involves all of the following enzymes **except**

(A) Phosphoglucomutase

(B) Phosphorylase$_a$

(C) α-1,4 $\rightarrow$ α-1,4 Glucan transferase

(D) α-Amylase

(E) Phosphorylase kinase

7. Which of the following processes is occurring after 1 week of starvation?

(A) Glucose is the primary source of energy for skeletal muscle.

(B) Ketone bodies are released from the liver into the blood.

(C) Protein is oxidized by the liver to provide energy for ATP synthesis.

(D) Fatty acids are transported from the liver to adipose tissue for storage.

(E) The ratio of insulin/glucagon in the serum is higher than after 12 hr of fasting.

8. Which of the following proteins is a useful marker for acute pancreatitis?

(A) Creatine kinase

(B) Haptoglobulin

(C) Lipase

(D) Transferrin

(E) Cholecystokinin (CCK)

9. Which of the following conditions would be seen in a patient with a thiamine deficiency?

(A) Pellagra

(B) Rickets

(C) Night blindness

(D) Lactic acidosis

(E) Increased clotting time

10. Which of the following statements about cAMP is correct?

(A) It is a 2′,3′-phosphodiester.

(B) Its synthesis is activated by the G_i protein.

(C) It activates protein kinase A.

(D) It is the second messenger for estrogen.

(E) Its concentration is decreased by caffeine.

11. All of the following statements about steroid hormones are true **except**

(A) They exert their effect in the nucleus of cells

(B) They are synthesized from acetyl CoA as the sole carbon source

(C) They are transported in the blood by proteins that are synthesized in the liver

(D) They require less time to exert their effect than peptide hormones

(E) They are synthesized in peripheral endocrine organs in response to stimulation by pituitary hormones

12. The phosphatidylinositol signal transduction pathway

(A) Is activated by hormones that bind to nuclear receptors

(B) Is inhibited by the action of Bordella pertussis toxin

(C) Generates diacylglycerol and inositol triphosphate

(D) Leads to the activation of protein kinase A

(E) Leads to the activation of hormone-sensitive lipase in adipose tissue

13. Which of the following enzymes and reaction products are correctly paired?

(A) 21-hydroxylase and cortisol

(B) 11-hydroxylase and aldosterone

(C) 1-hydroxylase and 1,25-dihydroxyvitamin D

(D) 20-22 desmolase and progesterone

(E) 17-20 lyase and estrogen

14. The action of which of the following hormones would be affected in a patient with a deficiency in the G_s protein?

(A) Thyroxine

(B) Cortisol

(C) Glucagon

(D) Insulin

(E) Angiotensin-II

15. Glucocorticoids

(A) Stimulate hepatic gluconeogenesis

(B) Stimulate protein degradation in skeletal muscle

(C) Stimulate fatty acid release from adipose tissue

(D) Inhibit the synthesis of prostaglandins

(E) All of the above

16. All of the following manifestations result from ethanol consumption **except**

(A) Hypoglycemia

(B) Lactic acidosis

(C) Decreased VLDLs

(D) Elevated HDLs

(E) Vitamin A deficiency

17. Which of the following metabolic patterns would be seen in a patient with a glucagon-secreting tumor?

(A) Decreased serum fatty acids

(B) Decreased blood glucose

(C) Elevated ratio of urea/NH_4^+

(D) Elevated phosphofrucokinase-1 activity in hepatocytes

(E) Decreased fructose-2,6-bisphosphate

18. Which of the following diseases occurs only in males?

(A) Homocystinuria

(B) Lesch-Nyhan

(C) Familial hypercholesterolemia

(D) Sickle cell disease

(E) Cystic fibrosis

19. Which of the following compounds is an allosteric effector of both pyruvate dehydrogenase and pyruvate carboxylase?

(A) Citrate

(B) NADPH

(C) Acetyl CoA

(D) ADP

(E) Pyruvate

20. Which of the following enzymes is expressed in brain only during prolonged fasting?

(A) Pyruvate dehydrogenase

(B) Phosphofructokinase-1

(C) Glucose-6-phosphatase

(D) Succinyl CoA:acetoacetate CoA transferase

(E) Fatty acyl CoA dehydrogenase

PART VI: ANSWERS AND EXPLANATIONS

1. **The answer is D.**

An increase in cAMP in hepatocytes increases the rate of gluconeogenesis, glycogenolysis, and fructose-2,6-bisphosphate degradation. A decrease in the rate of glycolysis, fructose-2,6-bisphosphate synthesis, and fatty acid synthesis occurs when cAMP concentration increases. An increase in cAMP levels in hepatocytes is stimulated by both glucagon and epinephrine.

2. **The answer is D.**

Dietary fructose is metabolized by the liver, where it sequentially undergoes phosphorylation at C-1, cleavage to dihydroxyacetone

phosphate (DHAP) and glyceraldehyde, and phosphorylation of glyceraldehyde to glyceraldehyde-3-phosphate. These reactions produce compounds that are intermediates in glycolysis. Synthesis of glycogen, glycoproteins, and glycolipids requires UDP-glucose as an activated donor of glucose. Synthesis of lactate requires UDP-glucose as a precursor of UDP-galactose.

3. **The answer is B.**

Insulin stimulates pathways that lead to glucose storage and inhibits pathways that lead to the glucose release into the blood. The pathways of glycogen degradation, gluconeogenesis, fructose-2,6-bisphosphate degradation, and lipolysis are all involved either directly or indirectly in the release of glucose into the blood. These pathways are inhibited when the ratio of insulin/glucagon is high. In contrast, insulin stimulates the conversion of glucose to fatty acids, a process that involves both glycolysis, the pyruvate dehydrogenase reaction, and fatty acid synthesis. Malonyl CoA is a key intermediate in fatty acid synthesis.

4. The answer is E.

In the untreated or poorly controlled diabetic, processes that are normally stimulated by glucagon are operating. Synthesis of muscle glycogen and fatty acids is not occurring because insulin is not present. Degradation of skeletal muscle protein is occurring and the amino acids are being used by the liver for gluconeogenesis. The mobilization of fatty acids from fat stores in adipose tissue is occurring and the fatty acids are being oxidized in an uncontrolled manner, resulting in excess acetyl CoA that is converted to ketone bodies by the liver. Fatty acids cannot be converted to glucose because there is no enzyme in mammalian cells that can convert acetyl CoA (the product of fatty acid oxidation) to pyruvate (an intermediate in glucose synthesis).

5. The answer is B.

Phagocytic cells synthesize superoxide by the NADPH-dependent reduction of O_2. This reaction is catalyzed by NADPH oxidase. The reactions in the pentose phosphate cycle that are catalyzed by glucose-6-phosphate dehydrogenase and 6-phosphogluconate dehydrogenase provide the NADPH for superoxide synthesis. Superoxide, and other toxic oxygen metabolites derived from superoxide (hydrogen peroxide and hypochlorous acid), kill foreign cells that are engulfed by the phagocytes.

6. The answer is D.

α-Amylase participates in the digestion of dietary starches by cleaving internal α-1,4 glycosidic bonds. Phosphorylase kinase and phosphorylase$_a$ are a part of the cascade of enzymes that degrade glycogen. Phosphorylase kinase is activated by the cAMP-dependent phosphorylation that is catalyzed by protein kinase A. The active form of phosphorylated kinase (phosphorylase kinase$_a$) catalyzes the phosphorylation of glycogen phosphorylase. The active form of glycogen phosphorylase is known as phosphorylase$_a$. Phosphorylase$_a$ sequentially releases glucose-1-phosphate from the nonreducing ends of the glycogen chains. Phosphoglucomutase converts glucose-1-phosphate to glucose-6-phosphate, and glucose-6-phosphatase hydrolyzes glucose-6-phosphate to glucose. Debranching of glycogen involves α-1,4 → α-1,4 glucan transferase.

7. The answer is B.

Fatty acids, released from adipose tissue, are oxidized by most tissues except the brain, which is impermeable to fatty acids. Excess acetyl CoA generated in the liver is used to synthesize ketone bodies (acetoacetate and β-hydroxybutyrate), which are transported to extrahepatic tissues for oxidation. Skeletal muscle protein is degraded to amino acids that are used by the liver for gluconeogenesis. The ratio of insulin/glucagon is much lower than it was after 12 hr of fasting.

8. The answer is C.

An increase in the plasma concentration of a particular protein can be used as a marker for inflammation or damage to the cell or tissue where the protein is normally synthesized or housed. Acute pancreatitis results in the release of pancreatic lipase and pancreatic amylase into the plasma. The major sources of creatine kinase are skeletal and cardiac muscle. Transferrin and haptoglobulins are normal plasma proteins that are synthesized by the liver and cholecystokinin is a hormone that is synthesized by the duodenum.

9. The answer is D.

Pyruvate dehydrogenase requires thiamine pyrophosphate as a coenzyme. A deficiency in thiamine results in the accumulation of pyruvate that is in equilibrium with lactic acid. Rickets results from a deficiency in vitamin D; pellagra results from a deficiency in niacin; night blindness results from a deficiency in vitamin A and increased clotting time results from a deficiency in vitamin K.

10. The answer is C.

Protein kinase A consists of two regulatory and two catalytic subunits that are inactive in the absence of cAMP. Binding of cAMP to the regulatory subunits results in the release of active catalytic subunits. cAMP is a 3′,5′-phosphodiester that functions as a second messenger for several peptide hormones. The hormone-receptor complex activates the G_s protein, which in turn activates adenylate cyclase. Estrogen is a steroid hormone that alters the rate of transcription of specific genes. Caffeine increases cAMP levels by inhibiting cAMP phosphodiesterase, the enzyme that hydrolyzes cAMP to AMP.

11. The answer is D.

The effect elicited by steroids requires more time and lasts longer than that for peptide hormones. The effect is exerted in the nucleus of cells where the hormone-receptor complex binds to DNA and alters the rate of transcription of specific genes. The steroid hormones are synthesized from cholesterol, which is synthesized entirely from acetyl CoA. The steroid hormones are hydrophobic and relatively insoluble and are transported in the blood by proteins that are synthesized in the liver. The synthesis of the most steroid hormones is stimulated by pituitary hormones that have receptors on peripheral endocrine organs. The exception is aldosterone, whose synthesis is stimulated by angiotensin II, a peptide hormone derived from angiotensinogen, a plasma protein.

12. The answer is C.

The phosphatidylinositol cascade is initiated by peptide hormones that bind to receptors on the plasma membrane, resulting in a hormone-receptor complex that activates the G_p protein that stimulates phospholipase C. Phospholipase C hydrolyzes phosphatidylinositol-4,5-bisphosphate to diacylglycerol and inositol triphosphate. Diacylglycerol activates protein kinase C and inositol triphosphate stimulates the release of Ca^{2+} from intracellular stores in the endoplasmic reticulum. Hormone-sensitive lipase is activated by protein kinase A. Pertussis toxin inhibits the G_i protein, resulting in an accumulation of cAMP, but has no effect on the G_p protein that is involved in the phosphatidylinositol signal transduction pathway.

13. The answer is C.

Vitamin D activation requires the sequential hydroxylation by 25-hydroxylase in the liver, followed by 1-hydroxylase in the kidney. The last step in the pathway of cortisol synthesis is catalyzed by 11-hydroxylase, whereas the last step in the synthesis of aldosterone is catalyzed by 18-hydroxysteroid dehydrogenase. The synthesis of progesterone requires the sequential action of 20-22 desmolase and 3β-hydroxysteroid dehydrogenase. The final step in estrogen synthesis is catalyzed by aromatase.

14. The answer is C.

The active form of the G_s protein stimulates adenylate cyclase and the production of cAMP. Glucagon is the only hormone listed that activates adenylate cyclase. Thyroxine and cortisol use signal transduction pathways that alter the rate of gene expression; these pathways do not involve G proteins. Angiotensin-II uses the G_p protein to activate the phosphatidylinositol signal transduction pathway. The action of insulin does not involve G proteins.

15. The answer is E.

Glucocorticoids stimulate gluconeogenesis by inducing the synthesis of phosphoenolpyruvate carboxykinase and several other liver enzymes involved in gluconeogenesis. The increased degradation of skeletal muscle protein provides amino acids that are used by the liver for gluconeogenesis. The synthesis of hormone-sensitive lipase in adipose tissue is stimulated by glucocorticoids, thereby stimulating the release of fatty acids from adipocytes. The fatty acids can be oxidized by the liver, resulting in the synthesis of ATP needed for gluconeogenesis. The synthesis of phospholipase A_2 is inhibited by glucocorticoids in various tissues, resulting in decreased release of arachidonic acid from membrane phospholipids and a decrease in the synthesis of all the eicosanoids derived from arachidonic acid.

16. The answer is C.

Ethanol consumption results in increased VLDL synthesis. Hypoglycemia, lactic acidosis, and vitamin A deficiency are associated with the elevated NADH/NAD$^+$ ratio that results from ethanol oxidation.

17. The answer is E.

This patient would have an increase in the glucagon/insulin ratio, resulting in the activation of fructose-2,6-bisphosphatase that leads to a decrease in the concentration of fructose-2,6-bisphosphate and a decrease in phosphofructokinase-1 activity. Release of fatty acids from adipocytes and increased hepatic gluconeogenesis would also occur. This person would have ketoacidosis. The increased H$^+$ concentration will shift the equilibrium between NH$_3$ and NH$_4^+$, resulting in a decrease in the relative concentration of NH$_3$ and a corresponding decrease in the production of urea.

18. The answer is B.

Lesch-Nyhan disease shows an X-linked recessive inheritance. Familial hypercholesterolemia has an autosomal dominant inheritance pattern, while homocystinuria, sickle cell disease, and cystic fibrosis are all inherited as autosomal recessive traits. Only males are affected in diseases that show X-linked recessive inheritance. In both autosomal recessive and autosomal dominant diseases, males and females are affected equally.

19. The answer is C.

Acetyl CoA is an allosteric activator of pyruvate carboxylase and an allosteric inhibitor of pyruvate dehydrogenase, thereby ensuring that pyruvate is not being decarboxylated and carboxylated simultaneously.

20. The answer is D.

The adaptation that allows the brain to oxidize ketones during prolonged fasting involves the synthesis of succinyl CoA:acetoacetate CoA transferase. This enzyme converts acetoacetate to acetoacetyl CoA, a reaction that allows acetoacetyl CoA to be cleaved to acetyl CoA and provide fuel for the tricarboxylic acid cycle. The absence of this enzyme in liver accounts for the fact that liver cannot oxidize ketone bodies.

Index